Praise for
Debunking the Bump

In this important book, Adler, a mathematician, management consultant, and self-proclaimed "numbers junkie," equips mothers with researched data behind recommendations for what to do (and not do) during pregnancy . . . She writes in a tone that is both authoritative and assuring—that of a mother rooting for all other mothers.

—*Publishers Weekly*

Ms. Adler has taken the time to research many of the top concerns of pregnant women and not simply give a recommendation for whether or not something is safe, but to talk about it in a manner that puts it in perspective . . . A valuable read.

—About.com

Adler spent three years examining thousands of studies before compiling her findings ... the result is a detailed, often surprising examination that puts accepted pregnancy precautions into perspective, and even occasionally overturns prevailing wisdom . . . an essential resource for any mothers-to-be who want to be more informed about the choices they make during pregnancy.

—*Nine in the Mirror*

Ms. Adler has done her homework. Her book is especially useful for those who teach pre-conception and early pregnancy classes and will help any birth educator answer many of the tough questions asked in childbirth classes about pregnancy issues.

—*The Family Way*

Debunking the Bump is a useful reference book for the research-minded parent and for the educator.

—Babble.com

Copyright © 2018 by Daphne Adler
All rights reserved.
Published by Familius LLC, www.familius.com

Familius books are available at special discounts for bulk purchases, whether for sales promotions or for family or corporate use. For more information, contact Familius Sales at 559-876-2170 or email orders@familius.com.

Note: The information in this book is true and complete to the best of our knowledge. This book is intended only as an informative guide for those wishing to know more about health issues relating to pregnancy. The author cannot be held responsible for any errors and omissions that may be found in the text or for the consequences of any actions or inactions by a reader as a result of reliance on the information contained in the text. In no way is this book intended to replace, countermand, or conflict with the advice given to you by your own physician. The ultimate decision concerning care should be made between you and your doctor. The author disclaims all liability in connection with the use of this book. Readers should also be aware that websites listed in this book may change.

Library of Congress Cataloging-in-Publication Data
2017962274

Print ISBN 9781945547805
Ebook ISBN 9781641700474

Printed in the United States of America

Edited by Katharine Hale
Cover design by David Miles
Book design by Brooke Jorden

10 9 8 7 6 5 4 3 2 1
Third Edition

DEBUNKING the BUMP

FAMILIUS

Many thanks to Blythe Adler and Kimberly Chase-Adler for their invaluable help and infinite patience in editing the many iterations of this book and to Tom Adler and Claudio Siniscalco for their practical assistance in bringing it to market.

DEBUNKING
the
BUMP

What the Data *Really* Say About Pregnancy's 165 Biggest Risks and Myths

Daphne Adler

CONTENTS

INTRODUCTION

What Are We Worried About?

The Soft-Serve Scandal, May 2008: *Beverly Hills 90210*'s Tori Spelling looked radiant, the picture of maternal health with her cropped blond hair and glossy candy-colored lipstick, a white-and-pink geometric print dress stretching across her eight-month bump. She had just arrived at Baskin Robbins, ready to promote the company's new soft-serve ice cream at an event called "First Swirl on Bump Day." Tori's job was to serve a few symbolic cones to other pregnant mothers, smile for the cameras, and attract a bit of publicity. She would be attracting plenty of publicity, but not the kind she had intended.

Tori was about to become the poster child for irresponsible motherhood, on a par with Michael Jackson, the baby dangler, and Britney Spears, the joyrider with an unbuckled baby in her lap. By promoting soft serve to pregnant women, she was apparently unwittingly encouraging them to put their unborn babies at risk. "Is Tori Baskin' in 31 flavors of bacteria?" crowed *TMZ*, an entertainment news website.

"Several sources in the know—including one pregnant OB/GYN—tell us that there are 'definite' health risks associated with soft-serve ice cream for expectant moms because of *Listeria* bacteria. Softie machines can be studded with bacteria that can cause all kinds of issues for newborns—in fact, it's pretty much forbidden for preggo women."[1]

Across internet chat rooms, the disbelief exploded: "Every day there is a new food that you're not supposed to eat . . . Good grief! . . . Maybe we shouldn't eat, breathe, or drink anything while pregnant, just get an IV drip and an oxygen mask, then we won't have to worry about anything." Or, as another woman complained, "If all pregnant women were as overly cautious in all other areas of our lives as we are expected to be about what we eat, we would wrap ourselves in bubble wrap (as long as there are no harmful chemicals in the plastic) and curl up into the fetal position until we deliver." Speaking of harmful chemicals in plastic . . .

The Case of the Undescended Testicles, October 2008: "Exposure to chemical may affect genitals of baby boys"[2] ran the headline in *USA Today*. A chemical leaching into women's wombs and causing genital deformities! What could this terrible chemical be? A persistent radioactive remnant of the Chernobyl disaster? A poison spewing out of factory smokestacks, afflicting a whole generation of unfortunate children in the Third World? Brace yourself. The chemical culprits being fingered were phthalates, commonplace ingredients in everyday plastics, found in virtually every American home. As the article explained: "Baby boys are more likely to have changes in their genitals—such as undescended testicles and smaller penises—if their mothers were exposed to high levels of a controversial chemical during pregnancy, a new study shows." Undescended testicles? Smaller penises?! It's more than enough to make any prospective mother (let alone father) shudder.

We don't need to be concerned about either soft serve or testicles (more on both later). But only a woman with nerves of steel could make it through an entire pregnancy without pausing to worry about the safety and health of her fetus; everywhere she looks, there are warnings about potential perils. Pregnancy books feature long lists of what is safe versus what is off limits. Babycenter.com has answers to 176 questions across eight different categories on the topic of *Is it safe?*, including *Is it safe to sit in a vibrating chair?*; *Is it safe to binge on Halloween candy?*; and *Is it safe to get Botox treatments?* (In case you're wondering, the answers respectively are Yes, Yes, and Yes, but you won't need it since you'll be retaining water and looking puffy anyway.)

In response to all of these unseen dangers, mothers-to-be across the country are heroically modifying their behavior during pregnancy, as a very first gesture of love and sacrifice on behalf of their unborn children. But there is still widespread worry and confusion about pregnancy.[3] When I was pregnant several years ago, I became fed up with the conflicting headlines and the scary rumors I heard traded over lunch with my expectant mothers' group. I decided to do some research to discover which threats were actually dangerous and which were merely red herrings. The result was this book.

I'm not a doctor, nor am I a scientist who conducts primary research. I'm a mathematician, management consultant, and numbers junkie who's obsessively interested in researching parenting topics. Such a background makes me uniquely qualified to write this book, because I've spent much of my professional career aggregating and interpreting information across a variety of fields, and many of the topics covered in this book span numerous fields of expertise.

Take "what foods to avoid," for example. Most websites and books quote doctors on what items should be avoided. While doctors are undoubtedly experts on the human body, they probably know less about which foods have most recently hit the top of the US Department of Agriculture's Food Safety and Inspection Service risk assessment reports; or if they do, they don't tend to mention it in their answers.

So why does everyone quote doctors? Because we're used to going to doctors for reassurance on matters related to the body. The agricultural inspectors who test foods for bacteria, the experts at the Centers for Disease Control who monitor annual rates of infection, and the researchers who study the effects of pathogens on pregnant women all have valuable contributions to make, but none can provide the whole picture. There's a need for someone who can bring together the insights from each of these fields into a cohesive answer, with actionable advice for parents. My professional background has prepared me well for such a task.

Before delving into specific threats, let's start with a basic question: Is all this tiptoeing around the little squirt necessary in the first place? Are unborn babies such fragile creatures that ordinary, everyday maternal behavior could cause terrible, irreversible damage? Let's investigate.

Below is a chart, "US pregnancies," showing the outcomes of the 5.2 million pregnancies in a given year in the United States.[4, 5, 6, 7, 8, 9, 10, 11] We start with total recognized pregnancies on the left, excluding elective abortions; we then lose some to miscarriage and fetal death before arriving at the lower number of total live births on the right.

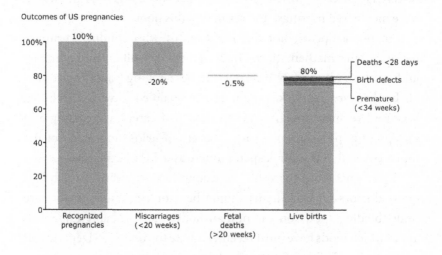

Outcomes of US pregnancies

About 20 percent of all pregnancies won't make it past 20 weeks;[12] an additional 0.5 percent (or 1 in 200) will die before delivery. Of those born alive, another 0.5 percent will die within 28 days of birth (such a small amount that it's virtually invisible on the chart above), 3 percent (or about 1 in 33) will have a birth defect such as cleft lip or Down syndrome, and 3.6 percent will be born very prematurely (6 or more weeks early).

The pessimist would look at these figures and say that there's plenty that can go wrong, so we're completely right to worry; a miscarriage rate of 20 percent is a shockingly high figure, and 5 percent of pregnancies will have some further complication. The optimist would frame it differently and counter that once you pass 20 weeks, you should really breathe a sigh of relief—at that point, you have a 92 percent chance of carrying a healthy baby to term.

But if your baby is born on its due date with ten fingers and ten toes, you can congratulate yourself on a successful pregnancy, right? Well, yes and no. Unfortunately, a chart like this doesn't really tell us everything we need to know about the ultimate consequences of pregnancy. Take a look at some of these disturbing news headlines:

- "Asthma Link to Pregnancy Stress"[13]
- "Scientists Find Link Between Maternal Diet and Diabetes"[14]
- "Excessive Weight Gain During Pregnancy Linked to Heart Disease Risk in Offspring"[15]
- "Smoking in Pregnancy Raises Child's Risk of Heart Disease in Later Life"[16]
- "Antidepressant Use in Pregnancy May Raise Autism Risk"[17]

Who could blame a mother for feeling stressed or needing an antidepressant in the face of all this bad news?

The difficulty with attempting to evaluate the risks to pregnancy is that the effects, both negative and positive, might only play out over the longer term. Not only do we have to wait until our child is a year old to diagnose autism, but we have to wait until our own hair is gray and our eyesight cloudy before we can discover that we may have unintentionally caused heart disease in our middle-aged offspring through our behavior while pregnant fifty years earlier. Even when parents face an obvious and immediate tragedy like miscarriage, they are rarely given a definitive diagnosis; doctors don't routinely perform autopsies or conduct genetic analyses on lost embryos. And nearly 70 percent of all birth defects have no known associated risk factor.[18]

So how can we have any idea about what causes problems in pregnancy? Researchers have to start with a hypothesis (like "Smoking causes birth defects") and then test whether that particular factor does indeed make a difference when studied across large groups of women (Do smokers actually have a higher rate of children with birth defects versus a similar group of nonsmokers? And is this correlation or causation?).

We have accumulated an impressive body of knowledge about pregnancy. Our knowledge will never be exhaustive; there could be culprits that we would never dream of testing in a million years. Maybe brushing your teeth or owning a hamster or eating artichokes increases your risk of miscarriage. As unlikely as they sound, we'll never know for sure unless someone makes a formal study of each activity. But in putting together this book, I did attempt to systematically think through the potential influences on the fetus to make sure I didn't miss anything important (see Appendix II for more detail).

My research uncovered a variety of answers, such as "eating deli meat gives you a small chance of something really nasty happening, while eating pesticides on your fruit gives you a high chance of something more minor happening." While true, this isn't very helpful. We have a limited amount of time and energy to devote to changing our behavior for the benefit of our fetuses, so we need a ranked list of the most important things to worry about and the key actions we should take.

I've therefore calculated a single "threat score" for every topic, which allows us to compare apples and oranges. Each score is based on three separate factors multiplied together: the likelihood that a worrying outcome will occur (is the chance one in a thousand, or one in a million?); a rating for the severity of the outcome (is the outcome death, a birth defect, or a minor decrease in IQ?); and a rating for the certainty (is the evidence rock solid, or is the topic still being researched?). I've then grouped the final threat scores into buckets representing the "threat level," from very high to very low. This is the known threat level, so if there's currently no evidence one way or the other, a threat will be ranked low on my scale until (if and when) further evidence comes to light. If you're interested in knowing more, Appendix I has further detail on my methodology, and the notes for each section provide the individual calculations.

Some threats I won't bother to address, since there's no point in worrying about things we can't control. No one wants to catch the flu while pregnant, but even if you wear a face mask and wash your hands constantly, you can hardly prevent someone sick from sneezing in your vicinity. Similarly, once you're pregnant, you can't exactly change your age or make any dramatic changes to your existing state of health. I'll also avoid giving medical advice (such as discussing specific health conditions or prescription drugs), as that's the rightful domain of doctors and pharmacists. Instead, I'll focus on what we can actually control—for example, what we eat.

Some of you may be so hungry for information that you devour every page, including appendices and endnotes. (I admit I have a lot of documentation! That's the point of the book.) Others may want to skim for chapters or items of particular concern. But if you can barely find time to read a magazine lately, the CliffsNotes of my years of research is contained in these five nuggets of advice:

1. Strive not to drive.
2. Feast on fish (and savor your sushi).
3. Opt for organic.
4. Heat your meat.
5. Request a lead test.

Yes, I'm actively recommending you eat sushi. According to my research, driving to a dinner party is more dangerous than eating blue cheese once you're there. You're better off going organic than cutting down on your coffee consumption. Danger may lurk in innocuous-looking deli sandwiches and restaurant chicken salads. And lead is a greater potential threat to your fetus than chemicals like phthalates.

I don't blame you for raising an eyebrow. If someone gave me this advice, I'd be inclined to dismiss it without watertight proof, too, since it directly contradicts the conventional wisdom. That's why I'll spend this whole book wading through potential pregnancy hazards and benefits one by one. I had no preconceived notion of what the results of my research would be and no ulterior motive except to debunk the hype, to discover the unvarnished truth, and to help women avoid unwarranted fear and enjoy healthy and relaxed pregnancies.

Notes

1. TMZ staff. (2008, May 21). Is Tori Baskin' in 31 flavors of bacteria? *TMZ.com*. http://www.tmz. com/2008/05/21/is-tori-baskin-in-31-flavors-of-bacteria/.

2. Szabo, L. (2008, October 2). Exposure to chemical may affect genitals of baby boys. *USA Today. com*. http://www.usatoday.com/news/health/2008-10-02-Boy-genitals_N.htm.

3. Browning, A. (2006, October 2). Confused, guilty and pregnant. *BBC News*. http://news.bbc. co.uk/2/hi/uk_news/5391718.stm.

4. Estimated pregnancy rates by outcome for the United States, 1990–2004. (2008). US Department of Health & Human Services, Centers for Disease Control and Prevention, National Center for Health Statistics. http://198.246.112.54/pub/Health_Statistics/NCHS/Publications/DVD/ DVD_3/National_Vital_Statistics_Reports/nvsr56/nvsr56_15.pdf.

5. US Department of Health & Human Services, Centers for Disease Control and Prevention, National Center for Health Statistics. (n.d.). Compressed mortality file (CMF) for 1999–2005 on CDC WONDER online database. http://wonder.cdc.gov/cmf-icd10.html.

6. MacDorman, M. F., Munson, M. L., & Kirmeyer, S. (2007). Fetal and perinatal mortality, United States, 2004. *National Vital Statistics Reports, 56* (3). http://198.246.124.29/nchs/data/nvsr/ nvsr56/nvsr56_03.pdf.

7. Silver, R. M., Varner, M. W., Reddy, U., Goldenberg, R., Pinar, H., Conway, D., . . . & Stoll, B. (2007). Work-up of stillbirth: a review of the evidence. *American Journal of Obstetrics and Gynecology, 196* (5), 433–444. www.ncbi.nlm.nih.gov/pmc/articles/PMC2699761/.

8. Fretts, R. C. (2005). Etiology and prevention of stillbirth. *American Journal of Obstetrics and Gynecology, 193* (6), 1923–1935. www.researchgate.net/publication/7442874_Etiology_and_ prevention_of_stillbirth/file/5046352249e3f25009.pdf.

9. Gray, R. H., & Wu, L. Y. (2000). Subfertility and risk of spontaneous abortion. *American Journal of Public Health, 90* (9), 1452. www.ncbi.nlm.nih.gov/pmc/articles/PMC1447624/pdf/10983206.pdf.

10. Martin, J. A., Hamilton, B. E., Sutton, P. D., et al. (2005). Births: final data for 2003. *National Vital Statistics Reports 52* (10). Hyattsville, MD: National Center for Health Statistics. www.cdc. gov/nchs/data/nvsr/nvsr54/nvsr54_02.pdf.

11. Martin, J. A., Hamilton, B. E., Sutton, P. D., Ventura, S. J., Menacker, F., & Kirmeyer, S. (2006). Births: final data for 2004. *National Vital Statistics Reports, 55* (1), 1–101. www.cdc.gov/nchs/ data/nvsr/nvsr55/nvsr55_01.pdf.

12. Martin, J. A., Hamilton, B. E., Sutton, P. D., et al. (2005). Births: final data for 2003. *National Vital Statistics Reports 52* (10). Hyattsville, MD: National Center for Health Statistics. www.cdc. gov/nchs/data/nvsr/nvsr54/nvsr54_02.pdf.

13. Asthma link to pregnancy stress. (2008, May 19). *BBC News*. http://news.bbc.co.uk/1/hi/ health/7404391.stm.

14. Bowdler, N. (2011, March 8). Scientists find link between maternal diet and diabetes. *BBC News*. www.bbc.co.uk/news/health-12668519.

15. Barclay, L. (2010, June 8). Excessive weight gain during pregnancy linked to heart disease risk in offspring. *Medscape.com*. www.medscape.com/viewarticle/723112.

16. Adams, S. (2011, June 22). Smoking in pregnancy raises child's risk of heart disease in later life. *The Telegraph*. www.telegraph.co.uk/health/8588914/Smoking-in-pregnancy-raises-childs-risk- of-heart-disease-in-later-life.html.

17. Hardin, A. (2011, July 6). Antidepressant use in pregnancy may raise autism risk. *CNN.com*. http://edition.cnn.com/2011/HEALTH/07/04/antidepressant.pregnancy.autism.risk/index.html.

18. Thulstrup, A. M., & Bonde, J. P. (2006). Maternal occupational exposure and risk of specific birth defects. *Occupational Medicine 56* (8), 532–543. http://occmed.oxfordjournals.org/ content/56/8/532.full.

1

LITTLE BEASTIES

Foodborne Pathogens

*I*n April 2009, panic gripped the nation. A new disease, ominously called swine flu, was rapidly spreading from its epicenter in Mexico around the world. Echoing the fears of Americans across the country, a CNN anchor breathlessly asked, "Is this the killer virus that we've all been fearing for decades? . . . Is this 1918, where 20 million people died worldwide?"[1]

We know now that swine flu did not turn out to be a killer virus. But admit it, I bet at the time you toyed with the idea of wearing a face mask. We have a tendency to overreact to potential threats, particularly those that capture our imagination. As CBS later reported, "On the network news last week, swine flu stories took up a whopping 43 percent of airtime . . . In China, more than 70 Mexicans were quarantined despite showing no signs of the flu, prompting charges of discrimination. In Egypt, more than 300,000 pigs were slaughtered despite the fact that no cases of the flu have been reported in the country—and that you can't get it from eating pork . . . And yet most cases

of the flu, outside an initial spate of fatalities in Mexico, have not been
life threatening. Just one American citizen has died from the disease.
Your standard everyday flu, by contrast, kills more than 100 people
a day, and yet it is largely treated as a fact of life, not a grave threat."[2]

Certain dangers steal more than their fair share of media limelight
while we ignore the daily hazards all around us. The fatal plane crash
attracts a zoo of media hoopla, while the fatal car crashes across the
world every day claim absurdly more lives but never make the headlines. Inevitably, the media skews toward stories that are exciting or
newsworthy, giving us a false sense of where the real risks lie. The
soft-serve ice cream scandal mentioned in the introduction is a prime
example. No one got sick, but Tori Spelling plus pregnancy plus the
potential for vicious bacteria made for a good story.

Plenty of parenting books and websites have come to the rescue,
filled with advice on how to avoid the potential perils of pregnancy.
Unfortunately, this advice is not always very helpful. To illustrate my
point, grab a pencil and paper, and then carefully read the following
list. It's provided courtesy of a popular parenting website, from an
article entitled "Foods and Beverages to Avoid During Pregnancy."[3]
They consider these foods forbidden during pregnancy:

- Raw or undercooked fish or shellfish (such as oysters and
  clams)
- Fish with high levels of mercury, including shark, swordfish,
  king mackerel, and tilefish (golden or white snapper)
- Unpasteurized, refrigerated smoked or pickled fish, unless
  heated until steaming
- More than six ounces of canned "solid white" or albacore
  tuna
- Raw or undercooked meat or poultry
- Refrigerated meat of any kind (ham, turkey, roast beef, hot
  dogs, bologna, prosciutto, pâté, etc.), unless heated until
  steaming (165 degrees Fahrenheit)
- Dry, uncooked sausages, such as salami and pepperoni,
  unless heated until steaming
- Runny or undercooked eggs

- Raw cookie dough or cake batter that contains raw eggs
- Homemade desserts or sauces that contain raw eggs (such as eggnog, ice cream, custard, chocolate mousse, hollandaise sauce, béarnaise sauce, mayonnaise, and caesar salad dressing)
- Unpasteurized soft cheese (such as feta, brie, camembert, blue-veined cheese, queso fresco, queso blanco, and queso panela)
- Prepared salads from the deli (especially if they contain eggs, chicken, ham, or seafood)
- Buffet or picnic food that's been sitting out for two or more hours (one hour on a hot day)
- Stuffing cooked inside a bird, unless heated to 165 degrees Fahrenheit
- Raw sprouts or any unwashed produce, especially lettuce and cabbage

Now turn away from this list and write down as many of these items as you can remember.

Couldn't remember all of them? Very worrisome—your unborn fetus may be destined to suffer from exposure to unnecessary food-borne danger. Remember all fifteen? Congratulations! Not only will your fetus likely emerge unharmed—he or she is bound to be blessed with a prodigious memory as well.

No mother wants to be responsible for harming her baby, so caution appears to be the sensible strategy while pregnant. But the list of forbidden foods is too long to remember, and it seems to grow longer every day. Even worse, not all sources agree on which foods make the cut. WebMD, the most popular American medical website, states that foods to avoid include:

- Unpasteurized milk and soft cheeses such as feta, brie, camembert, roquefort, queso blanco, and queso panela, unless the label says "made with pasteurized milk"
- Refrigerated meat spreads or pâtés
- Refrigerated smoked seafood (unless it is cooked in a casserole or other dish)

- Hot dogs and deli meats, unless they are heated until steaming
- Undercooked eggs, raw eggs, or eggnog made with uncooked eggs[4]

This list, at least, is shorter. But we're left to wonder why some foods are absent from the list. Are they not actually all that dangerous, or is WebMD simply editing the list to a digestible size? Their use of the word "include" at the beginning hints that perhaps the list isn't meant to be exhaustive.

To clear up the confusion, let's turn to the government for a definitive answer. Surely a government agency will provide a sensible view of which foods should be avoided, having taken into account all the most pertinent scientific evidence in order to guide the public appropriately. The chart on the right shows the foods to avoid listed by five different English-speaking national agencies: the US Food and Drug Administration,[5] the Public Health Agency of Canada,[6] the UK National Health Service,[7] the New South Wales (Australia) Food Authority,[8] and the New Zealand Food Safety Authority.[9]

This chart makes a lovely patchwork pattern, don't you think? There's not a lot of consistency here. Why does one source mention liver products while the others leave them off the list entirely? What are we supposed to conclude about hummus and raw sprouts? Is sushi safer in the UK than elsewhere in the world? More broadly, is the best approach to simply go with the most cautious common denominator and avoid all these foods, or are some agencies being overly conservative? The problem is that lists of forbidden foods tend to err on the side of cataloging any and every source of threat exhaustively rather than telling us where the substantive risks truly lie.

I decided it was time to look at the data on foodborne illnesses for myself. Uncovering the truth was not easy. After hours on Google Scholar, I had sore eyes but not a single report estimating how many pregnant women and fetuses are affected each year by different causes of food poisoning. I also couldn't find any exhaustive data on which foods were the riskiest for anyone, let alone pregnant women.

National Agency Food Recommendations

Food		US FDA	UK NHS	PHA of Canada	NSW Food Authority	New Zealand FSA
Dairy & Eggs	Unpasteurized cheese	Off-limits	Off-limits	Off-limits	Off-limits	Off-limits
	Raw eggs (cookie dough, eggnog etc)	Off-limits	Off-limits	Off-limits	Off-limits	Off-limits
	Soft serve ice cream	No mention	No mention	No mention	Off-limits	Off-limits
Meat & Poultry	Raw or under-cooked meat & poultry	Off-limits	Off-limits	Off-limits	Off-limits	Off-limits
	Poultry pre-cooked then chilled	No mention	No mention	No mention	Off-limits	Off-limits
	Deli meats (e.g. bologna, roast beef, turkey)	Off-limits	No mention	Off-limits	Off-limits	Off-limits
	Fresh patés / meat spreads	Off-limits	Off-limits	Off-limits	Off-limits	Off-limits
	Liver products	No mention	Off-limits	No mention	No mention	No mention
Sea-food	Raw fish / sushi	Off-limits	No mention	Off-limits	Off-limits	Off-limits
	Raw shellfish	Off-limits	Off-limits	Off-limits	Off-limits	Off-limits
	Large fish	Off-limits	Off-limits	No mention	No mention	Off-limits
	Unpasteurized juice	Off-limits	No mention	Off-limits	No mention	No mention
	Ready-made dressed salads (e.g. coleslaw)	No mention	No mention	No mention	Off-limits	Off-limits
Veg. & Fruit	Unwashed fruits & vegetables	Off-limits	Off-limits	No mention	No mention	Off-limits
	Raw sprouts	Off-limits	No mention	Off-limits	Off-limits	No mention
	Hummus	No mention	No mention	No mention	Off-limits†	Off-limits

† OK if eaten within 2 days

No wonder none of the typical parenting books and websites referenced real information. I would have to compile the research myself.
I started with a report on foodborne illness in the United States from
the Centers for Disease Control and Prevention (CDC) and researched
the effects during pregnancy of every pathogen listed. The results can
be found in Appendix IV. (If you suffer from intractable insomnia, I
recommend a careful slog through this particular appendix.)

It's not straightforward to estimate the number of fetuses affected
by a pathogen, for four reasons:

1. Some pathogens may make the mother sick but not the baby,
    as they don't pass through the placenta; therefore, there's no
    problem unless the mother becomes gravely ill and dies.
2. Some foodborne illnesses may make the baby sick but not the
    mother, as the immature fetus is more vulnerable than the
    mature mother if both are exposed.
3. Pregnancy itself can make a woman more susceptible to
    contracting certain foodborne illnesses, due to changes in
    her immune system during pregnancy to accommodate the
    foreign baby.
4. The treatment required could be harmful to the fetus.

Having worked my way through the full list of foodborne pathogens, here's what I discovered. First, it's completely impossible to
avoid foodborne illness (otherwise known as food poisoning) by cutting a list of forbidden foods out of your diet. A full 80 percent of cases
have an unknown cause. Why? People typically spend twenty-four
to forty-eight hours curled up by the toilet projectile-vomiting and
producing other noxious bodily fluids, but then the illness passes—so
they never bother to go to a hospital for a definitive diagnosis. Even
if they did, it can be tricky to work backward and pin the illness to a
specific food. Fortunately, a large-scale study of pregnant women has
shown that these cases of short, intense food poisoning rarely, if ever,
harm the fetus (see Appendix IV). Phew.

Second, only a handful of foodborne illnesses cause specific problems in pregnancy. *E. coli* infection can, in very rare cases, cause the

death of the fetus or mother, and *Campylobacter* can cause stillbirth, particularly if contracted during the second trimester. Then there are the truly nasty ones. The scare stories in the media about pregnancy and food tend to focus on *Listeria* (the bacteria potentially lurking in Tori's soft serve), and for good reason. *Listeria* infection is extremely rare, but the bacteria has a creepy predilection for infecting pregnant women, and unlike most bacteria, it can sneak past the protective barrier of the placenta and attack the fetus. So while it barely registers on the list of common pathogens (there are a full twenty-four other foodborne infectious diseases that are more common in the US than *Listeria*), it causes by far the most fetal deaths each year. Nearly as worrisome is *Toxoplasma gondii*. It doesn't cause as many deaths as *Listeria*, but it can cause serious complications like blindness and intellectual disability, which often don't show up until late childhood.

Surprisingly, all four of these pathogens tend to come from the same type of food. Contrary to popular perception, that source isn't unpasteurized cheese, sushi, or oysters. It's something far more commonplace.

Feral Pigs in the Spinach: *E. coli*

September 2006: Headlines ominously proclaimed that the national food supply was tainted with the deadly pathogen *E. coli*. First death struck in Wisconsin, then cases appeared in Utah, Oregon, Indiana, Idaho, New Mexico, and Connecticut, and no one knew where or when it would emerge next. Inspectors rushed to identify what factors the cases had in common. Before long, a likely culprit emerged: spinach, a vegetable previously upheld as the epitome of healthy eating. Bags and bags across the nation were possibly crawling with bacteria, forcing a recall on a grand scale. Taking a leadership role in a time of national crisis, the FDA issued a warning not to eat uncooked fresh spinach or products containing it. Sales of spinach immediately plummeted by 60 percent as consumers rushed to cut the offending vegetable from their diet.[10] By March 2007, the scare over spinach had reached such a level that the House of Representatives felt compelled to pass a spending bill with "a $25 million lifeline for spinach farmers reeling from the largest food recall in American history."[11]

A more detailed investigation was soon launched. Where exactly had the tainted spinach come from, and how had it become infected with E. coli? A bit of investigative journalism soon provided the answer: "The E. coli outbreak in the spinach crop was attributed to a group of escaped farm pigs that traipsed through a cow patch and wandered into a spinach field."[12] The true source of the E. coli was either pig or cow feces, not spinach. This virtuous leafy vegetable had been framed by a gang of dirty domestic farm animals! The spinach was merely an innocent bystander, implicated in a clear miscarriage of justice!

Well, yes and no. Those pigs could just as easily have wandered into any other patch of vegetables, so in some sense the spinach was in the wrong place at the wrong time. On the other hand, spinach belongs to a family of vegetables that grow above but close to the surface of the ground, are often consumed raw, and sometimes escape the vigorous scrubbing that vegetables such as carrots receive. For that reason, spinach is indeed a more likely vector for E. coli than, say, a turnip or an ear of corn. But it would be foolish to attempt to avoid E. coli by singling out spinach while continuing to eat other salad leaves with abandon.

Rather than looking at a single outbreak, let's look at outbreaks over time. What do the data actually say?[13] See the chart on the next page.

Beef is by far the largest culprit in E. coli outbreaks, significantly larger than all other categories combined. This is not particularly surprising, given that the primary vector for spreading E. coli is cow feces. But the FDA has never issued a warning not to eat beef. Spinach may be responsible for only a small fraction of E. coli outbreaks, and happens to be an extremely healthy source of iron and other good vitamins and minerals. But no, it's that dangerous spinach we should be watching out for, according to the FDA. Sadly, I suspect the beef industry can afford to hire more lobbyists than spinach farmers can.

If you do have the misfortune to contract E. coli, you'll suffer through a bout of diarrhea and will simply need to keep hydrated.[14] In a very small number of cases, E. coli infection can lead to a more

Number of *E. coli* outbreaks by source
(US 1982-2002)

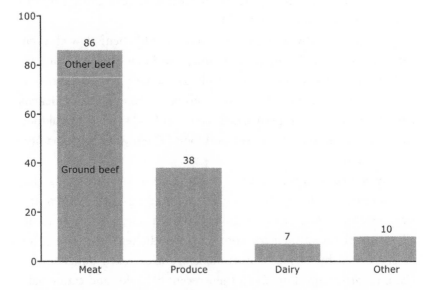

serious condition called hemolytic-uremic syndrome (HUS), which causes anemia, bleeding, and kidney failure. But even in this worst-case scenario, almost three quarters of pregnant women go on to successfully deliver a healthy baby (see Appendix IV for more detail). So please continue to eat your salad leaves without fear.

Threat level for *E. coli*: Low[15]

Twisted Bacteria: *Campylobacter*

Unless you're a strict vegetarian, I can tell you with almost 100 percent certainty that there is *Campylobacter* festering somewhere in your kitchen. It's culturing in invisible patches on your counter or your cutting board, hoping for an opportunity to reach your mouth, multiply rapidly in your gut, and cause a bout of severe intestinal distress.

The term *Campylobacter* literally means "twisted bacteria," and this bacteria is the leading cause of acute infectious diarrhea in most industrialized countries.[16] Like *E. coli*, almost everyone infected with *Campylobacter* recovers from their intestinal distress without requiring treatment, so this is not a serious disease.[17] But on very rare occasions, infection during the second trimester can cause stillbirth (see Appendix IV for more detail).

How do these twisty bacteria invade your kitchen? Raw chicken. "No, no," you say, "I buy only organic, free-range chicken." Doesn't matter—almost any healthy bird will have some *Campylobacter* hiding in its digestive tract.[18] In 2010, *Consumer Reports* tested chickens from more than 100 supermarkets, gourmet food stores, natural food stores, and mass merchandisers, and found *Campylobacter* in 62 percent of them.[19]

Given that *Campylobacter* is everywhere, it's unsurprising that the internet is filled with advice about avoiding pink chicken and washing cutting boards thoroughly. That's sensible, but we don't usually contract *Campylobacter* from our own kitchens. A recent study co-sponsored by various government agencies asked patients with *Campylobacter* infection about their recent behavior and eating habits.[20] Here's what the researchers concluded had caused the infections:

Percent of total *Campylobacter* cases attributable to each factor

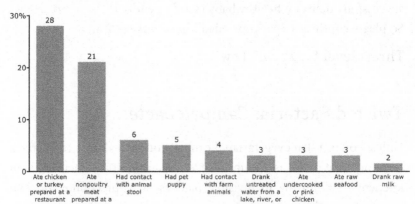

That's right: eating poultry or meat in a restaurant is by far the most likely way to infect yourself with twisted bacteria. Restaurants are responsible for almost half of all cases of *Campylobacter* infection.

Sometimes you really don't want to know what's going on behind those swinging doors. Hint: it's not the waiter spitting in your food that you should be worried about.

Threat level for *Campylobacter*: Low[21]

In Defense of Cat Litter: *Toxoplasma gondii*

The small ball of soft fur with the bright green eyes rolls around charmingly and purrs up at you, pleading, "Choose me, choose me!" You are smitten, and before you know it, you have arrived home with a new pet cat. Unfortunately, reality soon sets in. The couch has developed suspicious scratch marks down the front of the arm, your favorite rug now smells like pee, and then there's the relentless and thankless task of cleaning the litter box day after day. Fortunately, you soon have the perfect excuse: "I can't clean the litter box anymore, I'm pregnant!"

Many people have a notion that *Toxoplasma gondii* is related to cats, and that interacting with cats—or, more specifically, scooping cat litter—should be avoided during pregnancy. Popular pregnancy websites also frequently advise women to avoid changing cat litter.[22] This notion is perfectly logical: cats are indeed critical factors in the spreading of *Toxoplasma gondii*. Bizarrely, it's only in the gastrointestinal tract of cats that this specific type of parasite can sexually propagate, producing "oocysts," which are then excreted in the cats' feces and spread from there into the wider environment. It would therefore make sense to presume that humans could catch the parasite from cleaning cat litter.

The problem is that for many years, it was not known exactly how *Toxoplasma gondii* was transmitted to humans. Finally, a large-scale study was published in 2000.[23] The researchers screened hundreds of pregnant women for recent infection with *Toxoplasma gondii* and ran through a detailed questionnaire about diet, activities, and so on. They included as many questions to do with cats as they could think of to identify where the risk factors lay.[24]

To identify likely sources of *Toxoplasma gondii* infection, the researchers tested as many factors to do with cats as they could think of (kitten in home; adult cat in home; cat and kitten in home; any cat in home; cleaning litter tray; cat that hunts; cat fed raw meat; cat fed canned food). They also asked about consumption of raw/under-cooked meat and a number of other dietary and lifestyle factors. Here are the results:

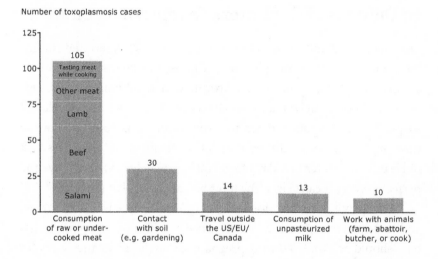

Number of toxoplasmosis cases

Conspicuously absent from this chart is anything to do with cats. In fact, the authors concluded that "contact with cats, kittens, cats' feces, or cats who hunt for food was not a risk factor for infection."[25]

How could that possibly be? The explanation lies in the life cycle of the parasite. Cats excrete oocysts for only two weeks when they first contract the parasite. The oocysts become infectious one to five days later and can survive for more than a year in the environment, getting spread around by surface water.[26] So, first of all, cats are rarely infectious—there's only a two-week window in their entire life. Second, most cat owners don't leave a full litter box to fester for days on end, which means that the infected cat feces would typically be long gone by the time the parasites are ready to creep out. Third, we certainly don't rub our hands around in the litter box as we do with soil when gardening, let alone let it come anywhere near our mouths, as with meat! So it should really be no surprise that scooping cat litter isn't the problem.

How does the virus typically reach humans, then? Oocysts in the water and soil infect domesticated animals, who then pass the parasite along to those humans who consume undercooked meat. In the words of the study authors: "The single most important health message for pregnant women is to avoid eating any meat that has not been thoroughly cooked."[27]

Unfortunately, the medical profession itself may be partly responsible for propagating the myth that toxoplasmosis comes from cats. The authors of a recent survey of 102 health professionals concluded: "Over one quarter of all participants inappropriately advised pregnant women to avoid all cat contact. Obstetricians, internists, and family practitioners were all likely to fail to identify undercooked meat consumption as the primary risk factor for toxoplasmosis transmission . . . Education of obstetricians and other healthcare providers is needed and may lower the rate of congenital toxoplasmosis, as well as decrease the frequency of cat abandonment during pregnancy."[28]

Health care providers are right to take toxoplasmosis seriously. A woman who contracts an infection for the first time while pregnant will typically have no symptoms herself, but her fetus is at risk of serious outcomes ranging from blindness to mental retardation and death.[29] *Toxoplasma gondii* is a nasty parasite. But you have to feel sorry for all the poor housecats thrown out of their comfortable homes to fend for themselves in the streets, when the real threat lies with good ol' dad, standing at the grill and cheerfully serving up plump, juicy, slightly undercooked hamburgers.

Threat level for *Toxoplasma gondii* from meat: Medium[30]

The Stinky Cheese Debate: *Listeria*

"In the early 1990s, word broke that the European Union was going to require all cheese to be pasteurized. It was a rumor. But it spread through France like a brush fire fanned by the mistral. Cheese makers, chefs, shop owners, and buyers panicked, and their Gallic pride kicked in. They signed petitions. They made noise in the news media. France's beloved cheeses made from raw milk—its Camembert, its

Chabichou—became symbols of cultural identity. 'If we had to pasteurize our cheeses,' said Jean Pierre Moreau, a cheese maker in the Loire Valley, 'there would have been a revolution.'"[31]

Across the Channel in London, a supermarket told one of its customers that she could not have unpasteurized Cheddar cheese because she was pregnant. She succeeded in buying the cheese only because she promised not to eat any of it herself.[32]

Cultural differences? Certainly. Differing attitudes toward risk? Perhaps. But the debate over cheese should be resolvable with recourse to the facts. Is cheese risky or not during pregnancy? If so, how risky?

Here's the conventional wisdom from a typical parenting website: "Is it safe to eat soft cheese during pregnancy? That depends on the cheese. If the cheese is made from pasteurized milk, it's fine. But some cheese is made with raw (unpasteurized) milk, and it's not safe to eat or drink anything made with raw milk during pregnancy. Most cheese sold in the United States—including soft cheese—is made with pasteurized milk and is therefore considered safe to eat. But some cheese made from raw milk also shows up on store shelves and at farmer's markets, so it's best to check the label before eating any."[33] This advice was offered by a genetic counselor. Next we'll be asking our pharmacist for help with buying a used car and our lawyer for gardening advice!

Let's turn instead to data from a report published by the US Food Safety and Inspection service (FSIS), which estimates the risk of contracting *Listeria* from various types of foods.[34] What have they concluded? The answers may surprise you:

Median *Listeria* risk per serving
(billionths)

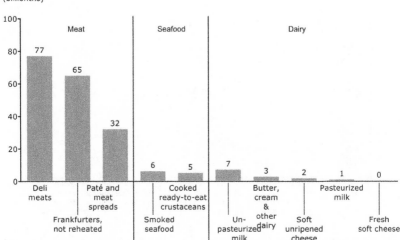

Note: *Soft unripened cheese includes cheeses such as cottage cheese, cream cheese, and ricotta. Fresh soft cheese includes queso fresco, queso de crema, and queso de puna. Many categories have been left off this chart, so low as to barely register; the list includes frankfurters (reheated), preserved fish, raw seafood, fruits, dry/semi-dry fermented sausages, semi-soft cheese (blue, brick, monterey, muenster), soft ripened cheese (brie, camembert, feta, mozzarella), vegetables, deli-type salads (fruit, vegetable, meat, pasta, egg, or seafood salads), ice cream & other frozen dairy products, processed cheese, cultured milk products (yogurt, sour cream, buttermilk), and hard cheese (cheddar, colby, parmesan)— all of which have a risk of less than one case per billion servings.*

Guess what? Deli meat tops the list. It's more than 10,000 *times* more dangerous than brie and camembert per serving. The results are even more striking when taking into account the typical frequency with which these foods are eaten by the average American, to reach a predicted number of cases of *Listeria* per year by food category (see chart on following page).

Deli meat emerges as THE single biggest hazard from *Listeria* facing the pregnant US population, absolutely dwarfing all others. No other food category comes close in terms of importance, with deli meat representing 89 percent of cases, or more than 8 times the risk of all other foods combined. So if you want to avoid *Listeria*, you simply need to heat any meat before eating it, including cold cuts.

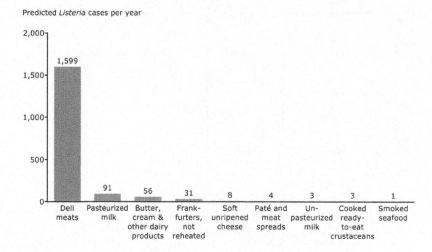

Predicted *Listeria* cases per year

As a final aside, the second most dangerous food is ordinary pasteurized milk. Milk has a relatively low risk per serving, but is consumed so frequently that cumulatively, the risk is higher than for less common foods. It should be your morning bowl of cereal, rather than the occasional restaurant cheese plate, that makes you think twice.

Threat level for *Listeria*: Medium[35]

Sinful, Slimy Seafood: Sushi

Following the advice about heating meat is all very well, but what if the whole point of a food is to eat it raw? Yes, there is one special category we need to discuss, and no, I'm not talking about steak tartare. I'm talking about sushi.

Sushi is typically the first item that pops to mind when you ask a pregnant woman what she's avoiding. A recent March of Dimes poll confirmed sushi and fish the number one food worry, with 61 percent of mothers-to-be concerned.[36] You can just picture the bacteria multiplying on the raw fish flesh, the tiny sea worms burrowing their way out of sight and curling up, awaiting their happy trip down your esophagus. (There's also a more general concern about mercury in fish, but we'll come to that later.)

The experts all agree: no sushi. But they can't get their story straight on what exactly is wrong with it. Here's the word from a popular parenting book: "Sorry to say, sushi and sashimi will have to go the way of sake (the Japanese wine often served with them) during pregnancy—which is to say, they're off the table . . . That's because when seafood isn't cooked, there's a slight chance that it can make you sick (something you definitely don't want to be when you're pregnant)."[37]

Sick from what, exactly? No one wants to be sick, but are the authors implying that sushi could harm the baby or merely sympathizing with the compounding misery of food poisoning on top of heartburn and puffy ankles? Maybe they're just trying to tone things down, since not everyone wants to read about the potential for creepy-crawlies in their food.

An expert on a popular parenting website explains: "Although the chances of getting a parasitic infection from eating sushi are slim, the consequences are severe enough that you wouldn't want to take the risk. Parasites live in the meat of raw fish. While sushi chefs are very careful, that doesn't mean they detect every single parasite . . . Some parasitic infections can lead to anemia or serious malnourishment in the mother or even cause miscarriage."[38] It's a "slim" chance, but with "severe" consequences like miscarriage, why gamble with the safety of your baby?

If you want to know which parasites, exactly, might be the problem, you can simply consult the "Fish and Fishery Products Hazards and Controls Guidance," a 476-page document you can download from the FDA website.[39] This weighty tome attempts to exhaustively describe every possible threat that might be lurking in the fish food chain. It's primarily aimed at "processors of fish and fishery products," although the document also claims it will "help consumers and the public generally to understand commercial seafood safety." (I have a sneaking suspicion that you haven't read this document.)

So what hazards might be festering in fish—in raw fish, in particular? Heating or freezing[40] would hardly affect toxins (we'll address those later), so if we're talking about the hazards of going raw, it's all about pathogens: "Pathogenic bacteria growth as a result of time and temperature abuse of fish and fishery products can cause consumer illness . . . Pathogenic bacteria can enter the process on raw materials. They can also be introduced into foods during processing from the air, unclean hands, unsanitary utensils and equipment, contaminated water, or sewage, and through cross-contamination between raw and cooked product."

In other words, sushi could theoretically be a vector for any of the nasty bacteria we've already covered simply by nature of being consumed raw. But that doesn't make eating sushi any more dangerous than eating, say, a green salad. In fact, it would be even less likely to be contaminated, since most sushi kitchens prepare primarily fish, as opposed to prepping a wide variety of animal products. And as we've seen, raw fish doesn't even register on the list of the common sources of bacterial food poisoning.

Instead, it's parasites that are the unique culprit when it comes to sushi. Here's the appetizing list from "Fish and Fishery Products Hazards and Controls Guidance": "Parasites (in the larval stage) consumed in uncooked or undercooked seafood can present a human health hazard. Among parasites, the nematodes or roundworms (*Anisakis, Pseudoterranova, Eustrongylides,* and *Gnathostoma*), cestodes or tapeworms (*Diphyllobothrium*), and trematodes or flukes (*Clonorchis sinensis, Opisthorchis, Heterophyes, Metagonimus, Nanophyetus salmincola,* and *Paragonimus*) are of most concern in seafood."

Ever heard of any of these? With the exception of tapeworms, I suspect not. I thought I'd become an expert on foodborne illnesses after spending hours with my head buried in the report described earlier, which purportedly covered all known causes of food poisoning in the United States. But not a single one of these little delights was mentioned in that report, which was published in 2011.

It turns out I wasn't the only one wondering whether these parasites were a real or imaginary threat. The FDA wondered as well. Could it be that eating sushi is such a newfangled trend that the national screening programs have yet to pick it up? To check, the FDA surveyed gastroenterologists in coastal states where people are likely eat more seafood to determine whether they were encountering a parasite problem. In the final report, the American Gastroenterological Association esti-mated the number of infections at 270 cases per year.[41] Given that approximately 30 million Americans eat raw fish on a regular basis,[42] this implies that regular sushi eaters have about a 1 in 100,000 chance of contracting a parasite. Are these odds infinitesimally small? No. But you're still four times less likely to become infected with a worm than to *die* in a car crash.

Unfortunately, statistics can only convince your brain, whereas the revulsion you're feeling about the prospect of unintentionally eating a parasite is probably originating in your gut. So perhaps the best way to reassure you is to make the case that even if you did have the extraor-dinarily bad luck to swallow a worm, nothing bad would happen to either you or the baby. Let's look at the three creepy-crawlies the gas-troenterologists had encountered.

The treatment for the most common parasite infection, *Anisakiasis*, is simply removing the worms with a help of a scope.[43] Similarly, *Pseudoterranoviasis* is treated by sending a scope down to remove the worm.[44] Unpleasant, undoubtedly, to have a tube put down one's throat, but hardly a threat specific to a pregnant woman—this is the digestive tract we're talking about, not the uterus. The treatment for *Diphyllobothriasis* is even easier: one can simply swallow some medi-cine,[45] which is safe during pregnancy according to the World Health Organization and the Extra Pharmacopoeia.[46, 47]

So please, just relax. Grab your ginger, your wasabi, and your chop-sticks, and chow down on that sashimi. As you'll see in a later chapter, you'll actually be doing your baby a favor by eating plenty of fish!

Threat level for sushi: Very low

Lemon, Tabasco, and a Dash of Sewage: Oysters

Would you feel comfortable sucking on the filter cartridge that had been sitting in your water pitcher for several weeks? What about licking the inside of your toilet bowl? If the thought of either of these turns your stomach, then you might want to consider skipping the raw oysters. Oysters (and other mollusks like clams, mussels, and scallops) are "filter feeders:" they eat by drawing in water and filtering out the nutrients as well as whatever pollutants or bacteria might be floating around. The average oyster filters between twenty and fifty gallons of water per day, depending on whose estimate you believe, and oyster beds have been proposed as a potential solution to clearing up water pollution in heavily polluted areas such as Chesapeake Bay. Discussion of oyster safety often centers on the level of fecal bacteria contamination, since we humans have an unfortunate tendency to spew sewage into the very coastal waters from which we then harvest seafood.

But could those little dollops of oyster flesh in their pretty iridescent shells actually be dangerous to you or your unborn baby? Here's the conventional wisdom found on typical parenting websites: "Though raw oysters are often safe to eat, they can also carry a virus called *Vibrio vulnificus*, which can lead to severe illness and even death in susceptible individuals. There's no way to know if these bacteria are present, so the prudent thing to do is to avoid raw oysters during pregnancy."[48] Risk of death!

In actual fact, the number of deaths reported to the Centers for Disease Control and Prevention each year from *Vibrio* infections is negligible, and cases are limited to "individuals with chronic underlying illnesses, such as liver disease."[49] So you're not going to die of *Vibrio* food poisoning anytime soon, even if you slurp down lots of Tabasco at the raw bar. Yes, a *Vibrio* infection can still make you sick. If you eat oysters, you have somewhere between a 1 in 100,000 and a 1 in 15,000 chance of infection, with a 40 percent chance of being hospitalized.[50, 51, 52] Unpleasant, yes, but there's no reporting of any pregnant women or fetuses being affected by *Vibrio* viruses.

Oysters can also harbor other nasties, such as *Salmonella, Shigella, Staphylococcus, Giardia, Campylobacter jejuni, Yersinia enterocolitica*, hepatitis A virus, and norovirus (all of which are covered in more detail in Appendix IV, on foodborne illnesses). Soon we'll be throwing out our Brita filters and cultivating pet mollusks instead! So your overall risk of getting sick from any kind of bacteria or virus from oysters works out to about 1 in 10,000 servings.[53] But besides *Campylobacter*, which we discussed previously, none of these infections poses a significant risk in pregnancy.

I've therefore come to the following conclusion after researching all about our slimy friends: oysters are disgusting if you think too hard about them. But eating a meat skewer at a wedding is actually more dangerous to your little one than slurping down the entire raw bar.

Threat level for oysters: Very low

Conclusions: Heat Your Meat!

Unfortunately, the message about which foods are truly dangerous tends to get completely lost in the long lists of forbidden foods found in most pregnancy books, pamphlets, and websites. Upon closer investigation, every single one of the dangerous foodborne pathogens in pregnancy, including *Listeria* and *Toxoplasma gondii*, are found primarily in infected meat. You can still eat that ham sandwich from the deli; it's just advisable to nuke it first. (No more cold cuts: when you're pregnant, think "hot cuts" instead.) So rather than banning fifteen foods and causing unnecessary panic about household pets, a better health message would scrap the list entirely, and instead scrawl a single message over it in large capital letters: when pregnant, "HEAT YOUR MEAT!"

The Most Dangerous Beasties of All: Cytomegalovirus and Parvovirus B19

I've saved the worst for last. The most dangerous little beasties during pregnancy don't lurk in food. If you want to avoid infection, here's the single most important thing you *shouldn't* be doing while pregnant: kiss your own child. (If you don't have small children already or spend time with anyone else's, you can skip this section.)

I'm not kidding. Here are the CDC's recommendations for how to protect yourself from your own small child while pregnant:

- Wash your hands often with soap and water for 15–20 seconds, especially after changing diapers, feeding a young

child, wiping a young child's nose or drool, or handling children's toys
- Do not share food, drinks, or eating utensils with young children
- Do not put a child's pacifier in your mouth
- Do not share a toothbrush with a young child
- Avoid contact with saliva when kissing a child
- Clean toys, countertops, and other surfaces that come into contact with children's urine or saliva[54]

If you're the parent of a typical baby or toddler, these guidelines are practically laughable. If you followed them, you'd be washing your hands every two minutes, not to mention the logistical impossibility of keeping every toy and surface constantly clean. Besides, how could your healthy little cherub possibly be the source of a dangerous virus that you don't already have yourself?

The problem lies in small children's tendency to leave behind a trail of drool and snot wherever they go. So if your child spends time with other small children—for example, in daycare or a playgroup—he or she is likely to chew on a toy that another baby has chewed on at some point, thereby contracting a harmless virus called cytomegalovirus (CMV).[55, 56, 57, 58] CMV often causes no symptoms at all, or at worst may cause a fever or sore throat. It's just your typical, run-of-the-mill virus that you'll get over very quickly. It's also ubiquitous in the population: 50–70 percent of adult women have already been exposed to it at some point. So most of us have antibodies to it and are therefore protected.

But if by some fluke you happen to have reached adulthood without being exposed, you could catch it for the first time from your small child.[59, 60] (You could also technically contract it through a sexual partner.) Children continue to shed the virus for months or even years after becoming infected.[61] And herein lies the problem, because this virus is not harmless to a fetus, who will sometimes catch it from you. According to the CDC, about 1 in 1000 children in the United States ends up suffering from permanent problems as a result of CMV infection in the womb.[62] These permanent problems include deafness, blindness, and, in the worst cases, even severe intellectual disability and death.

Have you ever heard of cytomegalovirus? I certainly hadn't. In a recent survey, only 22 percent of women were aware of CMV, and hardly anyone knew how it was spread. But CMV infection causes more long-term problems and childhood deaths than Down syndrome and fetal alcohol syndrome combined.[63]

It doesn't help that your doctor is likely to be in the dark, too. Although the American College of Obstetricians and Gynecologists recommends counseling women about CMV, only 44 percent of doctors actually discuss CMV with their pregnant patients.[64] Typical pregnancy books are no help either: "Many contain little information on CMV, and sometimes their information is inaccurate. For example, one popular pregnancy book states that 'Pregnant women with toddlers of their own need not worry about catching CMV; the possibility is extremely remote.'"[65] Pure misinformation.

CMV is not the only dangerous virus that can be caught from small children. There's another similar and equally obscure virus called parvovirus B19,[66] which is also ubiquitous in the population (50–60 percent of adults have been exposed),[67, 68] also harmless in general (a quarter of people have no symptoms; the rest feel like they have the flu),[69, 70, 71] and also spread by close contact, particularly with children.[72] And it can also cause miscarriage and stillbirth, with the highest risk before 20 weeks, although it's much less likely than CMV to cause birth defects.[73, 74, 75]

The good news is, advising women to be careful of toddlers and wash their hands frequently appears to help reduce the rate of CMV infection, according to preliminary studies.[76, 77] And there's strong evidence from studies of other infectious diseases that frequent handwashing can make a real difference to catching infections in general.[78, 79] The only caveat is that you have to wash your hands for a full 15–20 seconds to kill bacteria. (Antibacterial gel is slightly less effective than proper handwashing but more effective than typical cursory handwashing.)

Someday scientists will succeed in developing vaccines against CMV and parvovirus B19, and our little fetuses will be safe from these scourges. In the meantime, you can ask for a blood test to determine whether you already have immunity against them, in which case there's nothing to worry about.[80, 81] Otherwise, you'll just have to keep those hands clean and resist your overpowering urge to smooch Junior.

Threat level for viruses from small children: Medium[82]

Notes

1. Swine flu prompts EU warning against travel to US, Mexico. (2009, April 27). *CNN.com*. http://transcripts.cnn.com/TRANSCRIPTS/0904/27/ltm.03.html.

2. Montopoli, B. (2009, May 26). Did we overreact to swine flu threat? *CBSNEWS.com*. www.cbsnews.com/stories/2009/05/06/health/main4995966.shtml.

3. The BabyCenter Medical Advisory Board. (Last updated 2016, May). Foods and beverages to avoid during pregnancy. Babycenter.com. www.babycenter.com/0_foods-and-beverages-to-avoid-during-pregnancy_10348544.bc?showAll=true.

4. Eating right when pregnant. (n.d.). WebMD.com. www.webmd.com/baby/guide/eating-right-when-pregnant?page=2.

5. Food safety for moms-to-be. (Last updated 2017, November 6). US Food and Drug Administration. www.fda.gov/food/resourcesforyou/healtheducators/ucm081785.htm.

6. Food safety for pregnant women. (Last modified 2016, August 9). Health Canada. http://healthycanadians.gc.ca/eating-nutrition/safety-salubrite/pregnant-enceintes-eng.php.

7. UK National Health Service. (Last reviewed 2017, January 23). Foods to avoid in pregnancy. NHS Choices. www.nhs.uk/Planners/pregnancycareplanner/pages/Carewithfood.aspx.

8. Foods to eat or avoid during pregnancy. (Last updated 2016, January 5). The New South Wales Department of Primary Industry Food Authority. www.foodauthority.nsw.gov.au/foodsafetyandyou/life-events-and-food/pregnancy/foods-to-eat-or-avoid-when-pregnant.

9. New Zealand Food Safety Authority. (2013, January). List of safe food in pregnancy. Ministry for Primary Industries. https://www.mpi.govt.nz/food-safety/pregnant-and-at-risk-people/food-and-pregnancy/list-of-safe-food-in-pregnancy/.

10. Burros, M. (2006, December 27). You are what you eat: 2006 and the politics of food. *NYTimes.com*. www.nytimes.com/2006/12/27/dining/27food.html?scp=51&sq=e+coli+spinach&st=nyt.

11. Zeleny, J. (2007, March 15). House war bill: eat your spinach. *NYTimes.com*. http://thecaucus.blogs.nytimes.com/2007/03/15/house-war-bill-eat-your-spinach/?scp=2&sq=e%20coli%20spinach%20bailout&st=cse.

12. Brennan, T. (2006, December 11). *E. coli* outbreaks: too little being done? *CNBC.com*. www.cnbc.com/id/16157127/.

13. Rangel, J. M., Sparling, P. H., Crowe, C., Griffin, P. M., & Swerdlow, D. L. (2005). Epidemiology of *Escherichia coli* O157: H7 outbreaks, United States, 1982–2002. *Public Health Resources, 73*. http://digitalcommons.unl.edu/cgi/viewcontent.cgi?article=1069&context=publichealthresources.

14. *E. coli*: general information. (Updated 2015, November 6). Centers for Disease Control and Prevention. https://www.cdc.gov/ecoli/general/.

15. Threat score for *E. coli* in general is 0.27 (see Appendix IV for detail). Threat score for eating undercooked beef specifically is 0.27 x 86/(86+38+7+10) (proportion of outbreaks caused by beef, from the numbers on the chart) = 0.16. Note: this is the threat level for maternal exposure to foodborne *E. coli* during pregnancy rather than the threat level from *E. coli* caused by transmission to the baby during birth or soon thereafter.

16. McDonald, S. D., & Gruslin, A. (2001). A review of *Campylobacter* infection during pregnancy: a focus on *C. jejuni*. *Primary Care Update for OB/GYNS, 8* (6), 253–257.

17. *Campylobacter*. (Updated 2017, August 31). Centers for Disease Control. https://www.cdc.gov/campylobacter/index.html.

18. Centers for Disease Control. (2005). Foodborne illness—frequently asked questions. Atlanta: Coordinating Center for Infectious Diseases, Division of Bacterial and Mycotic Diseases.

19. Consumer Reports. (2010, January). How safe is that chicken? ConsumerReports.org. https://www.consumerreports.org/cro/2012/05/how-safe-is-that-chicken/index.htm.

20. The Centers for Disease Control and Prevention's National Center for Infectious Diseases, the US Department of Agriculture Food Safety Inspection Service, and the US Food and Drug Administration Center for Food Safety and Applied Nutrition; Friedman, Cindy R., Hoekstra, R. M., Samuel, M., Marcus, R., Bender, J., Shiferaw, B. . . . & Tauxe, R. V. (2004). Risk factors for sporadic *Campylobacter* infection in the United States: a case-control study in FoodNet sites. *Clinical Infectious Diseases, 38* (Supplement 3), S285–S296. http://cid.oxfordjournals.org/content/38/Supplement_3/S285.full.pdf.

21. Threat score for *Campylobacter* in general is 0.75 (see Appendix IV for detail). Threat score from eating chicken or turkey at a restaurant: 0.75 x 28% from the chart = 0.21. Threat score for eating (non-poultry) meat at a restaurant: 0.75 x 21% from the chart = 0.16.

22. Pregnancy and toxoplasmosis. (n.d.). WebMD.com. www.webmd.com/baby/toxoplasmosis.

23. Cook, A. J. C., Gilbert, R. E., Buffolano, W., Zufferey, J., Petersen, E., Jenum, P. A. . . . & Holliman, R. (2000). Sources of *toxoplasma* infection in pregnant women: European multicentre case-control study. Commentary: congenital toxoplasmosis—further thought for food. *British Medical Journal, 321* (7254), 142–147. http://www.ncbi.nlm.nih.gov/pmc/articles/PMC27431/?tool%3Dpubmed.

24. People are notoriously bad at accurately remembering how they have behaved in the past, particularly when new knowledge is available to retrospectively cloud their recollection. ["I have a parasitic infection! Hmm, I must have done something risky recently . . ."] A classic example was the cell phone study which seemed to conclude that holding your phone to one side of your head protects the other side from developing cancer. But "almost exactly the same decreased risk was seen on the other side of the head, leaving no overall increased risk of tumors for mobile phone users. Instead, they blamed biased reporting from brain tumor sufferers who knew what side of the head their tumors were on." (Mobiles 'don't raise cancer risk'. [2006, January 20]. *BBC News*. http://news.bbc.co.uk/1/hi/health/4628914.stm.) If there were no recall bias, the study results would obviously stretch the limits of credibility. In the case of this *Toxoplasma gondii* study, however, the researchers were prepared for such bias; in addition to asking about lifestyle factors, "women were first asked how they could avoid *Toxoplasma* infection to assess their knowledge about sources of infection." Interestingly, the women did indeed come in with preconceived notions of the sources of toxoplasmosis, but their notions ended up being the opposite of the conclusions reached from the data, which implies the conclusions are unlikely to have been bolstered by false recall.

25. Cook et al., Sources of toxoplasma infection in pregnant women.

26. Ibid.

27. Ibid.

28. Kravetz, J. D., & Federman, D. G. (2005). Prevention of toxoplasmosis in pregnancy: knowledge of risk factors. *Infectious Diseases in Obstetrics and Gynecology, 13* (3), 161–165. www.pubmedcentral.nih.gov/picrender.fcgi?artid=1784564&blobtype=pdf.

29. Smith, J. L. (1999). Foodborne infections during pregnancy. *Journal of Food Protection, 62,* 818–829. PubMed, CSA [article purchased].

30. Threat score from undercooked meat is 3.67 (threat score for *Toxoplasma gondii* in general; see Appendix IV for more detail) x 105/(105+30+14+13+10) = 2.24.

31. Hesser, A. (1998, May 20). The French resist again: this time, over cheese. *NYTimes.com.* www.nytimes.com/1998/05/20/dining/the-french-resist-again-this-time-over-cheese.html.

32. Store apology over cheese refusal. (2009, October 5). *BBC News.* http://news.bbc.co.uk/1/hi/england/beds/bucks/herts/8291536.stm.

33. Riordan, S. (Last updated 2015, October). Is it safe to eat soft cheese during pregnancy? Babycenter.com. http://www.babycenter.com/404_is-it-safe-to-eat-soft-cheese-during-pregnancy_3175.bc.

34. Quantitative assessment of the relative risk to public health from foodborne *Listeria monocytogenes* among selected categories of ready-to-eat foods. (2003, September). United States Department of Health and Human Services, Food and Drug Administration's Center for Food Safety and Applied Nutrition. www.fda.gov/downloads/Food/FoodScienceResearch/UCM197329.pdf.

The assessment was developed according to the following approach: "*Listeria* contamination data are based on 387 studies with over 346,000 samples . . . Expert advice on scientific assumptions was actively sought from leading scientists from academia, industry, and government . . . In addition, the risk assessment was initially published in draft form and public comments sought for six months." The authors of the report must have been anticipating some seriously heated debate, or perhaps this is simply how the government always conducts its research. At least we can conclude they have done their homework.

35. Threat score from unrefrigerated (e.g., deli) meat: 3.72 (threat score for *Listeria* in general; see Appendix IV for more detail) x 89% = 3.32.

36. Sushi & breastfeeding join birth defects & preterm birth as leading concerns of moms. (2009, December 9). March of Dimes. www.marchofdimes.org/news/sushi-and-breastfeeding-join-birth-defects-and-preterm-birth-as-leading-concerns-of-moms.aspx.

37. Murkoff, H., & Mazel, S. (2008). *What to expect when you're expecting* (4th ed). New York: Workman Publishing Company.

38. Johnson, M. (Last updated 2016, March). Is it safe to eat sushi while pregnant? Babycenter.com. www.babycenter.com/406_is-it-safe-to-eat-sushi-while-pregnant_1245280.bc. Accessed in 2014.

39. Fish and fishery products hazards and controls guidance. (2011, April). US Department of Health and Human Services, Food and Drug Administration, Center for Food Safety and Applied Nutrition. www.fda.gov/downloads/Food/GuidanceRegulation/UCM251970.pdf.

40. The Food and Drug Administration (FDA) was sufficiently concerned about the risk of parasites for the general population, let alone pregnant women, that it actually mandated that all fish be frozen prior to consumption. As reported in *The New York Times*: "If sushi has not been frozen, it is illegal to serve it in the United States. FDA regulations stipulate that fish to be eaten raw—whether as sushi, sashimi, ceviche, or tartare—must be frozen first, to kill parasites. 'I would desperately hope that all the sushi we eat is frozen,' said

George Hoskin, a director of the agency's Office of Seafood. Tuna, a deep-sea fish with exceptionally clean flesh, is the only exception to the rule." Why does our agency director have to merely hope rather than know with certainty? Isn't he the very man who should be monitoring this issue? This same article unfortunately continues: "The FDA does not enforce the frozen-fish rule, leaving that to local health officials. The agency says sushi fish can be frozen either by the wholesaler or in the restaurant, and each party likes to believe that the other is taking care of it." (Moskin, J. [2004, April 8]. Sushi fresh from the deep . . . the deep freeze. *NYTimes.com*. www.nytimes.com/2004/04/08/nyregion/sushi-fresh-from-the-deep-the-deep-freeze.html?pagewanted=all&src=pm.)

41. American Gastroenterological Association. (2000). Determination of the incidence of gastrointestinal parasitic infections from the consumption of raw seafood in the US. Bethesda, MD: Life Sciences Research Office, American Society of Nutritional Sciences, 9.

42. In *The Sushi Economy*, an exploration of the global sushi trade, journalist Sasha Issenberg has charted the rise of sushi to become one of America's favorite delicacies. He estimates that as of 2007, 30 million Americans were regularly consuming sushi. (Issenberg, S. [2007]. *The sushi economy: globalization and the making of a modern delicacy*. New York: Penguin.) This number might seem startlingly high, given that sushi was almost unheard of only a couple of decades ago. Anyone remember the students in *The Breakfast Club* mocking the high school princess for eating strange raw fish? But Americans truly have had a change of heart. As reported in the *Financial Times* in 2010, "Teenagers take sushi to school; prisons have introduced it; in California, it is served at trucker stops. Meanwhile, the National Sushi Association reports that there are now more than 5,000 sushi bars in American supermarkets, with the number continuing to rise fast." (Tett, G. [2010, December 3]. Land of the rising sushi. FT.com. www.ft.com/cms/s/0/e43c22ca-fcdc-11df-ae2d-00144feab49a.html-axzz1bu9x3pXq.)

43. Bouree, P., Paugam, A., & Petithory, J. C. (1995, February). "Anisakidosis: report of 25 cases and review of the literature." *Comparative Immunology, Microbiology and Infectious Diseases, 18* (2), 75–84. www.sciencedirect.com/science/article/pii/014795719598848C.

With misdiagnosed chronic infections that have lasted several weeks or months, surgery could be necessary, but this is rare.

44. Arizono, N., Miura, T., Yamada, M., Tegoshi, T., & Onishi, K. (2001, March). Human infection with *Pseudoterranova azarasi* roundworm. *Emerging Infectious Diseases, 17*, (3), 555. wwwnc.cdc.gov/eid/article/17/3/10-1350_article.htm.

45. According to Merck Manual, "treatment is with a single oral dose of praziquantel . . . alternatively, a single dose of niclosamide (4 tablets that are chewed one at a time and swallowed)." (Pearson, R. D. [Last reviewed 2016, August]. Diphyllobothriasis [fish tape worm infection]. *Merck Manual*. www.merckmanuals.com/professional/infectious_diseases/cestodes_tapeworms/diphyllobothriasis.html.)

46. Cestode (tapeworm) infection. (1995). *WHO model prescribing information: drugs used in parasitic diseases* (2nd ed.). Geneva: World Health Organization. http://apps.who.int/medicinedocs/en/d/Jh2922e/3.html.

47. Ofori-Adjei, D. (2004, February). Safety review of niclosamide, pyrantel, triclabendazole, and oxamniquine. Report prepared for Quality Assurance & Safety: Medicines, WHO/PSM for the Expert Committee on the Selection and Use of Essential Medicines meeting, March 7–11, 2005. http://archives.who.int/eml/expcom/expcom14/niclosamide/safety_review_08feb05.pdf.

48. Santerre, C. (Last updated 2016, March). Is it safe to eat smoked or raw oysters during pregnancy? Babycenter.com. www.babycenter.com/406_is-it-safe-to-eat-raw-oysters-during-pregnancy_1245282.bc.

49. 33 out of a population of ~300 million.

DePaola, A., Jones, J. L., Woods, J., Burkhardt III, W., Calci, K. R., Krantz, J. A. . . . & Nabe, K. (2010, May). Bacterial and viral pathogens in live oysters: 2007 United States market survey. *Applied and Environmental Microbiology, 76* (9), 2754–2768. www.ncbi.nlm.nih.gov/pmc/articles/PMC2863423/.

50. **1 in 100,000 chance:** Food and Agriculture Organization of the United Nations/World Health Organization. (2011). Risk assessment of *Vibrio parahaemolyticus* in seafood: interpretative summary and technical report. *Microbiological Risk Assessment Series, 16,* 2011, 193. www.who.int/foodsafety/publications/micro/MRA_16_JEMRA.pdf.

51. Hlady, W. G. (1997). Vibrio infections associated with raw oyster consumption in Florida, 1981–1994. *Journal of Food Protection, 60* (4), 353–357. http://www.jfoodprotection.org/doi/abs/10.4315/0362-028X-60.4.353?code=fopr-site.

52. **1 in 15,000 chance:** As referenced in an FDA report assessing the risk of *Vibrio parahaemolyticus* in raw oysters, the CDC has estimated that over 5 years, there were approximately 2,790 cases per year of *V. parahaemolyticus* illness, the most common type of *Vibrio* infection, attributable to oyster consumption in the US. (Quantitative risk assessment on the public health impact of pathogenic *Vibrio parahaemolyticus* in raw oysters. [2005, July]. Center for Food Safety and Applied Nutrition, Food and Drug Administration, and the U.S. Department of Health and Human Services. http://www.fda.gov/downloads/Food/ScienceResearch/ResearchAreas/RiskAssessmentSafetyAssessment/UCM196915.pdf.)

Assuming 20% of the population eats raw oysters out of a total US population at the time of ~280 million, that's 2,790 cases per 42 million people, or a risk of about 66 per 1,000,000, or ~1 per 15,000. (Food and Agriculture Organization of the United Nations/Word Health Organization. [2011]. Risk assessment of *Vibrio parahaemolyticus* in seafood: interpretative summary and technical report. *Microbiological Risk Assessment Series No. 16.* www.who.int/foodsafety/publications/micro/MRA_16_JEMRA.pdf.)

53. The answers here are less definitive. The US government and other research groups spend a lot of time publishing detailed reports evaluating the risk of the most common food/pathogen pairings; for example, *Vibrios* in shellfish, *Salmonella* in eggs, etc. But when it comes to more rare pairings (e.g., *Salmonella* in oysters), there's no special report we can turn to. However, there are plenty of testing and sampling data. For example, a group of researchers gathered oysters from 36 different bays on different coasts and discovered that "7.4% of all oysters tested contained *Salmonella*." (Brands, D. A., Inman, A. E., Gerba, C. P., Maré, C. J., Billington, S. J., Saif, L. A. . . . & Joens, L. A. [2005]. Prevalence of *Salmonella spp.* in oysters in the United States. *Applied and Environmental Microbiology, 71* [2], 893–897. http://www.ncbi.nlm.nih.gov/pmc/articles/PMC546685/pdf/0799-04.pdf.) But if 7 percent of everyone who ate raw oysters actually got sick with *Salmonella* food poisoning, we would have figured out pretty quickly not to eat oysters without cooking them first. In actual fact, we humans are remarkably robust and can down quite a few organisms without getting sick. It takes a whopping dose to overwhelm our immune systems and have any noticeable effect. So if sample testing isn't particularly informative, why can't we just look at how many people have actually gotten sick in the past? The CDC does publish data on total numbers of illnesses in the US population from different bacteria and viruses, but these are only estimates, and they're not tied to a specific type of food. When people get sick, many simply suffer through their bout of illness at home, so they never get counted; even if they do go to the hospital, they may have eaten a variety of different foods, most of which have already been fully consumed or thrown away. So teasing out what actually caused each case of sickness would be time consuming and costly. The best option is therefore to use outbreak data. An outbreak

is simply a case of food poisoning that affects at least two people. The CDC has decided it's worth the effort to track outbreaks, so there's a tool available online called FOOD (Foodborne Outbreak Online Database), which has a record of all foodborne disease outbreaks recorded in the United States over the last twelve years. (Centers for Disease Control and Prevention Foodborne Outbreak Online Datatabase [FOOD]: wwwn.cdc. gov/foodborneoutbreaks/Default.aspx.) Using these data as a starting point, we can estimate how many people fall ill each year from all bacteria and viruses in oysters; then, knowing the total volume of oysters eaten each year, we can calculate a risk of getting sick. Over 12 years, there were 123 outbreaks of illness in the database involving oysters (excluding the *Vibrio* cases, which we've already covered), with 1,905 people falling ill, or 159 per year. Clearly, outbreaks underestimate total illnesses, as there will be plenty of cases where just one person will get sick from a single bad oyster. So how much should we scale up these numbers to reach an estimate of total illnesses? We can't use other food items as a benchmark. Some commodities like eggs are used as ingredients in prepared dishes and are often pooled in large batches, so you could imagine one bad egg reaching many people; therefore outbreaks would be far more common with eggs than with oysters, which are consumed individually. Instead, we can use an oyster-specific disease such as *Vibrio parahaemolyticus*, which causes ordinary gastroenteritis, to calculate an appropriate scaling factor. Over 12 years, there were 816 people sick from outbreaks of *Vibrio parahaemolyticus* in oysters, or an average of 68 illnesses per year. As discussed previously, the CDC has calculated there are ~2,790 illnesses per year. That means our outbreak data underreports by a ratio of 41x. If we now apply this 41x scaling factor to our 159 outbreak illnesses, that's ~6,500 total illnesses per year. To understand the risk per oyster, we then need an estimate of how many oysters are eaten per year. From the report "Fisheries of the United States 2007," the US oyster supply (total domestic catch plus imports minus exports) was 58,082,000 pounds in 2001. (Van Voorhees, D. [2006]. Fisheries of the United States, 2007. NMFS Office of Science and Technology, Fisheries Statistics Division. www.st.nmfs.noaa.gov/st1/fus/fuso7/index.html.) About 50 percent of oysters are estimated to be consumed raw (FAO/WHO, Risk assessment of *Vibrio parahaemolyticus* in seafood), so that would be 29,041,000 pounds per year eaten raw. The average amount of raw oyster consumed at a single serving is 196 g (Ibid.), or .432 pounds, so that's ~67,225,000 servings of raw oysters consumed each year. (That figure seems reasonable; if 10–20 million people eat oysters regularly as referenced above, that would mean they eat on average between 3 and 6 servings per year.) Finally, taking 67,225,000 servings and 6,500 illnesses per year, we can calculate a risk per serving of ~1 in 10,000.

54. Cytomegalovirus (CMV) and congenital CMV infection. (n.d.). Centers for Disease Control and Prevention. www.cdc.gov/cmv/prevention.html.

55. About CMV. (Last updated 2016, June 17). Centers for Disease Control and Prevention. https://www.cdc.gov/cmv/overview.html.

56. Adler, S. P. (1988). Molecular epidemiology of cytomegalovirus: viral transmission among children attending a day care center, their parents, and caretakers. *The Journal of Pediatrics, 112* (3), 366–372. www.sciencedirect.com/science/article/pii/S0022347688803147.

57. Murph, J. R., Bale Jr, J. F., Murray, J. C., Stinski, M. F., & Perlman, S. (1986). Cytomegalovirus transmission in a Midwest day care center: possible relationship to child care practices. *The Journal of Pediatrics, 109* (1), 35–39. www.sciencedirect.com/science/article/pii/S0022347686805686.

58. Pass, R. F., Hutto, S. C., Reynolds, D. W., & Polhill, R. B. (1984). Increased frequency of cytomegalovirus infection in children in group day care. *Pediatrics, 74* (1), 121–126. http://pediatrics.aappublications.org/content/74/1/121.abstract.

59. Adler, S. P. (1991). Cytomegalovirus and child day care: risk factors for maternal infection. *The Pediatric Infectious Disease Journal, 10* (8), 590–594. http://journals.lww.com/pidj/abstract/1991/08000/cytomegalovirus_and_child_day_care__risk_factors.8.aspx.

60. Pass et al., Increased frequency of cytomegalovirus infection in children in group day care.

61. Pass, R. F., Hutto, C., Ricks, R., & Cloud, G. A. (1986). Increased rate of cytomegalovirus infection among parents of children attending day-care centers. *New England Journal of Medicine, 314* (22), 1414–1418. www.nejm.org/doi/full/10.1056/NEJM198605293142204.

62. Babies born with CMV (Congenital CMV Infection). (Last updated 2017, April 13). Centers for Disease Control and Prevention. https://www.cdc.gov/cmv/congenital-infection.html.

63. Jeon, J., Victor, M., Adler, S. P., Arwady, A., Demmler, G., Fowler, K. . . . & Cannon, M. J. (2006). Knowledge and awareness of congenital cytomegalovirus among women. *Infectious Diseases in Obstetrics and Gynecology,* (2006), article 80383, 1–7. http://downloads.hindawi.com/journals/idog/2006/080383.pdf.

64. Centers for Disease Control and Prevention. (2008). Knowledge and practices of obstetricians and gynecologists regarding cytomegalovirus infection during pregnancy—United States, 2007. *Morbidity and Mortality Weekly Report, 57* (3), 65. www.ncbi.nlm.nih.gov/pubmed/18219267.

65. Jeon et al., Knowledge and awareness of congenital cytomegalovirus among women.

66. **Also known as erythema infectiosum, this virus is called "fifth disease" when children catch it, and the rash it can cause on the face is known as "slapped cheek syndrome."**

    Corcoran, A., & Doyle, S. (2004). Advances in the biology, diagnosis and host-pathogen interactions of parvovirus B19. *Journal of Medical Microbiology, 53* (6), 459–475. http://jmm.microbiologyresearch.org/content/journal/jmm/10.1099/jmm.0.05485-0.

67. Anderson, L. J., Tsou, C., Parker, R. A., Chorba, T. L., Wulff, H., Tattersall, P., & Mortimer, P. P. (1986). Detection of antibodies and antigens of human parvovirus B19 by enzyme-linked immunosorbent assay. *Journal of Clinical Microbiology, 24* (4), 522–526. http://jcm.asm.org/content/24/4/522.full.pdf.

68. Cohen, B. J., & Buckley, M. M. (1988). The prevalence of antibody to human parvovirus B19 in England and Wales. *Journal of Medical Microbiology, 25* (2), 151–153. http://jmm.sgmjournals.org/content/25/2/151.full.pdf.

69. Snyder, M., & Wallace, R. (2011). Clinical inquiries: what should you tell pregnant women about exposure to parvovirus? *The Journal of Family Practice, 60* (12), 765–766. https://mospace.umsystem.edu/xmlui/bitstream/handle/10355/12452/WhatTellWomenParvovirus.pdf?sequence=1.

70. Harger, J. H., Adler, S. P., Koch, W. C., & Harger, G. F. (1998). Prospective evaluation of 618 pregnant women exposed to parvovirus B19: risks and symptoms. *Obstetrics & Gynecology, 91* (3), 413–420. http://journals.lww.com/greenjournal/abstract/1998/03000/prospective_evaluation_of_618_pregnant_women.18.aspx.

71. Corcoran, Advances in the biology . . . parvovirus B19.

72. Tuckerman, J. G., Brown, T., & Cohen, B. J. (1986). Erythema infectiosum in a village primary school: clinical and virological studies. *The Journal of the Royal College of General Practitioners, 36* (287), 267. www.ncbi.nlm.nih.gov/pmc/articles/PMC1960541/pdf/jroyalcgprac00150-0037.pdf.

73. **Miscarriage and stillbirth:** Vyse, A. J., Andrews, N. J., Hesketh, L. M., & Pebody, R. (2007). The burden of parvovirus B19 infection in women of childbearing age in England and Wales. *Epidemiology and Infection, 135* (8), 1354–1362. www.ncbi.nlm.nih.gov/pmc/articles/PMC2870696/.

74. **... with the highest risk before 20 weeks:** Mehta, S., Rajaram, S., & Goel, N. (Eds.). (2011). *Advances in obstetrics and gynecology*, vol. 3. New Delhi: Jaypee Brothers Medical Publishers Ltd., 46. https://goo.gl/vHrZpw.

75. **... much less likely to cause birth defects than CMV:** Miller, E., Fairley, C. K., Cohen, B. J., & Seng, C. (1998). Immediate and long term outcome of human parvovirus B19 infection in pregnancy. *British Journal of Obstetrics & Gynaecology, 105* (2), 174–178. http://onlinelibrary.wiley.com/store/10.1111/j.1471-0528.1998.tb10048.x/asset/j.1471-0528.1998.tb10048.x.pdf?v=1&t=ja80k3im&s=0e52877e8b4f9142ee3d7dfbd65ff4cfec50d67e.

76. Cannon, M. J., & Davis, K. F. (2005). Washing our hands of the congenital cytomegalovirus disease epidemic. *BMC Public Health, 5* (1), 70. www.biomedcentral.com/1471-2458/5/70.

77. Vauloup-Fellous, C., Picone, O., Cordier, A. G., Parent-du-Châtelet, I., Senat, M. V., Frydman, R., & Grangeot-Keros, L. (2009). Does hygiene counseling have an impact on the rate of CMV primary infection during pregnancy?: Results of a 3-year prospective study in a French hospital. *Journal of Clinical Virology,* (46) Suppl. 4, S49-S53. www.journalofclinicalvirology.com/article/S1386-6532(09)00419-3/abstract.

78. A review of studies over the last hundred years has concluded that handwashing is undoubtedly an effective way to reduce infection (Larson, E. [1988]. A causal link between handwashing and risk of infection? Examination of the evidence. *Infection Control, 9* [1], 28–36. http://europepmc.org/abstract/MED/3276640.) Another review concludes that handwashing can reduce the risk of contracting diarrhea by 47%. (Curtis, V. & Cairncross, S. [2003]. Effect of washing hands with soap on diarrhoea risk in the community: a systematic review. *The Lancet: Infectious Diseases, 3* (5), 275–281. www.hygienecentral.org.uk/pdf/CurtisHandwashing.pdf).

79. Cannon, Washing our hands of the congenital cytomegalovirus disease epidemic.

80. Unfortunately, according to the CDC, there's no way to tell midway through your pregnancy if your fetus has already been affected by CMV: "Maternal IgG antibodies pass through the placenta during pregnancy; thus, CMV IgG testing of infants may reflect maternal antibody status, and does not necessarily indicate infection in the infant." (Congenital CMV infection. [Last updated 2017, June 5]. Centers for Disease Control and Prevention. https://www.cdc.gov/cmv/clinical/congenital-cmv.html.)

81. Fifth Disease. (Last updated 2015, November 2). Centers for Disease Control and Prevention. www.cdc.gov/parvovirusb19/fifth-disease.html.

82. CMV: According to an estimate from the Institute of Medicine published in 2001, 40,000 infants are born annually with congenital CMV. 90% are asymptomatic at birth, and of these 36,000, 5,400 develop neurologic outcomes such as deafness for life. 10% are symptomatic at birth, and of the 4,000, 10% die (400). Of the 3,600 remaining, 90% or 3,240 have severe outcomes (severe mental retardation, reduced lifespan of 20 years, require long-term care), and 10% (or 360) have mild, lifelong outcomes (deafness, blindness, mild retardation). (Stratton, K. R., Durch, J. S., & Lawrence, R. S. [Eds.]. [2001]. Vaccines for the 21st century: a tool for decisionmaking. Washington, DC: The National Academies Press. https://www.nap.edu/read/5501/chapter/14.) In 2000, there were 4,059,000 live births. (Ventura, S. J., Abma, J. C., Mosher, W. D., & Henshaw, S. K. [2008, April 14]. Estimated pregnancy rates by outcome for the United States, 1990-2004. *National Vital Statistics Reports, 56* [15], 1–26. https://stacks.cdc.gov/view/cdc/13317.) Threat score: 400/4,059,000 (probability of death) x 100,000 (impact: death) x 1 (certainty: well proven) = 9.9.

3,240/4,059,000 (probability of severe outcomes) x (impact: significant impairment) x 1 (certainty: well proven) = 8.0.

(5,400 + 360)/4,059,000 (probability of mild outcomes) x (impact: minor impairment) x 1 (certainty: well proven) = 1.4.

Total threat score for CMV: 9.9 + 8.0 + 1.4 = 19.3.

Parvovirus B19: According to a study on parvovirus B19, "parvovirus infection in pregnancy was estimated to occur on average in up to 1 in every 512 pregnancies each year. This represents 1257 maternal infections, causing up to an estimated 59 fetal deaths and 11 cases of hydrops fetalis annually." (Vyse et al., The burden of parvovirus B19 . . . England and Wales.) Out of 51 newborns with hydrops fetalis, 32 died before age 1, and 4 had retardation. (Nakayama, H., Kukita, J., Hikino, S., Nakano, H., & Hara, T. [1999]. Long-term outcome of 51 liveborn neonates with non-immune hydrops fetalis. *Acta Paediatrica, 88* [1], 24–28. http://onlinelibrary.wiley.com/doi/10.1111/j.1651-2227.1999. tb01262.x/abstract.)

Threat score: 1/512 x (59 + 11 x 32/51)/1257 (probability of death) x 100,000 (impact: death) x 1 (certainty: well proven) = 10.24.

1/512 x 11/1257 x 4/51 (probability of retardation) x 10,000 (impact: significant impairment) x 1 (certainty: well proven) = 0.01.

Total threat score for parvovirus B19: 10.24 + 0.01 = 10.25.

Total threat score for viruses from small children (CMV and parvovirus B19): 19.3 + 10.25 = 29.5.

Handwashing can reduce infections by 47%, so assuming this applies to these viruses, the threat score for controllable virus exposure is 29.5 x 47% = 13.9, and the score for uncontrollable virus exposure is 29.5 x 53% = 15.6.

2

BOMBARDED

Environmental Toxins

n 2004, the Red Cross decided to test the umbilical cord blood of ten randomly selected American babies. Here is what they found: "Babies in utero had an average of 200 industrial chemicals and pollutants running through their veins. In total, 287 toxins were identified in the 10 babies tested, pollutants that are found in pesticides, stain repellents, flame retardants, waste from coal-burning power plants, gasoline, and garbage. Of these chemicals, 180 are known to cause cancer, 217 are poisonous to the brain and nervous system, and 208 have been linked to birth defects in animal studies."[1]

We all know the world is a polluted place: car exhaust fumes in the air, dust mites in the carpet, perhaps even lead in the wall paint. We do our best to protect our children from harm, knowing it's an almost impossible task. But *inside* the womb?

When I heard this news, I reacted first with denial: this couldn't possibly apply to me, a vegetarian who grew up in Vermont and rarely painted her toenails. Then realism set in. Most of these pollutants are ubiquitous in the environment, and having lived in cities from age seventeen, I could hardly have avoided being exposed. Eventually, defeatism took over: even if my baby were awash in toxic chemicals, there was probably nothing I could do about it, given my husband wasn't about to follow me back from New York or London to live in Vermont. Furthermore, even if I had an infinite amount of time on my hands, I'd be unable to research my way through the list of 287 chemicals, because most of them have never been studied thoroughly. Believe it or not, the government doesn't require any safety testing of commercially produced chemicals.

That's right. The vast majority of chemicals in use in the United States have never been tested on animals, let alone people. The 62,000 chemicals already in production when the US Toxic Substances Control Act was passed in 1976 were grandfathered in without any testing required. Since then, the number of commercially produced chemicals has grown to more than 84,000; that's about 760 new chemicals each year. And when companies introduce a new chemical, all they need to do is notify the Environmental Protection Agency.[2] No health and safety information is required, and typically none is provided. The agency reports that 67 percent of chemical registrations include no test data and 85 percent provide no health data.[3] Even worse, new chemicals can be submitted as trade secrets. Two out of every three new chemicals are classified as secret formulas, so their chemical compositions aren't accessible to the public.[4]

If you pause to consider, it's an astounding governmental black hole. To introduce a new drug, pharmaceutical companies have to jump through rigorous regulatory hurdles, including large human clinical trials to test for safety. This means your local pharmacy is a bizarrely divided place. On one side of the counter, you can feel pretty confident that the pharmacist won't hand you anything that has any chance of doing you serious harm. On the other side of the counter, the supposedly innocuous products you can pick up in the aisles could be another matter entirely.[5] Who knows what strange substances might be lurking in that antiperspirant or hair dye?

While everyday exposure to a random assortment of chemicals may not do an adult any noticeable harm, little Junior in the womb is uniquely vulnerable. Low levels of substances that would have no effect on an adult can cause permanent damage in the rapidly developing brain of a fetus.[6] But as dire as the situation sounds, maybe all of these chemicals are present in such trace amounts that they don't actually have any real impact. Most babies are born healthy and happy and grow up to live long, full lives.

So is the hoopla warranted? One way to attempt to answer that question is to look at what's been happening with pregnancies over time. Over the last several decades, the United States has been getting more prosperous and medical technology has been steadily improving. So overall, we would broadly expect our babies to be getting healthier or at least remaining equally healthy. If that's not the case—for example, if birth defects or miscarriages are on the rise—these chemicals could be partly to blame.[7]

By far, the most common problem in pregnancy is miscarriage, so let's start there. Taking a single ethnic group as an example, in 1990, the average national miscarriage rate among white 25–29-year-olds was 17.94 percent. By 2004, it was 17.91 percent.[8]

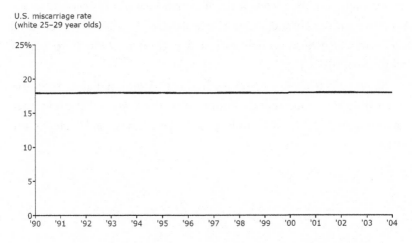

U.S. miscarriage rate
(white 25–29 year olds)

Fascinating, eh? The line technically slopes down a tiny bit, but that's barely visible on the chart. The miscarriage rate has been remarkably stable over time.

Let's move on to birth defects, which are sadly relatively common, affecting about one out of every thirty-three babies born in the

United States.[9] Here, there are plenty of scary headlines. For example, in May 2010, CBS News reported "an alarming increase in deformed sex organs." According to Dr. Howard Snyder, a pediatric urologist: "Thirty, forty years ago, the best data we had was that hypospadias occurred in about one in every 300 live male births. It's up to now about one in 100. So there's been a threefold increase."[10]

Hypospadias is a birth defect in which the urinary opening ends up somewhere along the underside of the penis instead of the tip. Not life threatening, but no parent wants their newborn baby boy to have a deformed penis. And a threefold increase sounds dramatic and scary. But is Dr. Snyder correct? Should we be panicking and rushing to protect our male offspring? To find out, we can turn to the city of Atlanta, home to the world headquarters of Coca-Cola, the site of the 1996 Olympics, and, most importantly for our purposes, the Metropolitan Atlanta Congenital Defects Program (MACDP).

Atlanta doesn't have its own special birth defects surveillance program because Atlantans are more likely to have malformed babies or because there's a nuclear waste disposal site hidden under the city. The government simply needed a single urban location to serve as representative for the United States. (Birth defects are not always recorded on birth certificates, which makes it extremely difficult to collect national statistics.)

So what's been going on with those Atlantan babes recently? According to a 2007 report, "Since 1973, the total defect prevalence has remained stable, with only year-to-year variation."[11] Here's the chart:

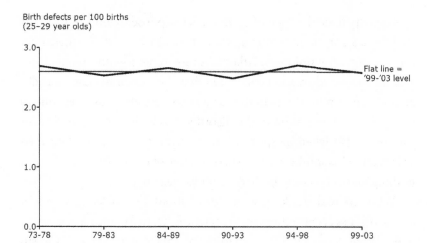

Birth defects per 100 births
(25–29 year olds)

Again, this is not very interesting-looking, which should be good news. But we can't relax yet, as this average line could be masking lots of interesting changes in individual defects. Maybe all those women obeying instructions and downing their daily folic acid pills have drastically reduced certain defects, masking big spikes in others. Here, then, is a chart with the most important defects broken down.[12] (Note that heart defects are only broken out as of 1984–89, when the medical community finally settled on a classification system for them.)[13]

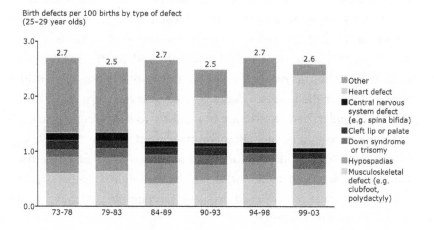

Birth defects per 100 births by type of defect
(25–29 year olds)

Hypospadias, the type of birth defect supposedly on the rise, was slightly *less* common in '99–'03 than it was in '73–'78. Furthermore, this finding is not unique to Atlanta. A researcher looking at data from around the world in 2000 concluded that the rate of hypospadias did go up in certain locations in the early 1980s, but this was likely due to changes in the definition of the disorder.[14] Whatever data Dr. Snyder was looking at when he spoke of the "alarming increase in deformed sex organs," his source wasn't representative of broader trends. There's nothing alarming going on here as far as we can tell.

While we're debunking scare stories about birth defects, we might as well discuss cryptorchidism, the scientific term for undescended testicles. What does the CDC have to say on this topic? "Cryptorchidism rates were available for 10 systems. Clear increases in this anomaly were seen in two US systems and in the South American system, but not elsewhere. Since 1985, rates declined in most systems." Again, not headline-grabbing news.

If birth defects aren't systematically rising, let's turn to our last direct indicator of problems in pregnancy, premature births, to find out if babies are increasingly getting booted out of the womb before their time. Unfortunately, it turns out that prematurity is not the most reliable statistic to measure, since knowing the age of the fetus requires knowing the date of conception, which isn't always possible for a variety of reasons. It's easier to look at low birth weight, which is related.

For very low birth weight infants (those born weighing less than 1.5 kg, or 3.3 lbs), the risk of dying in the first year of life is nearly 100 times that of normal-weight infants.[15] And for the majority of such babies who survive their first year, there are still ongoing health concerns. Over the past two decades, studies have shown that babies who were undersized at birth are more likely to suffer from a variety of problems as adults, including coronary heart disease,[16] diabetes,[17] stroke, hypertension, depression,[18] and schizophrenia,[19] among other conditions. But even babies with low birth weight (1.5–2.5 kg, or 3.3–5.5 lbs) are at risk for mild problems in cognition, attention, and neuro-motor functioning.[20]

So is low birth weight becoming more or less common? Here we have a chart showing the national percentage of babies born weighing less than 3 kg or 6.6 lbs:[21]

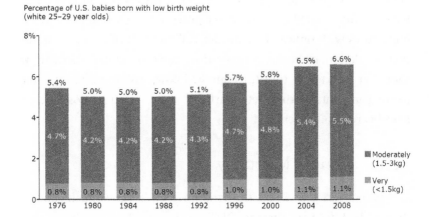

Percentage of U.S. babies born with low birth weight
(white 25–29 year olds)

Here, at last, is a trend that looks worrying. The report for the final year's bar proclaims this trend a "pronounced shift in recent years in the birth weight distribution toward smaller babies."

What are the possible explanations? According to the same report, "increases in the multiple birth rate, obstetric interventions such as induction of labor and cesarean delivery, older maternal age at child-bearing, and increased use of infertility therapies may have influenced the trends toward lower birth weights." This explanation is all well and good since it's describing the trend toward lower birth weights overall. But our chart is showing the trend just for 25–29-year-olds, so the influence of older mothers has been screened out. And we would expect some of the other factors mentioned, like the increase in multiple births and the use of infertility therapies, to go along with the trend toward older mothers. If more 25–29-year-olds are needing infertility treatment or having twins, that would be concerning in and of itself.

So maybe those 287 chemicals in the cord blood are something to worry about after all. While the number of babies with birth defects hasn't increased over the past forty years, the number of babies being born underweight has. Furthermore, the effects of toxins in the womb could be affecting our offspring in more subtle ways longer term, influencing their behavior or IQ. We'll never be able to unpack such trends in aggregate, given the vast number of other factors that influence children once they leave the womb. But a variety of eminent bodies have recently started opining on the potential dangers of bombarding our fetuses with untested chemicals, calling for further research, further regulation, or both.[22] So even if we can't investigate them all, we should at least take a tour through the known culprits when it comes to environmental toxins. Let's start with the one you're most likely to have heard about: mercury.

Fishy Advice: Mercury

Our parents grew up in blissful ignorance. Kids ate as much candy as they wished, farmers sprayed DDT on their fields, and when a thermometer broke, my mother and her friends would gather around to play with the liquid balls of mercury.

No one would ever make such a mistake nowadays. We all know mercury is highly toxic, ranking alongside lead and asbestos on the danger scale. And mercury poses a real threat during pregnancy.[23] In fact, even today, one in twenty American women has a level of mercury in her blood sufficient to put her unborn child at risk for ill health effects.[24]

In the concept of biomagnification, poisonous substances get increasingly concentrated up the food chain, with the largest predator, including large fish, containing the highest levels of toxins. As a result, warnings about fish consumption in pregnancy are everywhere. From popular parenting websites to government agencies like the FDA, the advice has been consistent: eat no more than two to three servings of fish per week.[25, 26] Mothers across the nation are heeding the advice. The average pregnant woman eats 36 percent less seafood than the average non-pregnant woman.[27] And in a recent Harvard study, many pregnant women said that they would rather avoid fish completely than risk harming themselves or their infants.[28] The advice these women are following is utterly misguided.

First, the level of mercury in your body builds up over long periods of time. The amount of mercury you're carrying around today is a function of how much contaminated fish you've been eating over the last couple of years, not the last week or month. According to the FDA, even if you were to stop eating fish today, it wouldn't necessarily make an appreciable difference: "Methylmercury is removed from the body naturally, but it may take over a year for levels to drop significantly."[29]

Second, and more important: despite the mercury, fish actually appears to be net beneficial during pregnancy. By limiting fish consumption, American mothers may be unwittingly lowering the average IQ of an entire generation of children. Below is a chart showing the relationship between maternal fish consumption during pregnancy and child IQ benefit:

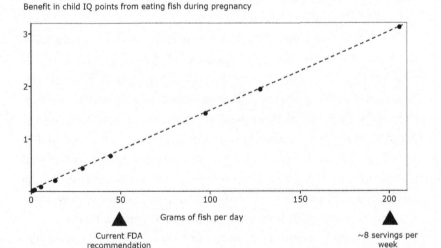

Benefit in child IQ points from eating fish during pregnancy

According to this chart, the more fish a woman eats, the higher the potential benefit to her child in terms of IQ. Less than one in 1,000 women (the 99.9th percentile) eat fish every day, but those who do have children who experience the highest benefit. Granted, the effects here are relatively small. Three IQ points wouldn't make the difference between a dunce and a genius. But if we could raise the average IQ of

Americans by a full three points simply by changing how we eat for a brief period of time, we should probably seize the chance.

This chart comes from the FDA—the very same agency that's currently officially cautioning women to limit their fish intake. In January 2009, the FDA published a new report re-examining the *net* effects of fish consumption in pregnancy,[30] taking into account not only the risk from pollutants such as mercury but the benefits from the other nutrients present in fish. Exposure to mercury indisputably interferes with fetal brain development, docking up to 0.87 of an IQ point at the very highest levels of exposure (the top 10th of 1 percent of the population in fish consumption).[31, 32] But the positive nutritional impact from eating fish appears to outweigh the negative impact of the mercury by several orders of magnitude.[33] For example, according to a research team from the National Institutes of Health, "We recorded beneficial effects on child development with maternal seafood intakes of more than 340 g per week, suggesting that advice to limit seafood consumption could actually be detrimental."[34]

But, as of 2011, the FDA had yet to revise its recommendation to pregnant women, in a classic example of the glacial pace at which new information makes its way through a government bureaucracy. Annoyed with the delay, two US senators formed a bipartisan coalition to kick the FDA out of its stupor.[35] In June 2014, a new draft recommendation about fish consumption during pregnancy was issued, but it took until January 2017 for the recommendation to be finalized and posted on the FDA's website. There was little accompanying media fanfare, so with each month that passes, thousands of women continue to "protect" their fetuses by limiting their seafood intake.

What should an expectant mother do? Those who eat the most seafood are those whose children experience the highest IQ benefits. But it's hard to forget that each bite is laced with a trace of heavy metal.

Let me therefore introduce you to the bane of the 19th- and early-20th-century child's existence: the daily spoonful of fish oil, which tasted "absolutely disgusting."[36] It turns out your great-grandmother was more fashionable than you realized. Fish oil is not only full of Vitamin D, which protected children from rickets in the era before

Vitamin D–fortified milk, it also could be the key to the brain-boosting benefits of fish,[37] perhaps because it's full of that trendy substance, omega-3.[38] Think what a powerful force Popeye could have been if he had drizzled a little cod liver oil on his spinach! Furthermore, fish oils themselves contain very little mercury.[39] And now that someone has invented those lovely gel caps that prevent us from having to actually taste the stuff on its way down, what's not to love?[40]

Unfortunately, it's premature to conclude that swallowing fish oil is equivalent to eating fish—there simply isn't enough evidence yet.[41] That's why the American Dietetic Association still recommends "a food-based approach" to getting your omega-3.[42] Besides, perhaps you're on vacation in the Caribbean and it would be criminal not to try the local fish. Or maybe you're addicted to your daily niçoise salad and an oil capsule balanced on top of your lettuce doesn't appeal. In that case, it would be helpful to know which fish are the most beneficial and least harmful. Here's some wisdom from a typical parenting book:[43]

- It's smart to avoid shark, swordfish, king mackerel, tilefish, and tuna steaks.
- Limit your consumption of canned tuna (chunk light tuna contains less mercury than white) and freshwater fish caught by recreational fishers to an average of 170 g (cooked weight) per week.
- Commercially caught fish usually has lower levels of contaminants, so you can safely eat more.
- Steer clear of fish from waters that are contaminated (with sewage or industrial runoff, for example).
- Avoid tropical fish, such as grouper, amberjack, and mahi-mahi.
- An average of 240 g of cooked fish per week is considered safe.
- Choose from salmon (wild caught is best), sole, flounder, haddock, tilapia, halibut, ocean perch, pollock, cod, and trout as well as other smaller ocean fish (anchovies, sardines, and herring) and seafood of all kinds.

This is like the list of forbidden foods we encountered earlier. Wait, how many grams of fish can I eat? Was it 170 of one type and 240 of the other? How much fish is 170 g anyway? A list like this puts your brain on overload, making you unlikely to remember any of it. And there's a lot of irrelevant information here. Tilefish is not even available in most supermarket chains, so warning us not to consume it is like warning us not to stand on our heads for prolonged periods during pregnancy. Could be quite harmful, but only the most obsessive yoga enthusiast would try it in the first place.

Let's turn, then, to the data on fish. This chart puts the various kinds of seafood in order, with the worst fish on the left and the best on the right. With the fish on the left, I've sorted by mercury level (i.e., the dark bars hanging downward); then, once we reach the lowest mercury category as defined by the FDA, the mercury content stops mattering as much, so I've sorted the rest of the fish on the right by omega-3 content (the bars sticking up). A caveat: the bottom and the top of the chart use different scales, so don't compare the heights of the mercury versus the omega-3 bars—what's important here is the ordering from left to right.

This chart probably requires a magnifying glass for you to read it, and most of these fish species are relatively obscure. I've included the full list here simply because you might want to look up a specific favorite fish before eating it.

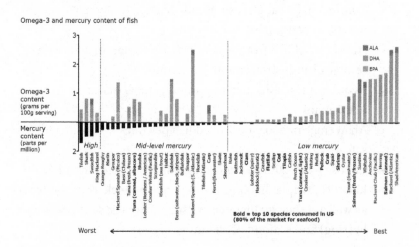

Omega-3 and mercury content of fish

Now let's look at the subset of fish that actually matter, the ones we eat on a regular basis:[44]

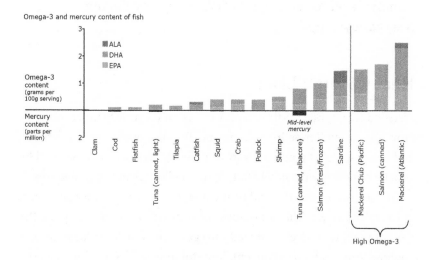

Omega-3 and mercury content of fish

Looking at this chart, only tuna falls into the mid-level mercury bucket, so that fish isn't the best choice. All the rest are low mercury, so there's not a lot to worry about. But it's clear that not all fish are created equal when it comes to omega-3 content. You'd have to eat ten servings of tilapia or seventeen servings of cod or haddock to get the omega-3 benefit of just one serving of canned salmon. In other words, you could eat cod every day for two weeks and still not get the benefit of eating salmon once.

Funny that all of these fish species appear as equals in the list from the parenting website above. I'd therefore like to make my own personal attempt to clear away the fog of confusion surrounding fish consumption during pregnancy. Paying homage to Michael Pollan, author of *In Defense of Food*, I propose a simple rule: "Eat lots of fish; eat salmon and mackerel in particular." Bet you can remember that one.

In conclusion, most women have it backward. They eat fish throughout their life and then suddenly abstain when they get pregnant. Instead, they should be flipping it around: theoretically avoiding fish a year or two before pregnancy but then binging on fish once pregnant. How's that for counterintuitive?

Threat level for prior accumulation of mercury: Medium[45]

Benefit level for eating oily fish every day during pregnancy: High[46]

Heavy Metal: Lead

Listened to any Black Sabbath or Van Halen recently? Didn't think so. How about Led Zeppelin? OK, maybe. But it's not the 1980s anymore, and heavy metal is going the way of many genres before it: beloved by a niche but otherwise slowly fading into collective cultural oblivion.

It's the same with the real heavy metal. Lead isn't trendy anymore. It's very old news. That's because most of us know the story. In the days of yore, we naïvely put lead into gasoline to help prevent our car engines from making inefficient "pinging noises."[47] Once the government wised up to the danger in 1973 and forced lead to be phased out, the level of lead in our blood has been steadily decreasing, helped by the ban on lead in paint that followed soon after. (Incidentally, there was never actually lead in pencils. That was just a confusion on the part of the residents of a hamlet town in England in 1565 who found a hard, dark substance and used it to mark their sheep, mistakenly thinking it was lead.)[48] So if lead has been all but phased out, problem solved, right?

If only it were that simple. If you're going to worry about toxins, you should forget all the recent scare headlines about weird chemicals in plastics such as BPA or PVCs. I'm not saying they're necessarily harmless; we'll come to them later. But really, we should still be worrying about that old favorite, Pb.

Just like mercury (not Freddy, the chemical element) and dioxins (which we'll come to next), lead has a tendency to hang around. Even if you were born well after 1973, you almost definitely have some heavy metal circulating in your blood. How do I know? Courtesy of the National Health and Nutrition Examination Survey (NHANES), a huge national health survey conducting interviews and physical examinations annually on a nationally representative sample of about 5,000 people.[49] And according to their data from 1999 to 2002, if you're a woman aged 20–59, you have about a 1 in 300 chance of having a blood lead level above 10 micrograms per deciliter.[50]

What does that mean, exactly? Well, a microgram is a minuscule amount. It's one millionth of a gram, and a gram is about the weight of a feather. So could 10 micrograms per deciliter possibly matter? Oh yes, indeed; maybe not to you, but to your baby. Lead crosses right through the placenta, so your fetus has almost the same blood lead level as you do.[51] And it's lead exposure in the womb that appears to matter the most to your child. A study at Harvard Medical School took a group of middle- and upper-middle-class infants and measured the level of lead in their cord blood and then in the children's own blood as they grew.[52] It was the amount of lead in their cord blood, rather than in their own blood later, that best predicted their mental development score at 12 months.

But would a trace 10 micrograms really make a difference? The answer is a resounding yes. According to a National Toxological Profile report on lead, there's sufficient evidence to conclude that even a blood level below 10 micrograms causes reduced fetal growth.[53] An author who reviewed many studies concluded that each increase of 10 micrograms per deciliter in children's blood causes a loss of 2.6 IQ points,[54] and several studies imply that measurable damage can occur at levels below 5 micrograms per deciliter.[55, 56, 57] Even worse, that same National Toxological Profile and the CDC warn that lead in low doses may increase the risk of miscarriage, based on evidence from a recent study of women in Mexico.[58, 59] As a result, the Association of Occupational and Environmental Clinics recommends intervention for pregnant women with blood lead levels above 5 micrograms per deciliter.[60]

Nope, doesn't apply to me, you say; *I don't have any micrograms in my blood. I live in a modern house with brand-new tiling and appliances, not a dilapidated fixer-upper with chips of suspicious paint everywhere. I go to work in an office building, not a construction site; and I live in the United States of America, not in China next to a factory.* Sadly, that's still no guarantee you're not carrying around a hefty dose of lead. The problem is, lead builds up in your bones and gets stored there, so it's your exposure over a lifetime that counts. And there continues to be lead everywhere, perhaps even in the plumbing bringing the water to your kitchen sink. As one author describes: "Women who were chronically exposed to environmental lead during infancy and adolescence may arrive at reproductive age with a significant bone lead burden. . . . Since approximately 95 percent of lead is stored in bone and mineralized tissues, and bone lead has a half-life of years to decades, women and their infants will continue to be at risk for exposure long after environmental sources of lead have been abated."[61]

All this talk about bones: you're probably wondering why lead in your skeleton has any relevance to the health of your baby. It's not as though there are lots of small bones floating around in your uterus that your fetus might happen to gnaw on. The answer is that babies are amazing little parasites. They have a terrible hunger for calcium as they grow their own skeletal structure. If they aren't getting enough calcium, they simply prompt you to suck it out of your own bones to deliver over to them. Calcium problem solved—but the lead gets released into your bloodstream along with the calcium, which is perversely why pregnancy is when your blood lead level is likely to be highest, just when it can do the most harm to your vulnerable baby.

So lead undoubtedly poses a potential risk to your fetus. But despite acknowledging this risk, the CDC and the American College of Obstetricians and Gynecologists currently stop short of recommending routine testing for all pregnant women in the United States. Instead they suggest that doctors run through a checklist to identify potential sources of lead exposure first, in what is presumably a pragmatic attempt to weigh societal costs and benefits.[62]

Did your doctor run through a lead assessment checklist at your very first prenatal checkup? There's a good chance the answer is no. Currently, states have inconsistent rules about assessing pregnant women for lead exposure.[63] But even if your doctor did ask you about lead, it's unlikely you knew all the answers. The checklist has factors like "women whose homes have leaded water pipes or source lines with lead." Do you happen to know off the top of your head what your pipes are made of? If you're living in a house or apartment that was built recently, you're probably OK, but if you're living in an older house, who knows? Presumably you could find out with a bit of effort, but what about all the houses you've lived in previously? It's very hard to know for sure if you've been exposed.

Returning to our statistic above, only 1 in 300 women has a true lead problem, and that number may not sound scary enough to spur you into action. I understand. You're sitting on your couch at home with your big pregnant belly, and the last thing you feel like doing is calling your water company, rushing off to a hardware store for a lead test kit, or getting down on your hands and knees to swab around for dust samples. Fortunately, the solution is much easier than that. Pregnant women get treated like gigantic pin cushions nowadays. (You thought your doctor was just going to listen to the baby's heartbeat, but instead the nurse comes in and lines up all those little vials and comes at you with that annoyingly tight arm band. I get woozy just thinking about it.) So if you're going to be stuck full of needles anyway, you might as well proactively ask your doctor to have the blood sample tested for lead. It may not be standard practice to test all pregnant women, but your doctor will likely comply if you're willing to pay for it.

The good news is that lead is a toxin you can do something about. If your levels are high, one solution may be to take calcium supplements to help keep your bones from releasing their lead stores.[64] Supplements can bring the level of lead in your blood down by about 15 percent, which is modest but better than nothing.[65, 66] More importantly, if you know lead is a problem, you'll have the motivation you need to have a proper snoop around your current home before your baby is born and starts crawling around putting paint chips in his or her mouth.[67] OK, your house may be new and immaculate, but have you considered your window blinds? If they're made of PVC, a common kind of plastic, they just might be shedding lead dust all over your carpet.[68] It's been thirty years, and we still haven't learned our lesson about using this highly toxic heavy metal. Go figure.

Threat level for lead: Medium[69]

Poisonous Produce: Pesticides

Snow White isn't the only one biting into poison apples. Ever eaten a piece of fruit and then remembered with a sinking feeling that you'd forgotten to wash it? Sometimes it's best not to think too hard about what kinds of chemical residues might be clinging to your fruits and vegetables.

Women of the twenty-first century at least have far less to worry about than our mothers did. In the 1970s, the EPA banned a dangerous group of pesticides called organochlorines, including the infamous DDT.[70] But despite the backlash against pesticides at the time, consumers weren't prepared to start buying produce full of worm holes, so farmers simply substituted their organochlorines with organophosphates, a new and improved class of pesticides that degraded into harmless substances after being exposed to air, water, and soil. Families even started using organophosphates at home to keep the cockroaches at bay.

If these new pesticides were so harmless, how did they actually kill pests? By being very, very toxic initially—and herein lay the next problem. It wasn't long before another wave of studies began to emerge, linking home use of organophosphates such as chlorpyrifos to all sorts of worrisome outcomes in children, including reduced head circumference at birth,[71] higher likelihood of ADHD,[72] and impaired IQ and cognitive development.[73,74,75] Not so nice. In response to the mounting proof that these chemicals were also dangerous for children, the EPA finally banned chlorpyrifos and its organophosphate brethren from residential use in 2001.[76] You'll note that this is all very recent history.

Never had to deal with a cockroach problem, you say? And anyway, now that these home poison bombs are off the market, the wider American population is finally safe from pesticides, right? Guess again. Agricultural use of chlorpyrifos is still allowed, and since we consumers still haven't overcome our aversion to pest-ridden food, farmers are still spraying chlorpyrifos on their crops.

The media occasionally takes notice and attempts to raise our indignation. Here's a recent report from CNN: "In a representative sample of produce, 28 percent of frozen blueberries, 20 percent of celery, and 25 percent of strawberries contained traces of one type of organophosphate. Other types of organophosphates were found in 27 percent of green beans, 17 percent of peaches, and 8 percent of broccoli."[77] This is a classic example of the kind of information I hate. It's a long list—too long to remember. Furthermore, it sounds scary, but it's not obvious what action to take. *Should I start avoiding strawberries from specific producers? Rinse my strawberries more carefully? Pay up for pricey organic ones? Or stop eating strawberries altogether? And if strawberries covered with chlorpyrifos are so dangerous, why do we allow them on supermarket shelves in the first place? And why haven't I noticed anyone suffering the consequences?* Rather than taking any action, I continue to cursorily rinse my vegetables but suffer from occasional pangs of worry that perhaps I haven't gotten all the chemicals off.

To get to the bottom of how dangerous our organophosphate exposure might be, I researched how much exposure the typical American is getting nowadays to these pesticides in aggregate and compared that to the level of exposure that has been linked to problems.[78] My conclusion is that almost 5 percent of American women have exposure levels high enough to dock 7 points off the IQ of their offspring. This is a shocking result, particularly given that the EPA is well aware of the dangers posed to children by organophosphates. Why they haven't banned this class of chemicals entirely is incomprehensible to me. Regardless, we now need to find out which foods are the culprits when it comes to these nasty poisons.[79]

On this topic, it's the US Department of Agriculture that has all the answers. They run the Pesticide Data Program (PDP), a massive testing program that has analyzed about 1.5 million food samples since 1991 and checked for more than 450 different pesticides. They do their best to reflect how people actually buy and use foods in their own kitchens, by washing and trimming the vegetables first just as you would at home.[80]

The next chart shows the data for some of the most common fruits and vegetables.[81]

Average organophosphate residues
(ug/kg Methamidophos equivalent)

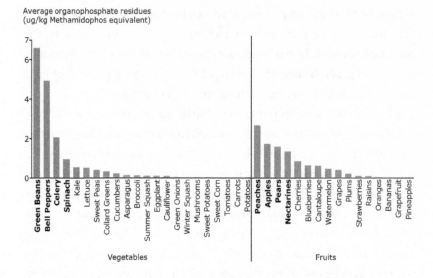

Parts of this chart make sense. Root vegetables like potatoes, sweet potatoes, and carrots grow under the ground, so they are unlikely to get covered in pesticide spray. Similarly, corn is protected by a husk, and cantaloupe, watermelon, oranges, bananas, and grapefruit all have thick rinds or peels that get thrown away, so it's no surprise they all appear fine. Beyond that, the results are not entirely intuitive. You wouldn't necessarily expect green beans to be so much worse than asparagus, when both are long, skinny vegetables. This is why it's important to rely on data rather than intuition when standing in the produce aisle.[82]

Given that most fruits and vegetables appear to be covered in pesticides, the obvious answer is to sling your eco-friendly linen shopping bag over your shoulder and go organic. The organic produce tested by the Pesticide Data Program above was virtually 100 percent free of organophosphates. Furthermore, a recent study found that switching children to an organic diet quickly eliminated their exposure.[83] The claim that eating organic is better for your health as well as the planet doesn't appear to be hype after all.[84, 85]

That answer would be perfectly fine if money were no object; unfortunately, I've estimated that the cost to go organic over the course of a full pregnancy is approximately 560 dollars, not an insignificant sum.[86] This is why looking at the data matters, not just consulting a list that ranks produce. Green beans, ranked at #1, are eight times worse than spinach, which is ranked at #4. And vegetable #2, bell peppers, are almost twice as bad as the worst-ranking fruit, peaches. So if going wholeheartedly organic is out of the question for budgetary reasons, keep in mind that not all produce is equal. If you want to get the maximum benefit with limited cost, you can look at the chart and see that you should mainly be splurging on buying organic green beans and bell peppers, by far the two worst offenders. Let's repeat that: beans and bell peppers. Beans and bell peppers. Beans and bell peppers. Say it a few times, and maybe it will come to mind the next time you find yourself at the grocery store.

Threat level for organophosphate pesticides on produce: Medium[87]

Skin Deep: Personal Care Products

What's the largest organ in your body? Hmm, could it be your liver? How about your brain? Nope, it's your skin. OK, skin is technically an organ *system*, not an organ. But regardless, we have a tendency to forget that our skin is a critical functioning part of our body. Instead, we treat it like an impermeable raincoat, covering it with all sorts of gunk. Putting aside the farcical nature of the question, would you spread glittery eye shadow or even foundation all over your liver without thinking twice? I thought not. Occasionally, we're reminded that skin is critical—like when Goldfinger's manservant murders a Bond girl by slathering her in gold paint—but in our daily lives, we disregard the fact that our skin is absorbent. Although the outer layer of skin forms a protective barrier, many chemicals can nevertheless penetrate this barrier.[88] Yet every day, the average woman covers her skin with twelve products containing 168 ingredients.[89]

Let's return to those 287 chemicals in the cord blood. Can I confirm that some of them are seeping in via your skin? And if so, can I prove that these are potentially harmful chemicals rather than just inert substances? Yes, I can, courtesy of a tool called the Skin Deep Database. A group of dedicated individuals at a nonprofit organization called the Environmental Working Group have compiled a database of close to 70,000 products and cross-referenced every ingredient against sixty toxicity and regulatory databases. They've then integrated all of this information for every product to produce a single hazard ranking on a scale of 0 (harmless) to 10 (worryingly hazardous). An enormous undertaking, but it's finished and available online at www.ewg.org/skindeep/. You type in a product name and brand, and out pops a score.

Take a guess: what kinds of personal care products do you think are the most likely to be hazardous? (To get your brainstorming started, the categories include sun protection, makeup, skincare, hair care, eyes/contact lens care, nails, fragrance, and oral care.) My very first thought was depilatory creams—if they can dissolve hair, they must be made out of some kind of strong acid, which can't be good for your skin. But then I thought about nail polish—pretty smelly, and those lacquer colors aren't exactly natural. Speaking of unnatural, who knows what ingredients they use to make metallic purple eye shadow or black lipstick...?

It was time to look at the data. This wasn't straightforward, as the Skin Deep Database is designed for looking at one product at a time, not summarizing information by category. I therefore worked through each category and manually counted the number of products in every rating bucket. The result is in the graph.

Breakdown of overall hazard scores for personal care products by category

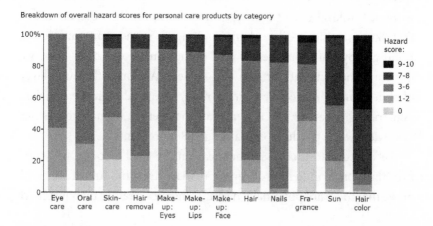

The shading shows what percentage of each type of product is bad. For example, if you look at the second bar, oral care, about 10 percent of products get a score of 0, 20 percent score 1 or 2, and the remaining 70 percent score in the 3–6 range; or, in other words, if you pick your toothpaste at random, about 70 percent of the time it will score a 3–6. One important caveat is that these are overall hazard ratings rather than specific to pregnancy, but they at least provide an indication.

You'll see the worst offenders appear to be hair dyes. If you'd rather wear a paper bag over your head for nine months than go out in public with a skunk stripe of gray, you might have preferred living in blissful ignorance. But take heart—although a few studies suggest that hairdressers themselves have a higher risk of having children with certain birth defects,[90, 91] other studies have not found an increased risk.[92] And although no one has ever directly studied occasional use of hair dye during pregnancy, an estimate of the absorption of the various chemicals through your scalp suggests the risk is minimal.[93] If the possibility still concerns you, you could always go natural. But watch out: even hair dyes labeled "natural" often still contain hazardous ingredients (these products are totally unregulated, remember?). If you look closely, there are a few products squeezed at the very bottom of the hair color bar on the chart that fall into the more harmless categories, including vegetable dyes like henna. Whether you'd look good as a redhead is, of course, none of my business.

Now take a look at the sun category. No one wears sunscreen to look beautiful or smell nice; it's supposed to be good for your health. The problem with sunscreens is that the majority of them contain a chemical called oxybenzone (otherwise known as benzophenone-3 or BP-3). This chemical has become so pervasive that 97 percent of Americans have some in their body,[94] and one study conducted in conjunction with the CDC has suggested that higher BP-3 exposure was associated with lower birth weight among female infants.[95] This is just a single preliminary result. Still, if you're going to be risk averse while you've got a bump, you can check out the Environmental Working Group's 2017 Sunscreen Report, which ranks the best and worst sunscreens.[96]

Returning one last time to our chart, you'll see that most categories have a spectrum. Some products are completely harmless, most fall in the midrange, and a few contain ingredients that might be worrisome. If you want to transform yourself into a totally alternative nature-chick while pregnant, it's easy enough. You can simply type each of your favorite products into the database and find out how they score. I apologize in advance for interfering with your makeup routine; whoever thinks that "pregnancy glow" is all natural probably hasn't looked closely enough.

Threat level for hair dye: Low[97]

Threat level for oxybenzone in sunscreen: Low[98]

Threat level for chemicals in personal care products: Low[99]

Secret Scents: Perfume

What if I told you that you're constantly being exposed to potentially hazardous chemical fumes? Most of us breathe in whiffs frequently throughout the day: in the bathroom, on the bus to work, at the office, on the street, at cocktail parties and nightclubs. I'm not referring to cigarette smoke; these fumes are invisible. Nor am I referring to carbon monoxide; there are no detectors you can scatter around your house to warn you, although this problem is far more ubiquitous. What is this potentially toxic vapor, and how could it be so pervasive if you've never heard about it before? Actually, you have heard of it: it's called perfume.

Perfume. *Parfum. Eau de Toilette.* Fragrance. These are all euphemisms for what might more accurately be described as an undisclosed soup of volatile chemicals that happen to smell nice. Now let's pause here for a second. The confusion is that perfume smells good. It's easy to get your head around the idea that something noxious like paint thinner or cigarette smoke might be harmful, because that would match your unpleasant experience. But it requires considerable mental effort to believe that perfume might be worrisome—unless you're allergic and hate the smell, knowing it will lead to a bad headache. (Companies have caught on to that persuasive power of smell. You know the scent of cinnamon buns you encounter at malls and airports? That's not the smell of anything baking—it's a synthetic chemical being pumped into the environment to entice you to eat those gooey pastries.[100] In the quest to avoid synthetic scents while pregnant, it's important to realize that lots of the smells you encounter daily are fake!)

Why do I call perfume an "undisclosed" soup of chemicals? Because companies can register their scent formulations as trade secrets, granting them the same protected status as the mythical recipe for Coca-Cola. This makes for absurd ingredients labels, which list "aqua" and "parfum" as the first two most important ingredients and then give you the detailed rundown on all the other harmless items found in trace quantities in the product. That means that we have very little knowledge about what we're breathing in or dabbing on our wrists. As described by the Environmental Working Group, the same nonprofit we encountered earlier: "The parallels between secondhand smoke and synthetic fragrance use are many. At its core, both are battles over indoor air quality. In the 1960s, when a few people began complaining about secondhand smoke and possible negative effects on health, the general public and business considered this a fringe movement that was unlikely to gain steam . . . The US consumer is as uneducated about the dangers and health risks associated with constant exposure to the chemicals used in synthetic fragrance products as the average non-smoker was to the risks of secondhand smoke. When ignorance is replaced with knowledge, a large segment of the population will respond with a demand for clean and safe air in the workplace."[101]

My first reaction here was mild skepticism. These folks at the EWG clearly mean well, but perhaps they've worked themselves up into a lather of righteous indignation simply because that's their mission as environmentalists. Just because we don't know what's in perfume doesn't mean it's necessarily harmful. And anyway, few of us have the misfortune to work behind a department store perfume counter. So what's the evidence that casually dabbing perfume is bad?

In fairness to the environmentalists, they have done their home-work. Rather than just hypothesizing that the chemicals in perfumes might be bad, they decided to test them. They chose seventeen popular brands of fragrance, including Coco Chanel and Calvin Klein Eternity, and conducted a battery of laboratory tests to identify secret ingre-dients. Their conclusions? The average fragrance tested contained fourteen secret chemicals not listed on the label. More important, 70 percent of the total ingredients found across all the perfumes had never been assessed for safety by anyone, either in industry or academia.[102]

That's the point: the safety of most perfumes is unknowable. So if you're someone who's uncomfortable with uncertainty, you should put your perfume, air fresheners, scented candles, and probably even dishwashing liquid, fabric softener, and laundry detergent aside and use essential oils as a safer alternative to perfume. If, on the other hand, you can't live without your signature scent, you can at least feel comfortable that there's no direct evidence (yet) that you're doing your baby any harm.[103]

Am I worried that the hormone disruptors found in many com-mon perfumes can cause reproductive abnormalities in turtles[104] and enlarged uteruses in rats,[105] among other examples? Yes, I admit I've gone perfume-free. But that's probably just my overprotective preg-nancy hormone system kicking in.

Threat level for perfume: Low[106]

The Swan Study: Phthalates

ABC News, 2009: "Could Plastics Chemicals 'Feminize' Boys' Play? Researchers surveyed parents about the kids' preferences during play-time: Did they play masculine games like 'cops and robbers' or feminine games like 'house'? Boys whose mothers had the highest levels of phthalates in their urine while they were in the womb had masculinity 'scores' that were 8 percent lower than those whose mothers had the lowest levels . . . Shanna Swan, a University of Rochester professor of obstetrics and gynecology and environmental medicine, said it's clear that 'these common chemicals have the ability to alter the development of the male fetus.'"[107]

Phthalates, found in a wide variety of plastics, were leaching into homes and potentially causing young boys to become emasculated. From a journalist's perspective, this little piece of research was almost too good to be true. Even nonparents would read on simply out of morbid curiosity. Even better, the lead author was a woman with an unusual name. "The Swan Study" was both memorable and slightly salacious—research at its most marketable.[108]

In fact, this was the second time Dr. Swan had made the headlines. Just four years before, she had published the results of a study measuring the "anogenital distance" of newborn boys (that's the distance from the anus to the base of the genitalia)[109] and was quoted in the *San Francisco Chronicle*'s article "Parents needn't wait for legislation to shield kids from toxins in products," saying, "Children are highly vulnerable [to phthalates] long before they are even born. In-utero exposures to phthalates can lead to birth defects and genital malformations, as numerous studies have shown in laboratory animals and, as suggested most recently, in a study of baby boys."[110] The headlines quickly proliferated: "Study links plastics to small genitals" (Fox News);[111] "Chemicals in plastics harming unborn boys: scientists say chemicals have gender bending effect" (*The Guardian*).[112]

Parents read these articles with dismay. Plastic was no longer a miracle of convenience; it was a source of hormone-mimicking chemical pollution. As they looked around their homes at the baby bottles, the shower curtains, the toothbrushes, and the colorful toys strewn around the living room, they realized danger was everywhere. Sensing the tidal wave of indignant public sentiment, the government leapt into action. In 2008, the Consumer Product Safety Improvement Act was passed, banning children's toys containing high levels of certain phthalates.

The scientific community also leapt into action. The number of research papers on phthalates soared; Swan's original article has now been cited a whopping 619 times. We've moved beyond a small, preliminary study (which should never have made headlines) to reach a state of robust scientific consensus. So are boys being born with smaller genitals because of phthalates?[113] Drumroll, please . . . According to two reviews from 2009 and 2010, the evidence against phthalates is unconvincing and "for the most part lacks coherence and physiological plausibility."[114, 115] And in April 2010, a report to the government's Chronic Hazard Advisory Panel concluded that only two types of phthalates, DEHP and DBP, appear to pose any risk to unborn babies.[116] What kind of risk? Deformed testicles? Shrunken penises? Nope. Slightly lower birth weight[106] and slightly earlier delivery.[118, 119, 120]

No one wants to risk their baby being born slightly prematurely, but we probably shouldn't be losing sleep over phthalates compared to other potential threats. In 2008, a hefty document (146 pages and 850 citations) attempted to exhaustively summarize all the known links between environmental chemicals and pregnancy/child outcomes, and phthalates didn't even make the cut.[121] The CDC[122] and the Center for the Evaluation of Risks to Human Reproduction (CERHR)[123] have both concluded there's no direct evidence of any reproductive or developmental threat from exposure to DBP. So, while a trendy villain, phthalates are hardly top of the list. And as we've seen, the world is full of chemicals that have never been tested—let alone subjected to 619 separate studies.

On the other hand, the scientific community has yet to agree on a way to add up total phthalate exposure (like in the pesticide example we looked at), and very few studies have looked at the effects of exposure to multiple phthalates simultaneously. The EPA has promised to eventually publish one of its "cumulative risk assessments." But until then, our answer on phthalates will remain slightly unsatisfying.

For those of you who can't stand the idea of taking even unproven risks, you may be wondering how to go phthalate-free. For an answer to that question, let's turn to a little book called *The Toxic Sandbox*.[124] Given to me by a kind friend during my first pregnancy, it has a picture on the cover of a pail emblazoned with a radioactivity symbol sitting in a sandbox. It argues that our children are in significant danger from environmental toxins and has an entire chapter dedicated to phthalates.

The author is a big proponent of going natural. She "strongly urges" us to remove any plastics in our homes that might contain phthalates. Fortunately, she also provides some advice on how to do so: "It is easy to identify the offending plastics and keep them out of your home . . . What products contain the big three? DEHP: vinyl products, floor tiles, upholstery, shower curtains, cables, garden hoses, rainwear, car parts and interiors, packaging film, sheathing for wire and cable, some food containers, toys, and medical devices. DBP: nail polish, cosmetics, and insecticides. BBP: adhesives, paints, sealants, car-care products, vinyl flooring, and some personal care products."

Sure, it's easy to get rid of phthalates. Here's how: you just have to rip up the floor tiles in your kitchen, throw away your upholstered living room couch and armchair, throw away the cables for your computer, telephones, and television, avoid buying any food that comes in containers, and purchase secondhand cars from now on. And avoid going to the hospital, where there might be medical devices. As I said, easy.

Luckily, this is overcomplicating matters. Most of the items on this long list are culprits because they contribute to phthalates in household dust. Small children are indeed at risk from dust, because they spend a lot of time close to the floor, putting their hands and other assorted objects into their mouths. But it's safe to assume that you as a pregnant adult do not spend time crawling around your house, or chewing on your computer cables, for that matter. (Once the baby is born, you might want to consider throwing out your smelly plastic shower curtain, but that's a topic for a later book.)

In fact, the top culprit for adult exposure to phthalates is only indirectly included on the list above, and that is . . . food. Yes, we return to food once again. There's yet another chemical lurking in your dinner. Food represents ~95 percent of the total exposure of adults to both DEHP and DBP, the most worrisome phthalates.[125, 126] The problem with cans, plastic wrap, and food containers (some which have been left out entirely from the list) is that they leach phthalates—particularly when heated or cooled, which is what we spend a lot of time doing to food.

But even having narrowed down the problem to food, it's not a trivial task to avoid phthalates. One team of researchers made a valiant attempt: they recruited five families from the San Francisco Bay area and convinced them to spend three days eating only foods that had been specially prepared for their consumption. These families were not exactly heavy users of plastic to begin with: they didn't use plastic water bottles, eat frozen prepared foods, or microwave their food in plastic. But the team wanted to ensure that every possible source of plastic had been eliminated: "Foods were prepared almost exclusively from fresh and organic fruits, vegetables, grains, and meats. Preparation techniques avoided contact with plastic utensils and non-stick-coated cookware, and foods were stored in glass containers with BPA-free plastic lids. Containers were filled to below the top so foods did not contact the lids. Participants received stainless steel water bottles and lunch containers. Coffee drinkers were advised to use a French press or ceramic drip rather than using a plastic coffee maker or buying coffee from a café." As a result of these elaborate rules and restrictions, the families' exposure to DEHP (as measured in their urine) went down by ~50 percent.[127]

Why not more than 50 percent? There was no plastic anywhere near the food! Sadly, there's only so much you can control in your own kitchen, because phthalates are ubiquitous in the food chain. As the researchers went on to explain, cows are milked using PVC tubing, and whole eggs can even contain phthalates. So there's plastic residue in almost everything we eat.

That's not even the end of the bad news: women of childbearing age are getting an extra dose of these chemicals. According to a recent study, women age 20–40 years have levels of DBP 50 percent higher than the rest of the population.[128] Here, at least, there's a clear explanation: our vanity. The additional dose of DBP is coming from nail polish. The only products in the Skin Deep Database that contain DBP are nail products, with about 1 in 5 containing this chemical.

Phthalates are everywhere, so here's what I conclude. If you want to earn your A+ in parenting, skip the nail polish, avoid PVC plastic wrap, and transfer your food to a glass bowl or ceramic plate before microwaving it, as these are likely to be the biggest sources of phthalate exposure in your life. Canned food, restaurant food, and bottled/canned drinks are other likely culprits you could try to avoid if you want to be heroic. But don't kid yourself that you've really gone plastic-free; if you want to do that, you'll need to move to a small organic farm somewhere. With your unpolished nails, you'll fit right in.

Threat level for phthalates: Low[129]

An Ode to Elbow Grease: Cleaning Products

"May be fatal or cause permanent damage. Causes severe burns which may not be immediately painful or visible. Will penetrate skin and attack underlying tissues and bone. Wear gloves, safety goggles and a face mask." Is this a highly regulated industrial chemical? A bottle on the very back shelf of your high school chemistry teacher's locked cabinet? No. It's a household cleaning product called Whink Rust Stain Remover that anyone can buy for $10.50 at Walmart and store under the kitchen sink.

No longer do we need to spend hours down on our hands and knees scrubbing at stains with a bristle brush, Cinderella-style: magic cleaning products have come to the rescue. And we're so delighted with the performance of these products ("Look, the stain is really gone! My blouse isn't ruined after all!") that we rarely stop to think about what interesting substances might be inside our spray bottles. But just as with personal care products, companies at the moment aren't required to test their ingredients at all. In fact, as reported by *The New York Times*, "if the EPA does not take steps to block the new chemical within 90 days . . . the chemical is by default given a green light. The law puts federal authorities in a bind. 'It's the worst kind of Catch-22,' said Dr. Richard Denison, senior scientist at the Environmental Defense Fund. 'The EPA can't even require testing to determine whether a risk exists without first showing a risk is likely.'"[130]

At least journalists are finally catching on to the absurdity of this situation, and perhaps you'll feel shocked enough to write an indignant letter to your congressional representative. But there's inevitably a delay between dawning public awareness and substantive governmental action. In the meantime, the Environmental Working Group has once again leapt in to fill the public information void. They've compiled the EWG Cleaners database, an online tool listing hazard ratings for 2,000+ cleaning products, from mildew remover to pet deodorizer.[131] In addition to an overall hazard score (which will steer you away from the delightfully corrosive Whink product), each product has a specific rating for "Developmental and Reproductive Toxicity." The chart shows the breakdown of the data I compiled for each product category, showing what percentage of products get what rating for developmental and reproductive toxicity:

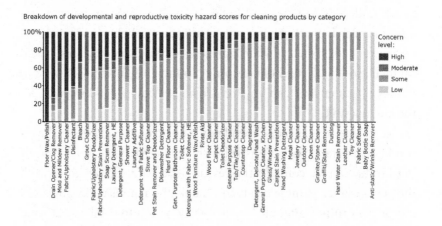

Breakdown of developmental and reproductive toxicity hazard scores for cleaning products by category

This chart is not entirely surprising. Floor polish on the far left does smell disgusting; drain clog remover and bleach are clearly not products you want to be messing around with; and it's nice to see that toy cleaner and baby bottle soap are on the more harmless side of the spectrum. But how about ordinary products we use all the time, like laundry detergent? A full ~40 percent of regular laundry detergents are ranked of moderate or high concern! Why would a soap for cleaning clothes be so potentially harmful to a fetus? To find out, let's take an example: Tide Liquid Detergent, Original, which has a rating of "high concern." This detergent contains one specific ingredient of high concern: sodium borate. (It also has seven more ingredients of moderate concern, but let's focus on what's most important.)[132]

Companies put boric acid and/or sodium borate, a salt of boric acid, in detergent (as well as in fabric/upholstery cleaner, deodorizer, bleach, disinfectant, and soap scum remover) because it converts some water molecules to hydrogen peroxide and bonds with other particles to keep ingredients dispersed evenly in a mixture, which maximizes the surface area of active particles.[133] There's little doubt this chemical can be harmful to animals in large doses during pregnancy: in rats, rabbits, and mice, boric acid has been shown to affect fetal skeletal development and birth weight.[134] However, as of 2010, the European Chemicals Agency (ECHA) concluded that "it is not known whether there are significant differences . . . between humans and laboratory animal models," because "investigations of potentially reproductive effects in humans have not been specifically focused on boric acid alone," although "there are indications that boric acid is able to cross human placenta."[135] In other words, this chemical could very well be harmful to our babies, but there's no direct proof (as least yet).

How exposed to this chemical are we, anyway? It's not like we're drizzling detergent on our food and eating it. Fortunately, the European Chemicals Bureau, part of the Institute for Health and Consumer Protection, did an in-depth analysis of our practical exposure to boric acid in detergents, considering both inhalation of dust released and skin exposure from improperly using detergent for handwashing.[136] They ultimately concluded that cleaning staff who work in laundries, canteens, restaurants, or hospitals might be at risk from continuous repeated exposure, but for the rest of us, exposure is "negligible." For the record, I'm not trying to say that the Environmental Working Group is being paranoid. This is undoubtedly a nasty chemical, and future studies may very well show it causes harm. By all means, avoid it if you can. But it's not going to jump to the top of my hazards list just yet.

What other ingredients get ratings that are particularly ominous? There's sodium hypochlorite, otherwise known to you and me as bleach, which appears in many products, including mold and mildew remover, drain opener/clog remover, disinfectant, and grout cleaner. But according to a UK government agency, "There are no data indicating that sodium hypochlorite, without severe maternal toxicity, is associated with adverse effects on reproductive function, pregnancy, or lactation in humans."[137] Floor polish gets a bad score for containing our familiar phthalate, DBP. Some fabric and upholstery deodorizers contain silicon compounds, at least one of which is suspected of being a hormone disruptor, although this hasn't been proven yet in humans.[138] Some degreasers contain ingredients like methoxydiglycol,[139] which shows developmental toxicity in animals,[140, 141] and as a result has been banned from paints and cleaning products in the European Union since 2008.[142] This is clearly not a chemical you want to be spraying liberally around your house every day.

None of these ingredients individually has been put on the stand, had a fair trial, and been found guilty of harming human fetuses— at least not yet. But cumulatively, the chemical soup we surround ourselves with every day could be doing some harm. Preliminary studies suggest that cleaners and housekeepers may have higher risks of birth defects like cleft palate[143, 144] and spina bifida,[145] among others.[146] Keep in mind, though, that cleaning your house occasionally is not the same as working with cleaning products all day, every day.

What to do? A brochure on the CDC website helpfully suggests "it's easy and cheap to make effective, non-toxic cleaners. You can use common items like vinegar and baking soda."[147] That's all very well in theory. But if you've never tried it, cleaning with baking soda requires some real scrubbing effort. And no matter what the eco websites claim, it's never going to take away the worst stains. Watch out, too: trusty old Arm & Hammer has expanded its brand into all manner of additional cleaning products, but don't assume they're all as harmless as the original.[148]

So what's my recommendation? Take ten minutes one day to check the contents of your kitchen cabinet against the EWG database, and throw out the truly toxic products. Then if you want to be really careful, buy some rubber gloves and keep the windows open when you're using anything with a strong smell. Even better, abdicate responsibility for cleaning entirely and hand the cleaning products over to some other lucky member of your household. You have the perfect excuse.

Threat level for working as a cleaner: Low[149]

Threat level for using household cleaning products: Low[150]

The Painting Instinct: Organic Solvents

"In human females, the nesting instinct often occurs around the fifth month of pregnancy, but can occur as late as the eighth, or not at all. It may be strongest just before the onset of labor. It is commonly characterized by a strong urge to clean and organize one's home."[151]

Call it what you like. When I was six months' pregnant with my first child, I looked around the small room that had been functioning as our home office and decided a drastic makeover was in order. This was going to be the bedroom of my firstborn! Not only did the printer and the filing cabinets and the miles of miscellaneous computer cables have to go, but the room itself needed to be transformed from a hub of stressful activity into a space of zen-like serenity. I'd spent a few guilty hours poring over baby magazines, and I had just the decorative palette in mind. A subtle taupe for the walls to contrast with the cream furniture, with perhaps a few slate blue throw pillows for accents here and there . . . and so, a couple of months before my son was due, I waylaid a friendly painter working on a renovation project a few houses down and persuaded him to come apply a coat of paint.

The next morning, I showed the painter my carefully chosen wall color then skipped off merrily to work, eager to return home to see the transformation that evening. When I walked into the room, I realized, to my horror, that I had turned our lovely study into a small, claustrophobic dungeon. Perhaps I exaggerate, but as some of you may have the good sense to already know, dark-colored walls do not work in small rooms. The taupe had looked subtle in small patches, but it was mud-colored when applied in large swaths across a room. A second coat of lighter paint did little to improve the situation, which is how I ended up spending a large sum of money on three complete paint jobs to ultimately finish with a room almost exactly the same cream color as it had been before I started!

It was only in researching topics for my book that it occurred to me: not only had I wasted money with my little home-makeover project gone wrong, I had probably unnecessarily exposed myself to several nights' worth of breathing paint fumes as well. As it turns out, I'm not alone in having painting instincts during pregnancy. Some researchers in Denmark called 19,000 pregnant women and found that a full 45 percent of them had been exposed to paint fumes at home while pregnant.[152] Fortunately, that study also concluded that the fumes were harmless or at least insufficiently harmful to have had a noticeable effect on fetal growth. And another study found that household use of solvent-containing products (e.g., oil paints and paint thinners) didn't have any strong association with miscarriage.[153]

That doesn't mean you're completely off the hook, you there wearing the smock over your belly and brandishing a wet paintbrush. Occupational (in other words, significant and prolonged) exposure to organic solvents[154] has been linked to problems such as miscarriage,[155, 156] birth defects,[157, 158, 159, 160] lowered IQ, and behavioral problems,[161, 162, 163] as has maternal exposure to solvent-contaminated drinking water.[164] Similarly, purposefully sniffing those solvents to get high (otherwise known as "glue sniffing") is clearly not a good plan when you're pregnant, again causing all sorts of abnormalities and birth defects.[165, 166, 167] I bring this up not because I suspect you work in a nail polish plant or choose to sniff glue in your spare time. I'm merely making the point that if a lot of something is bad, it stands to reason that a small amount of it may still be bad, just not bad enough to detect in small sample populations.

Moreover, there is one worrying study that found that using household paint during pregnancy appears to increase the odds of your child developing a type of leukemia later in childhood by 20 percent.[168] Keep in mind this is quite a rare disease,[169] and this was only one study. But it fits with the intuitive possibility that paint fumes aren't so healthy. Then again, the odds of this leukemia appear to go up by ~40 percent for paint exposure after birth. So if you have a real compulsion to paint Junior's room blue, you might as well get the paint job over with now.[170]

Threat level for breathing household paint fumes: Low[171]

Healthy Hot Dogs: Nitrates and Nitrites

It's a key ingredient in dynamite. Its synthesis is considered by some to be the single most important invention of the 20th century, more important than electricity, cars, and computers.[172, 173] It's found in large quantities in human saliva. It keeps hot dogs red. And it might be causing birth defects or brain tumors in your unborn baby.

I'm talking about nitrogen. Nitrogen-based fertilizers (nitrates) averted a global famine during the twentieth century and are currently estimated to be responsible for sustaining about a third of the earth's population.[174] But like all such great leaps forward, there's a dark side to the story: nitrate runoff from cropland is contaminating our drinking water (and causing algal blooms and dead zones in our oceans, but that's another story). Nitrate is the only substance the government feels the need to regulate with a national drinking-water standard,[175] and the EPA "urges owners of private wells to have their well water tested annually and more often if someone in the household is pregnant or nursing."[176] This sounds serious. We've heard that pesticides are toxic, so fertilizers seem unlikely to be much better. Is there any true cause for alarm?

On balance, probably not. First, it's unlikely you're being exposed to dangerously high levels in your water, unless you live surrounded by crops (in which case, you should probably consider buying bottled water). A US Geological Survey analyzed 34,000 water samples from across the United States and found that while 16 percent of samples in agricultural areas exceeded the drinking-water standard for nitrates, only 1 percent of public-supply wells had nitrate levels above the guideline.[177]

Second, the impact of drinking nitrate-contaminated water during pregnancy is still not definitively proven. A variety of studies have investigated a link between nitrate levels in water and effects such as miscarriage[178] and an increased risk of birth defects.[179, 180, 181, 182] But a review of the field from 2006 that considered these studies, as well as others, concluded there's insufficient evidence to prove that nitrates in water cause reproductive effects.[183]

Furthermore, water might not even be your biggest source of exposure to nitrogen. Once taken into the body, nitrates are converted by bacteria into nitrites.[184] And nitrites might just ring a bell for their notorious role as an additive in hot dogs (and all other cured meat and fish). Although they may make your meat look rosier, that's not their primary purpose—it's to prevent the growth of bacteria, those same bacteria we were worrying about in Chapter 1.

Here again, researchers have poured time and energy into studying a possible link between maternal consumption of nitrites (e.g., in lunch meat) and later childhood brain cancer.[185, 186, 187, 188, 189] But the International Agency for Research on Cancer, an international body tasked with analyzing the risks posed by potential carcinogens, isn't convinced, concluding that there's "inadequate evidence in humans for the carcinogenicity of nitrate in food and drinking water" and "limited evidence in humans for the carcinogenicity of nitrite in food (associated with an increased incidence of stomach cancer)."[190] And the EPA and the CDC agree.[191] So that's the evidence, and it's not particularly worrisome in the end. In fact, some researchers are now hypothesizing that nitrates/nitrites might even be beneficial to human health, which would help explain why they're naturally present in our saliva.[192]

But we've vilified nitrites for so long, I can still imagine you vacillating in front of the meat section at the grocery store and ultimately grabbing the pricier organic sausages with "no nitrites added" just in case. You're wasting your money: those organic sausages are still full of nitrites.[193] As reported by The New York Times: "Current rules bizarrely require products that derive the preservatives from natural sources to prominently place the words 'Uncured' and 'No nitrates or nitrites added' on the label even though they are cured and do contain the chemicals. A study published earlier this year in The Journal *of Food Protection* found that natural hot dogs had anywhere from one-half to 10 times the amount of nitrite that conventional hot dogs contained."[194]

Furthermore, the amount of nitrite in meat has gone down substantially over the last thirty years due to improvements in curing methods, so there's a good chance nowadays that neither meat nor water is your main source of exposure.[195] Nope, the primary culprit is more likely to be . . . vegetables. That's right. "The majority of exposure to nitrite and nitrate in most people is through dietary intake of vegetables,"[196] leafy vegetables in particular. If you don't believe it, here's a little graph, courtesy of the International Agency for Research on Cancer we mentioned before,[197] showing your potential exposure levels in different scenarios.[198]

Average amount of nitrites consumed per day
(mg nitrite equivalent)

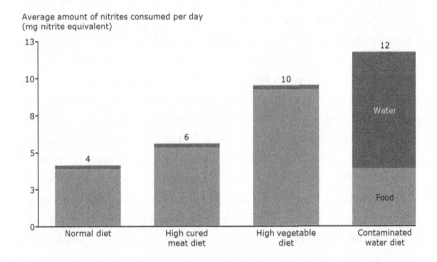

I hope you won't jump to the conclusion that you need to stop eating leafy vegetables, although giving them a good wash to clear away the fertilizer never hurts. The main point is that the hoopla over cured meat appears to be unfounded. So go ahead and eat that hot dog (as long as it's thoroughly cooked); it may not be so good for your own health, but it's unlikely to harm Junior.

Threat level for nitrates and nitrites: Very low[199]

A Breath of Fresh Air: Pollution

January 2013: "In China's capital, they're calling it the 'airpocalypse,' with air pollution that's literally off the charts. The air has been classified as hazardous to human health for a fifth consecutive day, at its worst hitting pollution levels 25 times that considered safe in the US. The entire city is blanketed in a thick grey smog that smells of coal and stings the eyes, leading to official warnings to stay inside."[200]

Take a moment to breathe a quick sigh of relief: that breath you just took probably isn't going to poison either you or your baby. Then again, it's all relative: compared to our ancestors who grew up in small villages, the outdoor air most of us breathe is probably filthy. Almost 80 percent of the US population lives in urban areas, and almost 60 percent of us live in cities with populations greater than 200,000.[201] So if you happen to be reading this in New York or LA, you might be wondering whether the car exhaust belching in your direction as you cross the street might be harming your unborn baby.

The answer is: possibly, but it's tough to say how much. This topic is being actively studied by research teams in both California and upper Manhattan[202, 203, 204, 205, 206, 207] as well as in other countries like Poland and China,[208, 209, 210, 211, 212, 213] where exposure to air pollution is high. According to a 2011 review, "evidence that poor air quality can adversely affect birth outcomes is increasing. A small number of review articles[214] have summarized existing studies and concluded that there is likely an adverse effect of air pollution on pregnancy outcome. However, estimated associations between these outcomes and air pollutant exposures over the whole pregnancy and during specific time windows (e.g., trimester) have been inconsistent, making definitive conclusions difficult."[215] Or in the words of another review, "research exploring the effects of air pollution on human reproduction is a young field."[216]

If relocating to Wyoming isn't a feasible option, you might be tempted to buy an indoor air filter. The gold standard of filters is the "high-efficiency particulate absorption," or HEPA filter, which can clean the air of many smaller particles as well as larger ones. There's no doubt that HEPA filters reduce indoor air pollution levels.[217] There's also preliminary evidence that they can improve health outcomes; one study found that elderly people living near a major road showed improvements in their blood vessel health after two days of living with indoor HEPA air filters running continuously in their bedrooms and living rooms.[218] And according to the American Academy of Allergy, Asthma, & Immunology, "portable room air cleaners with HEPA filters, especially those that filter the breathing zone during sleep, appear to be beneficial" for those suffering from asthma.[219] Unfortunately, there don't appear to be any studies yet on the effects of HEPA filters on pregnancy outcomes.

There is one other way you can reduce your exposure, which surprisingly has nothing to do with improving air quality. Air pollution contains a mixture of polycyclic aromatic hydrocarbons—PAHs for short—which are released into the air when we burn things like coal, gasoline, wood, garbage, or tobacco. But they also form in grilled meat. According to the CDC, "The average total daily intake of PAHs by a member of the general population has been estimated to be 0.207 µg from air, 0.027 µg from water, and 0.16-1.6 µg from food."[220] In other words, some people may be getting eight times as much exposure to these chemicals from eating chargrilled meat than from breathing polluted air. (Grilling vegetables doesn't create a similar threat. PAHs are formed when fat and juices from meat drip onto a fire, creating flames containing PAHs, which then adhere to the surface of the meat.) If you're grilling inside your home, the effects are potentially magnified even further, as grilling is a source of indoor air pollution if it produces smoke.[221] Preliminary research supports a link between grilled meat consumption and pregnancy outcomes,[222] although this result will need to be validated with further studies. So if buying a HEPA filter will blow the budget, you might consider putting the barbecue grill in storage instead.

Threat level for PAHs: difficult to calculate for now

The Microwave Strikes Back: Non-Ionizing Radiation

"Could microwaves [used during pregnancy] be associated with children's asthma?"[223] queried the headline in *Time* in 2011. Not again. We'd finally overcome our societal fear of microwaves ("They use radiation! They'll give us cancer!"). The term "nuking" now conjures up banal mental images of TV dinners rather than spectacular mushroom clouds or power plants. For many families, abandoning the microwave would require a complete rethink of how to prepare meals. But here was yet another reason to worry about our kitchen appliance.

Is it really necessary for pregnant women to return to the dark ages of cooking with pots and pans? Fortunately, the answer, as far as I can tell, is no. But before we go too far, let's start with a quick primer for anyone who doesn't work in radiology. There are two broad categories of radiation. Non-ionizing radiation (as opposed to ionizing radiation, which we'll address in the next section) is the lower-energy, more harmless end of the spectrum. Starting from the lowest energy, it includes five subcategories:[224]

1. Extremely low frequency (ELF) radiation, produced by power lines and household appliances
2. Radio-frequency (RF) radiation, produced by radios, TVs, cell phones, and wireless devices
3. Microwaves, produced by microwave ovens and heating lamps
4. Infrared, produced by remote controls
5. Visible light

Let's discuss each of these categories in turn, except visible light (for obvious reasons).

Extremely low frequency (ELF) radiation

Whenever electricity flows, it produces a magnetic field that causes electromagnetic radiation. This radiation can create currents within the human body, which could theoretically cause stimulation of nerves and muscles or affect other biological processes.[225] Fortunately, it's unlikely that we have anything to fear from this type of radiation during pregnancy. The World Health Organization's International Electromagnetic Field Project concluded that "exposure to fields at typical environmental levels does not increase the risk of any adverse outcome such as miscarriage, malformations, low birth weight, and congenital diseases."[226]

Let's say you happen to fall in the one percent of the population living close to a power line.[227] According to a study cited by the WHO, "the exposure of people living in the vicinity of high voltage power lines differs very little from the average exposure in the population."[228] In addition, there's no research to indicate that power lines have any specific effects on pregnancy outcomes,[229] although the jury is still out on the longer-term health impacts for children.[230]

When it comes to the radiation generated by electrical appliances, there's similarly little reason for concern. First, on average, only about one-third of your total exposure to EMFs is estimated to come from appliances. The rest comes from the so-called "background field," which you can't do anything about.[231] Second, "appliances are not a significant source of whole-body exposure," even if they're the main source of exposure for your extremities, so your bump is probably not affected.[232] Third, the fields generated by household appliances all fall far below the WHO recommended limit of 100 microteslas (μT).[233] See the following page for a chart of the fields produced by various common household appliances.[234]

Before we leave this topic, it turns out that headline about asthma is actually referring to the magnetic field produced by the microwave rather than the microwaves themselves. But the authors caveat that "as with any epidemiological study, these findings need to be replicated."[235] It's simply too soon to know whether future studies will reproduce the same findings or if researchers will be able to show that it's the magnetic fields that are causing the asthma rather than, say, both being related to another factor like spending time indoors. Anyway, as you can see from the chart, it's your vacuum cleaner that's the worst culprit, not your microwave.

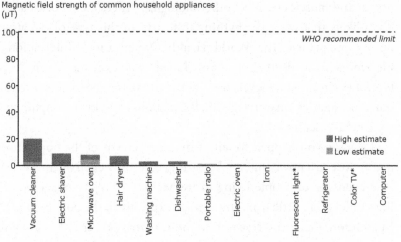

Magnetic field strength of common household appliances (µT)

*Note: all measurements from a distance of 30cm away, except TV and fluorescent light from a distance of 1m

High-frequency or radio-frequency (RF) fields

The potential concern with RF fields is that exposure can heat up the body. But here, there's even less evidence that these waves can harm your baby,[236, 237] although the topic hasn't been studied extensively given our exposure to these fields is a relatively recent phenomenon. Several studies have examined physiotherapists who frequently use machines that emit RF fields ("short-wave diathermy" machines that produce heat to relieve joint stiffness and relax muscles) to treat their patients, but there have been no consistent findings of harm to their offspring thus far.[238]

Microwaves

This type of radiation generates heat, which is why we use it to heat up food.[239] According to the WHO, "microwave energy can be absorbed by the body and produce heat in exposed tissues. Organs with a poor blood supply and temperature control, such as the eye, or temperature-sensitive tissue like the testes, have a higher risk of heat damage. However, thermal damage would only occur from long exposures to very high power levels, well in excess of those measured around microwave ovens." Furthermore, "effective shielding reduces leakage outside the ovens to almost non-detectable levels."[240] So there's no risk to the fetus here.

Infrared

This type of radiation does not penetrate very deeply into biological tissue, so it doesn't have the potential to reach the fetus.[241]

I wouldn't worry about exposure to non-ionizing radiation from magnetic fields. Both the National Research Council[242] and the International Commission for Non-Ionizing Radiation Protection[243] agree there's no good evidence linking such radiation to pregnancy outcomes. On the other hand, if you happen to dislike cleaning, you now have a vaguely legitimate-sounding excuse to hand the vacuum over along with those cleaning chemicals. Who thought being pregnant would be this easy?

Threat level for magnetic fields: Very low[244]

Galactic Beams: Ionizing Radiation

The beams of galactic cosmic radiation stream out of the exploding star, sail through space, and rain down on the unsuspecting pregnant female, bombarding her unborn fetus and catalyzing a raft of spontaneous, potentially harmful cellular mutations. This woman is not the heroine of the latest sci-fi novel—she's you.

We are all constantly being pelted with galactic cosmic radiation and many other kinds of radiation as well. This may sound concerning. As one researcher describes in deadpan academic fashion, "The term radiation evokes emotional responses both from lay persons and from professionals."[245] But does our "emotional response" have any basis in fact? Can radiation hurt our fetus?

Ionizing radiation is radiation that has sufficient energy to produce ions that can cause DNA damage.[246] This is the category that includes medical X-rays, radon gas, and nuclear reactions. This type of radiation is most definitely harmful in any quantity. According to both the American College of Radiology and the American College of Obstetricians and Gynecologists, no single diagnostic X-ray results in radiation exposure to a degree that threatens a developing embryo or fetus, so if a single test is needed for health, that's fine.[247, 248] But multiple X-rays or any X-rays that are less than essential should be postponed until after delivery. Thankfully, we figured this out a long time ago, and by now we understand the risks quite well: according to a review addressing pregnancy, "in the field of ionizing radiation, we have a better comprehension of the biologic effects and the quantitative maximum risks than for any other environmental hazard."[249]

The average American receives a non-negligible dose of ionizing radiation every year.[250] But a full 68 percent comes from exposure to radon gas, which fortunately doesn't reach the fetus (although it's not great for you).[251, 252] The remaining exposure comes from radioactive material in the ground (9 percent), radioactive material in body tissues (14 percent), and galactic cosmic radiation (another 9 percent). (Galactic cosmic radiation, rather than the villain in a sci-fi movie, is the very real and constant stream of radiation emanating from sources in outer space.)[253] The increased lifetime risk of fatal cancer from radiation received during prenatal development is about 3 in 10,000.[254] So there's a certain level of risk to your fetus that you simply can't control.

No one knows the risks of ionizing radiation to the fetus better than the folks at the Federal Aviation Administration (FAA), the government agency with responsibility for protecting our safety in the air. That's because air travel can be a major additional source of radiation exposure. It's not the airport security scanners, which don't appear to pose any risk in pregnancy.[255] As you fly higher, there's less atmosphere to shield you from those cosmic rays.[256]

So what if you live like George Clooney's character from *Up in the Air*? Let's say you have a punishing work schedule that requires you to fly all the way across the entire country and back once a week. The dose of additional radiation you'd receive would be 0.028 per flight x 2 flights per week x 36 weeks of pregnancy (airlines won't let you fly in the last 4 weeks) = 2.02 millisieverts.[257] So the probability your child will someday get cancer as a result of all your globetrotting is still very small (~2 in 10,000), although it's not zero. You could theoretically buy a lead apron to carry on with you; they retail for about $200 on the internet.[258] But I suspect you might face a few delays going through security.

Threat level for weekly long-haul air travel: Medium[259]

Threat level for a single long-haul flight: Very low[260]

Threat level for unavoidable exposure to background radiation: Low[261]

Professor Plum in the Library with the Rice Cereal: Arsenic

It was Agatha Christie's favorite poison: a colorless, odorless powder, as easily procured as rat poison or flypaper.[262] It remained undetectable at twenty to sixty times the lethal dose when dissolved in hot cocoa, tea, or milk and soon caused convulsions and death.[263] So why was this potent murder weapon suddenly making headlines associated with baby food?

In November 2012, *Consumer Reports* published a report claiming that baby rice cereal and other rice products in the United States contained unacceptable levels of arsenic.[264] This was not a case of a mass murderer targeting innocent children. Inorganic arsenic (the more harmful kind) is naturally present in the groundwater of a number of countries, including the United States,[265] although there's also speculation that historic use of arsenic as a pesticide on cotton may have further contaminated our soil.[266]

Fortunately, despite its deserved reputation as a fearsome poison, and despite the recent hype it's been attracting in the news, arsenic doesn't appear to pose a significant health risk during pregnancy. In animal studies, effects in fetuses are typically seen only at doses that also affect the mothers.[267, 268] In humans, there's evidence of danger to the fetus from acute exposure,[269, 270] as well as from chronic exposure.[271] This evidence is mostly based on studies of women in Bangladesh,[272] where approximately half the population is at risk of drinking arsenic-contaminated well water.[273] But according to the CDC, evidence of the effects from lower-level exposure is less definitive.[274] And two different reviews both suggest that arsenic is unlikely to pose a risk during pregnancy at current levels found in the environment in the United States.[275, 276] After extensive testing of rice samples, the FDA concurs, saying "Consumers can certainly eat rice as part of a well-balanced diet . . . we encourage pregnant women to eat a variety of foods, including varied grains."[277]

So as long as you're not drinking suspiciously delicious hot cocoa offered to you before bed by the recently added beneficiary of your last will and testament, you should be fine.

Threat level for arsenic: Very low

Conclusions: Detox

Our babies are being marinated in a complex soup of chemicals and heavy metals before they leave the womb. Some of these substances are harmless, some are mysterious, and some appear to be deleterious. And although there aren't any alarming trends in birth defects or miscarriages, low birth weight is on the rise, and there might also be more subtle effects playing out over the longer term. Most of our exposure we can't control, at least for now, but a few of the more noxious substances we could avoid if we were aware of the threat they posed.

We understandably rely on physicians to shepherd us through the unfamiliar territory of pregnancy. They're the experts on the inner world of the fetus, and we feel safe in their hands. But they tend to know very little about environmental pollutants. A nationwide survey of 2,600 obstetricians and gynecologists found that most don't warn their pregnant patients about chemicals that could endanger their fetuses. More than half said they don't discuss mercury, and hardly any give advice about lead, pesticides, air pollution, or chemicals in plastics or cosmetics.[278] And while official bodies may recommend that doctors take a patient history during the first prenatal visit to identify any potential sources of hazardous exposure, my physician didn't do so, and I suspect yours didn't either.[279]

We can hope that someday Congress will adopt new legislation to update the archaic Toxic Substances Control Act, moving us closer to a more sensible world in which chemicals are tested for safety before being allowed into our cabinets.[280] The government is at least pouring significant funds into research to better understand how chemicals may be affecting the health of our children.[281] In the meantime, the best we can do is avoid the known culprits, most importantly lead and pesticides. If you want to protect Junior by cleansing the toxins out of your system, don't bother with a trendy "detox diet"; three days of drinking green juice isn't going to flush the lead out of your bones or the mercury out of your system. But a trip to the organic produce section of the grocery store and a blood test for lead just might help.

Notes

1. Body burden: the pollution in newborns. (2005, July 14). Environmental Working Group. www.ewg.org/research/body-burden-pollution-newborns#.WdIL1MIm7jY.

2. Basic information for the review of new chemicals. (n.d.). US Environmental Protection Agency. www.epa.gov/reviewing-new-chemicals-under-toxic-substances-control-act-tsca/basic-information-review-new#newchemical.

3. Overview: Office of Pollution Prevention and Toxics Programs. (2003, December 24). US Environmental Protection Agency. http://www.chemicalspolicy.org/downloads/TSCA10112-24-03.pdf.

4. Ibid.

5. The safety of prescription drugs falls outside of the scope of this book, being the rightful domain of the medical profession. However, it's worth noting that 98% of drugs all approved by the FDA between 2000 and 2010 have an "undetermined" risk of causing birth defects in pregnancy, with 73% having no data available at all regarding safety in pregnancy. And of the 640 prescription drugs approved since 1980, only 9% have been evaluated for the risk of causing birth defects, with only half of those evaluated ultimately deemed safe for use in pregnancy. (Adam, M. P., Polifka, J. E., & Friedman, J. M. [2011, August]. Evolving knowledge of the teratogenicity of medications in human pregnancy.

American Journal of Medical Genetics Part C: Seminars in Medical Genetics, 157 [3], 175-182. http://onlinelibrary.wiley.com/doi/10.1002/ajmg.c.30313/abstract]. So while prescription drugs are unlikely to harm you personally if used correctly, it's worth caveating that it's hard to know what effect they might be having on your fetus.

6. Grandjean, P., & Landrigan, P. J. (2014). Neurobehavioural effects of developmental toxicity. *The Lancet Neurology, 13* (3), 330–338. www.farmlandbirds.net/sites/default/files/Grandjean%20Landrigan%20Lancet%202014_0.pdf.

7. "Are fetal outcomes getting worse nowadays?" is not actually a straightforward question to answer, because so many other factors besides chemical exposure have changed over the years. Women are waiting longer to have families, and older mothers are more likely to have problems. Demographics in the United States are also changing, and recent immigrant populations might change the statistics. These two factors are fortunately ones we can control—the US National Vital Statistics department conveniently breaks down data about births by age group and race. That's why you'll see "White 25–29-year-olds" written at the top of most of the charts in this section. But there are lots of other factors we can't strain out—for example, improvements in our ability to diagnose conditions might falsely make those conditions appear to be increasing; our ability to save premature babies who might have died otherwise could make rates of associated problems appear worse; pregnancy tests allow earlier recognition of pregnancies, which might make the miscarriage rate look worse; and other health issues affecting pregnancy such as obesity are on the rise, to name a few. In addition, we would ideally want to look back over several decades. But it's easy to forget that forty years ago, the computer as we know it didn't exist, so gathering national data on birth outcomes wasn't a feasible task. That's why most of the data in this section aren't ideal; the data on miscarriage only go back to 1990, the data on birth defects come only from Atlanta, etc.

8. Ventura, S. J., Abma, J. C., Mosher, W. D., & Henshaw, S. K. (2008). Estimated pregnancy rates by outcome for the United States, 1990–2004. *National Vital Statistics Reports, 56* (28), 1–25. www.cdc.gov/nchs/data/nvsr/nvsr56/nvsr56_15.pdf.

9. Correa, A., Cragan, J. D., Kucik, J. E., Alverson, C. J., Gilboa, S. M., Balakrishnan, R., Strickland, M.J., Duke, C. W., O'Leary, L.A., Riehle-Colarusso, T., Siffel, C., Gambrell, D., Thompson, D., Atkinson, M., & Chitra, J. (2007). MACDP 40th anniversary edition survelliance report—reporting birth defects surveillance data 1968–2003: executive summary. *Birth Defects Research Part A: Clinical and Molecular Teratology, 79*, 66–93. http://onlinelibrary.wiley.com/doi/10.1002/bdra.v79:2/issuetoc.

10. Phthalates: are they safe? (2010, May 21). *CBSnews.com*. www.cbsnews.com/stories/2010/05/21/60minutes/main6506892.shtml.

11. Correa et al., Executive summary.

It's technically possible that an increase in the rate of birth defects could have been masked by an increase in prenatal screening resulting in more fetuses with birth defects being aborted. Unfortunately, the data are insufficient to investigate this question further.

12. Correa, A., Cragan, J. D., Kucik, J. E., Alverson, C. J., Gilboa, S. M., Balakrishnan, R., Strickland, M.J., Duke, C. W., O'Leary, L.A., Riehle-Colarusso, T., Siffel, C., Gambrell, D., Thompson, D., Atkinson, M., & Chitra, J. (2007). MACDP 40th anniversary edition survelliance report—reporting birth defects surveillance data 1968–2003: appendix A. *Birth Defects Research Part A: Clinical and Molecular Teratology, 79*, 94–177. http://onlinelibrary.wiley.com/doi/10.1002/bdra.v79:2/issuetoc.

13. According to the authors of the report, "the ability to diagnose heart defects through bedside echocardiography in the newborn improved dramatically during the period of MACDP surveillance."

14. Paulozzi, L. J. (1999). International trends in rates of hypospadias and cryptorchidism. *Environmental Health Perspectives, 107* (4), 297. www.ncbi.nlm.nih.gov/pmc/articles/ PMC1566511/pdf/envhper00509-0089.pdf.

E.g., how far back does the opening have to be before it officially becomes a defect rather than normal variation? In the words of the author, "Severe hypospadias is much less likely to be affected by changes in definition because it has clearer anatomical boundaries . . . Severe hypospadias in the Atlanta system increased from 1982 to 1985 and then leveled off. Rates from the California Birth Defects Monitoring Program for severe hypospadias showed no upward trend."

15. Martin, J. A., Hamilton, B. E., Sutton, P. D., Ventura, S. J., Menacker, F., & Kirmeyer, S. (2006). Births: final data for 2004. *National Vital Statistics Reports, 55* (1), 23.

16. Barker, D. J. (1995). Fetal origins of coronary heart disease. *British Medical Journal, 311* (6998), 171–174. www.ncbi.nlm.nih.gov/pmc/articles/PMC2550226/pdf/bmj00601-0037. pdf.

17. Hales, C. N., Barker, D. J., Clark, P. M., Cox, L. J., Fall, C., Osmond, C., & Winter, P. D. (1991). Fetal and infant growth and impaired glucose tolerance at age 64. *British Medical Journal, 303* (6809), 1019. www.ncbi.nlm.nih.gov/pmc/articles/PMC1671766/pdf/ bmj00150-0019.pdf.

18. Thompson, C., Syddall, H., Rodin, I. A. N., Osmond, C., & Barker, D. J. (2001). Birth weight and the risk of depressive disorder in late life. *The British Journal of Psychiatry, 179* (5), 450–455.

19. Wahlbeck, K., Forsén, T., Osmond, C., Barker, D. J., & Eriksson, J. G. (2001). Association of schizophrenia with low maternal body mass index, small size at birth, and thinness during childhood. *Archives of General Psychiatry, 58* (1), 48–52. http://jamanetwork.com/journals/ jamapsychiatry/fullarticle/481697.

20. Hack, M., Klein, N. K., & Taylor, H. G. (1995, Spring). Long-term developmental outcomes of low birth weight infants. *The Future of Children, 5* (1), 176–196. www.jstor.org/discover/ 10.2307/1602514?uid=3738032&uid=2&uid=4&sid=21102905178893.

21. Martin, J. A., Hamilton, B. E., Sutton, P. D., Ventura, S. J. Mathews, T. J., & Osterman, M. J. K. (2010, December 8). Births: final data for 2008. *National Vital Statistics Reports, 59* (1), 1–72. www.cdc.gov/nchs/data/nvsr/nvsr59/nvsr59_01.pdf.

22. According to a clinical opinion published in the *American Journal of Obstetrics & Gynecology*, "Rapidly accumulating scientific evidence documents that widespread exposure to environmental chemicals at levels that are encountered in daily life can impact reproductive and developmental health adversely. Preconception and prenatal exposure to environmental chemicals are of particular importance because they may have a profound and lasting impact on health across the life course. Thus, prevention of developmental exposures to environmental chemicals would benefit greatly from the active participation of reproductive health professionals in clinical and policy arenas." (Sutton, P., Woodruff, T. J., Perron, J., Stotland, N., Conry, J. A., Miller, M. D., & Giudice, L. C. [2012]. Toxic environmental chemicals: the role of reproductive health professionals in preventing harmful exposures. *American Journal of Obstetrics and Gynecology, 207* [3], 164–173. http://www.sciencedirect.com/science/article/pii/S0002937812000658.) According to the Endocrine Society, "For reproductive function in both humans and animals, fetal life is most vulnerable because there are rapid structural and functional events . . . As endocrinologists, we suggest that The Endocrine Society actively engages in lobbying for regulation seeking to decrease human exposure to the many endocrine-disrupting agents." (Diamanti-Kandarakis, E., Bourguignon, J. P., Giudice, L. C., Hauser, R., Prins, G. S., Soto, A. M., Zoeller, R. T., & Gore, A. C. (2009, June). Endocrine-disrupting chemicals: an Endocrine Society scientific statement. *Endocrine Reviews, 30*

(4), 293–342. www.cancersupportinternational.com/July%202009%20Endocrine%20 Society%20EDC%20Scientific%20Statement.pdf.) According to the American Congress of Obstetricians and Gynecologists (ACOG), "The evidence that links exposure to toxic environmental agents and adverse reproductive and developmental health outcomes is sufficiently robust, and the American College of Obstetricians and Gynecologists and the American Society for Reproductive Medicine join leading scientists and other clinical practitioners in calling for timely action to identify and reduce exposure to toxic environmental agents while addressing the consequences of such exposure."(American College of Obstetrics and Gynecology. [2013, October]. Exposure to toxic environmental agents. Committee opinion no. 575. *Obstetrics and Gynecology, 122,* 931–935. www.acog.org/Resources_And_Publications/Committee_Opinions/Committee_on_ Health_Care_for_Underserved_Women/Exposure_to_Toxic_Environmental_Agents.) According to the participants at the International Conference on Fetal Programming and Developmental Toxicity, "The accumulated research evidence suggests that prevention efforts against toxic exposures to environmental chemicals should focus on protecting the embryo, foetus, and small child as highly vulnerable populations. Given the ubiquitous exposure to many environmental chemicals, there needs to be renewed efforts to prevent harm."(Grandjean, P., Bellinger, D., Bergman, Å., Cordier, S., Davey-Smith, G., Eskenazi, B., Gee, D., Gray, K., Hanson, M., Van Den Hazel, P., Heindel, J. J., Heinzow, B., Hertz-Picciotto, I., Hu, H., Huang, T. T. K., Kold Jensen, T., Landrigan, P. J., McMillen, I. C., Murata, K., Ritz, B., Schoeters, G., Skakkebæk, N. E., Skerfving, S., & Weihe, P. [2008]. The Faroes statement: human health effects of developmental exposure to chemicals in our environment. *Basic & Clinical Pharmacology & Toxicology, 102* [2], 73–75. http://onlinelibrary.wiley.com/doi/10.1111/j.1742-7843.2007.00114.x/full.) And according to a recent publication in *The Lancet*, the exposure of our fetuses to such a wide variety of chemicals represents a "silent pandemic." (Grandjean, Neurobehavioural effects of developmental toxicity.)

23. The term "mercury" is used throughout this section to indicate organic mercury, also known as methylmercury, which is the type of mercury found in fish and the type which has been proven to be harmful to fetal neurodevelopment. Women are also exposed to other types of mercury—for example, inorganic mercury, which is used in dental amalgams—but this type of mercury has not been proven to be harmful in pregnancy. For more detail on this topic, see Appendix VI under "amalgam." According to the EPA, "Children who are exposed to low concentrations of methylmercury prenatally are at increased risk of poor performance on neurobehavioral tests, such as those measuring attention, fine motor function, language skills, visual-spatial abilities (like drawing), and verbal memory." From https://books.google.co.uk/books?id=ALV66PbKE3cC&print-sec=frontcover#v=onepage&q&f=false, citing: Grandjean, P., Weihe, P., White, R. F., Debes, F., Araki, S., Yokoyama, K., Murata, K., Sørenson, N., Dahl, R., & Jørgensen, P. J. (1997). Cognitive deficit in 7-year-old children with prenatal exposure to methylmercury. *Neurotoxicology and Teratology, 19* (6), 417–428.

24. 5.8 parts per billion.

   US Environmental Protection Agency (EPA). (2011, March 10). Human exposure to environmental contaminants; U.S. Environmental Protection Agency. (2001). Integrated Risk Information System (IRIS) Risk Information for Methylmercury (MeHg). Washington, DC: National Center for Environmental Assessment. https://cfpub.epa.gov/ ncea/iris/iris_documents/documents/subst/0073_summary.pdf.

25. Santerre, C. (Last updated 2016, March). Is it safe to eat fish and other seafood when I'm pregnant? Babycenter.com. www.babycenter.com/406_is-it-safe-to-eat-fish-and-other-seafood-when-im-pregnant_1380503.bc.

26. US Food and Drug Administration. (2004, March). What you need to know about mercury in fish and shellfish. Brochure. FDA.gov. https://www.fda.gov/food/foodborneillness contaminants/metals/ucm351781.htm.

27. Choiniére, C. J., Timbo, B., Street, D., Trumbo, P., Fein, S. (2008, August 3–6). Fish consumption by women of childbearing age, pregnant women, and mothers of infants. Presented at the International Association for Food Protection Annual Meeting, Columbus, Ohio.

28. Bloomingdale, A., Guthrie, L. B., Price, S., Wright, R. O., Platek, D., Haines, J., & Oken, E. (2010). A qualitative study of fish consumption during pregnancy. *The American Journal of Clinical Nutrition, 92* (5), 1234–1240. http://ajcn.nutrition.org/content/92/5/1234.full.

29. US Food and Drug Administration, What you need to know about mercury in fish and shellfish.

It's difficult to estimate the potential reduction in fetal brain mercury levels from a woman reducing fish consumption once already pregnant. A wide variety of studies have estimated that in adults, the half-life for methylmercury in the blood is on average approximately 50 days (National Research Council. [2000]. *Toxicological effects of methylmercury.* Washington, DC: National Academy Press. https://www.nap.edu/catalog/9899/toxicological-effects-of-methylmercury; US Food and Drug Administration. [2009, January 21]. Report of quantitative risk and benefit assessment of consumption of commercial fish, focusing on fetal neurodevelopmental effects (measured by verbal development in children) and on coronary heart disease and stroke in the general population, and summary of published research on the beneficial effects of fish consumption and omega-3 fatty acids for certain neurodevelopmental and cardiovascular endpoints; availability. *Federal Register, 74* [12]. https://www.gpo.gov/fdsys/pkg/FR-2009-01-21/pdf/E9-1081.pdf; Centers for Disease Control and Prevention. [n.d.]. Biomonitoring summary: mercury. CDC.gov. www.cdc.gov/biomonitoring/Mercury_BiomonitoringSummary.html), and the amount in fetal blood is likely to be proportional to that in the mother's (Counter, S. A., & Buchanan, L. H. [2004]. Mercury exposure in children: a review. *Toxicology and Applied Pharmacology, 198* (2), 209–230. http://www.sciencedirect.com/science/article/pii/S0041008X04000432). But the whole-body half-life is likely to be longer, closer to 70–80 days (National Research Council, Toxicological effects of methylmercury) with a very wide variance—35 to 189 days (Al-Shahristani, H., & Shihab, K. M. [1974]. Variation of biological half-life of methylmercury in man. *Archives of Environmental Health: An International Journal, 28* [6], 342–344. www.tandfonline.com/doi/abs/10.1080/00039896.1974.10666505). And the half-life in the brain may be substantially longer than that: "Methylmercury readily crosses the blood-brain barrier. . . . Methylmercury accumulates in the brain where it is slowly converted to inorganic mercury. Whether central nervous system damage is due to methylmercury per se, to its biotransformation to inorganic mercury, or to both is still controversial. . . . Both adult and fetal brains are vulnerable. . . . Both methylmercury and elemental mercury are converted to mercuric mercury in the brain, where it is trapped. The biological mechanisms for removing mercuric mercury from the brain are limited. . . . Risk-assessment models for methylmercury in humans are complicated because of inadequate data regarding the cumulative neurotoxic effects of methylmercury per se and its biotransformation product mercuric mercury, which has a very long half-life in the brain . . . inorganic mercury in the brain for years following early methylmercury intake is possibly related to the latent or long-term neurotoxic effects reported. The long half-life of inorganic mercury in the brain following methylmercury intake should be considered in risk assessment of methylmercury." (National Research Council, Toxicological effects of methylmercury.) Another study echoes that the half-life of mercury in brain tissue is measured in years (Hightower, J. M., & Moore, D. [2003, April]. Mercury levels in high-end consumers of fish. *Environmental Health Perspectives, 111* [4], 604. https://www.ncbi.nlm.nih.gov/pmc/articles/PMC1241452/pdf/ehp0111-000604.pdf). It's therefore unclear how much mercury would accumulate in a fetal brain during the earliest stages of pregnancy and how much of that could be influenced by later reductions in blood levels. Finally, a study of women in Sweden who followed government guidelines and reduced their fish consumption when pregnant found that "cord blood methylmercury was almost twice that in maternal blood in late pregnancy and was probably influenced by maternal methylmercury exposure earlier and before pregnancy" (Vahter, M., Åkesson, A., Lind, B., Björs, U., Schütz, A., & Berglund, M. [2000]. Longitudinal study of methylmercury and inorganic mercury in blood and urine of pregnant and lactating women, as well as in umbilical cord blood. *Environmental Research, 84* [2], 186–194. www.sciencedirect.com/science/article/pii/S0013935100940982). This supports the FDA's statement that it may be too late to dramatically reduce fetal blood mercury levels once pregnant. A medical treatment called chelation therapy can be used in situations of acute mercury and other heavy metal poisoning to draw the metal out of the body. But this form of treatment is only used in serious cases of poisoning and is not appropriate during pregnancy. "Chelation therapy may produce toxic effects, including kidney damage, irregular heartbeat, and swelling of the veins. It may also cause nausea, vomiting, diarrhea, and temporary lowering of blood pressure. Since the therapy removes minerals from the body, there is a risk of developing low calcium levels (hypocalcemia) and bone damage. Chelation therapy may also impair the immune system and decrease the body's ability to produce insulin. . . . Women who are pregnant or breastfeeding should not use this method." (Chakrabarty, N. [Ed.]. [2016]. *Arsenic toxicity: prevention and treatment.* Boca Raton, FL: CRC Press.)

30. US Food and Drug Administration. (2009). Draft report of quantitative risk and benefit assessment of consumption of commercial fish, focusing on fetal neurodevelopmental effects (measured by verbal development in children) and on coronary heart disease and stroke in the general population. Center for Food Safety and Applied Nutrition, 15, Section V, Table V-8, 81–82. https://wayback.archive-it.org/7993/20170406180738/https://www.fda.gov/Food/FoodborneIllnessContaminants/Metals/ucm088794.htm.

31. Axelrad, D. A., Bellinger, D. C., Ryan, L. M., & Woodruff, T. J. (2007, April). Dose-response relationship of prenatal mercury exposure and IQ: an integrative analysis of epidemiologic data. *Environmental Health Perspectives, 115* (4), 609–615. www.ncbi.nlm.nih.gov/pmc/articles/PMC1852694/pdf/ehp0115-000609.pdf.

32. Cohen, J. T., Bellinger, D. C., & Shaywitz, B. A. (2005). A quantitative analysis of prenatal methyl mercury exposure and cognitive development. *American Journal of Preventive Medicine, 29* (4), 353–365. www.ajpm-online.net/article/S0749-3797(05)00248-5/abstract.

33. A variety of studies have demonstrated a positive effect from eating fish:

Daniels, J. L., Longnecker, M. P., Rowland, A. S., Golding, J., and the ALSPAC Study Team–University of Bristol Institute of Child Health. (2004, July). Fish intake during pregnancy and darly cognitive development of offspring. *Epidemiology, 15* (4), 394–402. http://journals.lww.com/epidem/Abstract/2004/07000/Fish_Intake_During_Pregnancy_and_Early_Cognitive.4.aspx; Oken, E., Østerdal, M. L. M., Gilman, M. W., Knudsen, V. K., Halldorsson, M. S., Bellinger, D. C., Hadders-Algra, M., Michaelsen, K. F., Olsen, S. F. (2008). Associations of maternal fish intake during pregnancy and breastfeeding duration with attainment of developmental milestones in early childhood: a study from the Danish National Birth Cohort. *American Journal of Clinical Nutrition, 88* (3), 789–796. http://ajcn.nutrition.org/content/88/3/789.full; Gale, C. R., Robinson, S. M., Godfrey, K. M., Law, C. M., Schlotz, W., & O'Callaghan, F. J. (2008). Oily fish intake during pregnancy—association with lower hyperactivity but not with higher full-scale IQ in offspring. *Journal of Child Psychology and Psychiatry, 49* (10), 1061–1068. https://www.researchgate.net/profile/Wolff_Schlotz/publication/5429230_Oily_fish_intake_during_pregnancy-Association_with_lower_hyperactivity_but_not_with_higher_full-scale_IQ_in_offspring/links/0c960521b6f5c26bbd000000/Oily-fish-intake-during-pregnancy-Association-with-lower-hyperactivity-but-not-with-higher-full-scale-IQ-in-offspring.pdf; Lederman, S. A., Jones, R. L., Caldwell, K. L., Rauh, V., Sheets, S. E., Tang, D., Viswanathan, S., Becker, M., Stein, J., Wang, R., & Perera, F.

P. (2008). Relation between cord blood mercury levels and early child development in a World Trade Center cohort. *Environmental Health Perspectives, 116* (8), 1085. https://www.ncbi.nlm.nih.gov/pmc/articles/PMC2516590/; Boucher, O., Burden, M. J., Muckle, G., Saint-Amour, D., Ayotte, P., Dewailly, E., Nelson, C. A., Jacobson, S. W., & Jacobson, J. L. (2011). Neurophysiologic and neurobehavioral evidence of beneficial effects of prenatal omega-3 fatty acid intake on memory function at school age. *The American Journal of Clinical Nutrition, 93* (5), 1025–1037. http://ajcn.nutrition.org/content/93/5/1025.full; Sagiv, S. K., Thurston, S. W., Bellinger, D. C., Amarasiriwardena, C., & Korrick, S. A. (2012). Prenatal exposure to mercury and fish consumption during pregnancy and attention-deficit/hyperactivity disorder–related behavior in children. *Archives of Pediatrics & Adolescent Medicine, 166* (12), 1123–1131. www.centerforthedevelopingmind.com/sites/default/files/2C_S_archpediatrics.pdf.

For example, one study of ~12,000 pregnant women found that eating plenty of fish during pregnancy ultimately gave their children higher IQs as well as better motor, communication, and social skills (Hibbeln, J. R., Davis, J. M., Steer, C., Emmett, P., Rogers, I., Williams, C., & Golding, J. [2007]. Maternal seafood consumption in pregnancy and neurodevelopmental outcomes in childhood [ALSPAC study]: an observational cohort study. *The Lancet, 369* [9561], 578–585. www.lancet.com/journals/lancet/article/PIIS0140-6736(07)60277-3). And another set of studies at Harvard Medical School found that maternal fish intake more than twice a week during pregnancy was associated with improved performance on tests of language and visual motor skills in infants (Oken, E., Wright, R. O., Kleinman, K. P., Bellinger, D., Amarasiriwardena, C. J., Hu, H., & Gillman, M. W. [2005]. Maternal fish consumption, hair mercury, and infant cognition in a US cohort. *Environmental Health Perspectives, 113* [10], 1376. www.ncbi.nlm.nih.gov/pmc/articles/PMC1281283/) and 3-year-olds (Oken, E., Radesky, J. S., Wright, R. O., Bellinger, D. C., Amarasiriwardena, C. J., Kleinman, K. P., Hu, H., & Gillman, M. W. [2008]. Maternal fish intake during pregnancy, blood mercury levels, and child cognition at age 3 years in a US cohort. *American Journal of Epidemiology, 167* [10], 1, 171-1, 181. http://aje.oxfordjournals.org/content/167/10/1171.full.pdf). However, not all studies have found an effect (Makrides, M., Gibson, R. A., McPhee, A. J., Yelland, L., Quinlivan, J., & Ryan, P. [2010]. Effect of DHA supplementation during pregnancy on maternal depression and neurodevelopment of young children: a randomized controlled trial. *JAMA, 304* [15], 1675–1683. http://jama.jamanetwork.com/article.aspx?articleid=186750). It's also worth noting that some of the "fish effect" could theoretically be driven by correlation rather than causation, given that women with higher socioeconomic status, healthier lifestyles, etc. are more likely to consume fish, and it can be difficult to completely eliminate the effects of such confounders.

34. Hibbeln, Maternal seafood consumption in pregnancy and neurodevelopmental outcomes in childhood.

35. Senators urge more fish for women, children. (2011, March 14). VitalChoice.com. www.vitalchoice.com/shop/pc/articlesView.asp?id=1329.

36. Cryer, Pat. (n.d.). 1940s war-time health care for children: food supplements for children. *Join me in the 1900s.* www.1900s.org.uk/1940s-edgware-health.htm.

37. In a study cited by the FDA report, 10 ml of cod liver oil daily in pregnancy led to a 4% point advantage in children's scores on an intelligence test at age four (Helland, I. B., Smith, L., Saarem, K., Saugstad, O. D., & Drevon, C. A. [2003]. Maternal supplementation with very-long-chain n-3 fatty acids during pregnancy and lactation augments children's IQ at 4 years of age. *Pediatrics, 111* [1], e39–e44. http://pediatrics.aappublications.org/cgi/reprint/111/1/e39).

38. As reported in a BBC article in 2010, "The interest in omega-3 has snowballed over the past decade. . . . Over the past 10 years, about 12,500 scientific studies on the benefits of omega-3 have been published, both reflecting and reinforcing the fashion for consuming

this apparent super-food. Today, everything from loaves of bread to frozen fish fingers come with a 'RICH IN OMEGA-3' tag. . . . Dr. Lee Hooper, lead author of one of the most thorough studies on the apparent benefits of omega-3, urges people not to get 'carried away.' Dr. Hooper says she believes the fashion for omega-3 betrays our herd-instinct: how, as a group, we periodically get overexcited about certain foodstuffs. There always seems to be some 'new food panacea' to our problems, she says. Another doctor, Michael Fitzpatrick, says . . . that today there is almost a 'cult of omega-3'" (O'Neill, B. [2010, March 1]. The cult of omega-3. *BBC News Magazine*. http://news.bbc.co.uk/1/hi/magazine/8543172.stm). The positive effect of eating fish during pregnancy is undeniable; whether it's the omega-3 fatty acids that are causing the effect remains to be definitively proven.

39. Survey of mercury in fish oil supplements. (n.d.). Food Standards Agency. http://webarchive.nationalarchives.gov.uk/20101210122850/http://www.food.gov.uk/news/pressreleases/2005/oct/fishrelatedsurveyspub.

40. Cod liver oil does contain high levels of vitamin A, and vitamin A in sufficiently large quantities can cause birth defects. But you would need to be swallowing ten 100 g capsules a day before reaching the threshold at which problems begin to occur, according to a study of 22,748 pregnant women (Rothman, K. J., Moore, L. L., Singer, M. R., Nguyen, U. S. D., Mannino, S., & Milunsky, A. [1995]. Teratogenicity of high vitamin A intake. *New England Journal of Medicine, 333* [21], 1369–1373. http://content.nejm.org/cgi/content/full/333/21/1369). And cod liver oil is actually the outlier—other fish and plant oils contain only trace amounts of vitamin A, according to the USDA National Nutrient Database (United States Department of Agriculture. [Revised 2016, May]. Fats and oils food group. National Nutrient Database for Standard Reference, Release 28. https://ndb.nal.usda.gov/ndb/search/list?SYNCHRONIZER_TOKEN=0fb9d97b-49d8-4f83-8a67-2b99ef1a35a3&SYNCHRONIZER_=%2Fndb%2Fsearch%2Flist&qt=&ds=Standard+Reference&qlookup=&fgcd=Fats+and+Oils&manu=). For vegetarian women, the options aren't currently obvious. Alpha-linolenic acid (ALA), which is found in plant foods such as flaxseed, walnuts, and canola oil, is partially converted by the body into EPA and DHA, the two biologically important omega-3 acids. Unfortunately, according to a recent review, trying to obtain sufficient omega-3 fatty acids from plant-based oils would require ingestion of too many fat calories. Therefore, "in order to make up the omega-3 fatty acid deficit in the diet, pregnant women are left with essentially 2 choices: fish oil supplements supplying EPA and DHA, or algae-derived DHA. Meaningful vegetarian sources of DHA are essentially limited to algae-derived DHA from Martek Biosciences (Columbia, MD) . . . [but] the oils do not contain any EPA and data demonstrating the benefits in pregnancy of DHA alone are lacking" (Greenberg, J. A., Bell, S. J., & Van Ausdal, W. [2008]. Omega-3 fatty acid supplementation during pregnancy. *Reviews in Obstetrics and Gynecology, 1* [4], 162. www.ncbi.nlm.nih.gov/pmc/articles/pmc2621042/). Note: there may still be benefit from taking DHA supplements despite the fact that the IQ benefits of DHA alone are unproven, since one study has suggested that visual acuity is improved in infants whose mothers take DHA supplements (Innis, S. M., & Friesen, R. W. [2008]. Essential n−3 fatty acids in pregnant women and early visual acuity maturation in term infants. The *American Journal of Clinical Nutrition, 87* [3], 548–557. http://ajcn.nutrition.org/content/87/3/548.full). There is also preliminary evidence that omega-3 supplements could subtly improve pregnancy outcomes (Szajewska, H., Horvath, A., & Koletzko, B. [2006]. Effect of n−3 long-chain polyunsaturated fatty acid supplementation of women with low-risk pregnancies on pregnancy outcomes and growth measures at birth: a meta-analysis of randomized controlled trials. The *American Journal of Clinical Nutrition, 83* [6], 1337–1344. http://ajcn.nutrition.org/content/83/6/1337.full; Horvath, A., Koletzko, B., & Szajewska, H. [2007]. Effect of supplementation of women in high-risk pregnancies with long-chain polyunsaturated

fatty acids on pregnancy outcomes and growth measures at birth: a meta-analysis of randomized controlled trials. *British Journal of Nutrition, 98* [02], 253–259. http://journals. cambridge.org/action/display Abstract?fromPage=online&aid=1208476; Olsen, S. F., Secher, N. J., Tabor, A., Weber, T., Walker, J. J., & Gluud, C. [2000]. Randomised clinical trials of fish oil supplementation in high risk pregnancies. *BJOG: An International Journal of Obstetrics & Gynaecology, 107* [3], 382–395. www.ncbi.nlm.nih.gov/pubmed/10740336), but the data are not yet sufficiently robust to reach firm conclusions (Makrides, M., Duley, L., & Olsen, S. F. [2006]. Marine oil, and other prostaglandin precursor, supplementation for pregnancy uncomplicated by preeclampsia or intrauterine growth restriction. *Cochrane Database of Systematic Reviews, 3.* http://onlinelibrary.wiley.com/doi/10.1002/14651858.CD003402. pub2/full).

41. Gould, J. F., Smithers, L. G., & Makrides, M. (2013). The effect of maternal omega-3 (n–3) LCPUFA supplementation during pregnancy on early childhood cognitive and visual development: a systematic review and meta-analysis of randomized controlled trials. *The American Journal of Clinical Nutrition, 97* (3), 531–544. http://ajcn.nutrition.org/content/97/3/531.long.

42. Kris-Etherton, P. M., Innis, S., & Ammerican, D. A. (2007). Position of the American Dietetic Association and Dietitians of Canada: dietary fatty acids. *Journal of the American Dietetic Association, 107* (9), 1599–1611. http://europepmc.org/abstract/MED/17936958.

43. Murkoff, H., & Mazel, S. (2008). *What to expect when you're expecting.* (4th ed). New York: Workman Publishing.

44. Gibbons, Gavin. (2008). Shrimp, canned tuna lead NFIs Top 10 Most Popular list. AboutSeafood.com. https://www.aboutseafood.com/press_release/shrimp-canned-tuna-lead-nfis-top-10-most-popular-list/.

The top ten fish species represent over 80% of the market for seafood. In addition, I've also thrown in any other types of fish that are very commonly accessible. Walmart is the largest national grocery store chain. In addition to the top 10, Walmart also sells mackerel, squid, and sardines in its online store.

45. Threat score is 6% (probability of having a blood mercury level of 5.8 parts per billion, the level linked to cognitive impairment) x 1,000 (impact: minor impairment) x 1 (certainty: well proven) = 6.

46. Benefit score is 99.9% (probability you eat less than 8 servings of oily fish per week) x 100 (impact: statistically detectable improvement) x 1/10 (certainty: preliminary) = 9.999.

47. Gasoline. (n.d.). Wikipedia. http://en.wikipedia.org/wiki/Gasoline.

Lead increased the "octane rating" of gasoline, i.e., enabled it to be compressed more without combusting.

48. Pencil. (n.d.). Wikipedia. http://en.wikipedia.org/wiki/Pencil.

49. Centers for Disease Control and Prevention. (Last reviewed 2015, September 17). About the National Health and Nutrition Examination Survey. National Center for Health Statistics. www.cdc.gov/nchs/nhanes/about_nhanes.htm.

50. Centers for Disease Control and Prevention. (2005). Blood lead levels—United States, 1999-2002. *Morbidity and Mortality Weekly Report, 54* (20), 513. www.cdc.gov/mmwr/preview/mmwrhtml/mm5420a5.htm.

51. Goyer, R. A. (1990). Transplacental transport of lead. *Environmental Health Perspectives, 89*, 101. www.ncbi.nlm.nih.gov/pmc/articles/PMC1567784/pdf/envhper00422-0101.pdf.

52. Bellinger, D., Leviton, A. N. H. L., Needleman, H. L., Waternaux, C., & Rabinowitz, M. (1986). Low-level lead exposure and infant development in the first year. *Neurobehavioral Toxicology and Teratology, 8* (2), 151–161. https://www.researchgate.net/profile/

David_Bellinger/publication/20732005_Low-level_lead_exposure_and_infant_development_in_the_first_year/links/0c96051bf67580d21c000000.pdf.

53. US Department of Health and Human Services (2012, June). NTP monograph: health effects of low-level lead. National Toxicology Program. http://ntp.niehs.nih.gov/ntp/ohat/lead/final/monographhealtheffectslowlevellead_newissn_508.pdf.

54. Schwartz, J. (1994). Low-level lead exposure and children's IQ: a meta-analysis and search for a threshold. *Environmental Research, 65* (1), 42–55. www.rachel.org/files/document/Low-Level_Lead_Exposure_and_Childrens_IQ_A_Met.pdf.

55. Miranda, M. L., Kim, D., Galeano, M. A. O., Paul, C. J., Hull, A. P., & Morgan, S. P. (2007). The relationship between early childhood blood lead levels and performance on end-of-grade tests. *Environmental Health Perspectives, 115* (8), 1242–1247. www.ncbi.nlm.nih.gov/pmc/articles/PMC1940087/pdf/ehp0115-001242.pdf.

56. Miranda, M. L., Kim, D., Reiter, J., Overstreet Galeano, M. A., & Maxson, P. (2009). Environmental contributors to the achievement gap. *Neurotoxicology, 30* (6), 1019–1024. www.ncbi.nlm.nih.gov/pmc/articles/PMC2789840/.

57. Needleman, H. L., & Landrigan, P. J. (2004). What level of lead in blood is toxic for a child? *American Journal of Public Health, 94* (1), 8–9. www.cdc.gov/NCEH/lead/ACCLPP/supplementalMar04/AJPHlessthantenfinal.pdf

58. Centers for Disease Control and Prevention. (Last updated 2016, December 27). Biomonitoring summary: lead. National Biomonitoring Program. www.cdc.gov/biomonitoring/Lead_BiomonitoringSummary.html.

59. Borja-Aburto, V. H., Hertz-Picciotto, I., Lopez, M. R., Farias, P., Rios, C., & Blanco, J. (1999). Blood lead levels measured prospectively and risk of spontaneous abortion. *American Journal of Epidemiology, 150* (6), 590–597. http://aje.oxfordjournals.org/content/150/6/590.full.pdf.

    According to this study, the odds ratios for miscarriage for 5–9 and 10–14 μg/dL blood lead levels were 2.3 and 5.4, respectively, vs. lead levels below 5 μg/dL. To calculate the baseline incidence of miscarriage in the population: according to National Vital Statistics Reports, in 2004 there were 1,056,000 fetal losses of all gestations (Estimated pregnancy rates by outcome for the United States, 1990-2004. [2008]. US Department of Health & Human Services and Centers for Disease Control and Prevention National Center for Health Statistics. http://stacks.cdc.gov/objectView!getDataStreamContent.action?pid=cdc:13317&dsid=DS1&mimeType=application/pdf) and 25,655 fetal deaths >20 weeks, which implies 1,030,345 miscarriages <20 weeks. There were 6,390,000 pregnancies minus 1,222,000 induced abortions, or 5,168,000 wanted pregnancies (MacDorman, M. F., Munson, M. L., & Kirmeyer, S. [2007]. Fetal and perinatal mortality, United States, 2004. *National Vital Statistics Reports, 56* [3]. https://pdfs.semanticscholar.org/02ec/9107597bf5cf7207e2dcf3aa7db8c238c1e3.pdf), implying a miscarriage rate of 19.9%. So applying the appropriate conversion formula (Higgins, J. P. T., & Green, S. [eds.]. [2011, March]. Computing absolute risk reduction or NNT from an odds ratio [OR]. *Cochrane Handbook for Systematic Reviews of Interventions* 12.5.4.3. http://handbook.cochrane.org/chapter_12/12_5_4_3_computing_absolute_risk_reduction_or_nnt_from_an_odds.htm), this equates to absolute increases in miscarriage of 16.5% and 37.4% attributable to these levels of lead exposure.

60. Wedeen, R., Goldman, R., Headapohl, D., Hipkins, K., Hu, H., & Kosnett, M. (2007). Medical management guidelines for lead-exposed adults. The Association of Occupational and Environmental Clinics. www.aoec.org/documents/positions/mmg_final.pdf.

61. Ettinger, A. S., Hu, H., & Hernandez-Avila, M. (2007). Dietary calcium supplementation to lower blood lead levels in pregnancy and lactation. *The Journal of Nutritional Biochemistry, 18* (3), 172–178. www.ncbi.nlm.nih.gov/pmc/articles/PMC2566736/pdf/nihms18750.pdf.

62. The American Congress of Obstetricians and Gynecologists. (2012, August). Committee opinion 533: lead screening during pregnancy and lactation. *Obstetrics and Gynecology, 2012* (120), 416–420. www.acog.org/Resources_And_Publications/Committee_Opinions/ Committee_on_Obstetric_Practice/Lead_Screening_During_Pregnancy_and_Lactation.

63. Joelving, F. (2012, July 23). OB-GYNs say no to routine lead testing in pregnancy. Reuters. com. www.reuters.com/article/2012/07/23/us-mothers-lead-idUSBRE86M1B920120723.

64. Wedeen et al., Medical management guidelines for lead-exposed adults.

65. Ettinger et al., Dietary calcium supplementation to lower blood lead levels in pregnancy and lactation.

66. Lamadrid-Figueroa, H., Téllez-Rojo, M. M., Mercado-García, A., Hu, H., Hernández-Avila, M., Ettinger, A. S., & Schwartz, J. D. (2008). Effect of calcium supplementation on blood lead levels in pregnancy: a randomized placebo-controlled trial. *Environmental Health Perspectives, 117* (1), 26–31. http://dash.harvard.edu/bitstream/handle/1/5978622/2627861. pdf?sequence=1.

67. Checking for sources of lead is a job best left to the professionals, since it turns out home testing kits aren't very accurate. You can contact the National Lead Information Center (NLIC) at (800) 424-5323 (424-LEAD) or visit the NLIC website to find a qualified professional.

68. Schaller, K. E., & Arreola, P. (1999). Imported mini-blinds: a potential source of lead exposure for young children. *Journal of Environmental Health, 61* (10). www.questia.com/ googleScholar.qst?docId=5002319855.

69. Threat score: 1/300 * 37% (probability: 1/300 is the chance of having a blood lead level above 10 micrograms per deciliter times the probability of miscarriage at that level based on the study in Mexico described in a previous footnote) x 100,000 (impact: death) x 1/10 (certainty: preliminary) = 12.5. Since calcium supplements can only reduce lead levels by 15%, the threat score for controllable lead exposure is 12.5*15% = 1.87, for uncontrollable lead exposure is 12.5*85% = 10.6 + 1/300 (probability of having a blood lead level above 10 micrograms per deciliter) * 100 (impact: statistically detectable impairment—lowered IQ) x 1 (certainty: well proven) = 0.3. Total: 12.5 + 0.3 = 12.8.

70. As part of the wider ban on persistent organic pollutants, discussed previously.

71. Berkowitz, G. S., Wetmur, J. G., Birman-Deych, E., Obel, J., Lapinski, R. H., Godbold, J. H., Holzman, I. R., & Wolff, M. S. (2004). *In utero* pesticide exposure, maternal paraoxonase activity, and head circumference. *Environmental Health Perspectives, 112* (3), 388. www. ncbi.nlm.nih.gov/pmc/articles/PMC1241872/pdf/ehp0112-000388.pdf.

72. Rauh, V. A., Garfinkel, R., Perera, F. P., Andrews, H. F., Hoepner, L., Barr, D. B., Whitehead, R., Tang, D., & Whyatt, R. W. (2006). Impact of prenatal chlorpyrifos exposure on neurodevelopment in the first 3 years of life among inner-city children. *Pediatrics, 118* (6), e1845–e1859. www.ncbi.nlm.nih.gov/pmc/articles/PMC3390915/.

73. Rauh, V., Arunajadai, S., Horton, M., Perera, F., Hoepner, L., Barr, D. B., & Whyatt, R. (2011). Seven-year neurodevelopmental scores and prenatal exposure to chlorpyrifos, a common agricultural pesticide. *Environmental Health Perspectives, 119* (8), 1196. http:// ehp03.niehs.nih.gov/article/info:doi/10.1289/ehp.1003160.

74. Engel, S. M., Wetmur, J., Chen, J., Zhu, C., Boyd Barr, D., Canfield, R. L., & Wolff, M. S. (2011). Prenatal exposure to organophosphates, paraoxonase 1, and cognitive development in childhood. *Environmental Health Perspectives, 119* (8), 1182–1188. https://www.ncbi. nlm.nih.gov/pmc/articles/PMC3237356/.

75. Rauh, V., et al., Seven-year neurodevelopmental scores and prenatal exposure to chlorpyrifos, a common agricultural pesticide.

One point that may have occurred to you: if a mother is exposed to pesticides during pregnancy, her child might also be exposed to those same pesticides after birth and throughout childhood from living in the same household. So how do we know that the exposure during pregnancy actually matters and isn't just a red herring? Two different studies have examined that very question (Marks, A. R., Harley, K., Bradman, A., Kogut, K., Barr, D. B., Johnson, C., Calderon, N., & Eskenazi, B. [2010]. Organophosphate pesticide exposure and attention in young Mexican-American children. *Environmental Health Perspectives, 118* [12], 1768–1774. www.ncbi.nlm.nih.gov/pmc/articles/PMC3002198/ pdf/ehp-118-1768.pdf; Eskenazi, B., Marks, A. R., Bradman, A., Harley, K., Barr, D. B., Johnson, C., Johnson, C., Morga, N., & Jewell, N. P. [2007]. Organophosphate pesticide exposure and neurodevelopment in young Mexican-American children. *Environmental Health Perspectives, 115* [5], 792–798. www.ncbi.nlm.nih.gov/pmc/articles/PMC1867968/ pdf/ehp0115-000792.pdf), and both concluded that it's the prenatal exposure to the pesticides that seems to count by far the most. And another study looking at the link between use of a professional pest-control service and childhood leukemia found that the highest risk to the child was from exposure during pregnancy (Ma, X., Buffler, P. A., Gunier, R. B., Dahl, G., Smith, M. T., Reinier, K., & Reynolds, P. [2002]. Critical windows of exposure to household pesticides and risk of childhood leukemia. *Environmental Health Perspectives, 110* [9], 955. www.ncbi.nlm.nih.gov/pmc/articles/PMC1240997/ pdf/ehp0110-000955.pdf). There are at least two possible explanations: one is that in the womb, the brain is growing at such a rapid pace that it may be particularly vulnerable to disruption; the second is that in early development, fetuses have very low levels of the enzymes used to break down these pesticides, so they are particularly vulnerable to being flooded with them.

76. In case you think I oversimplify, organophosphates aren't the only type of pesticide that can do harm to a fetus, but I've concluded based on my research that they are by far the most important. If you're insatiably curious, you can read about the other kinds of pesticides in Appendix V.

77. Klein, S. (2010, May 17). Study: ADHD linked to pesticide exposure. CNN.com. http:// edition.cnn.com/2010/HEALTH/05/17/pesticides.adhd/index.html, citing: United States Department of Agriculture. (2009, December). Pesticide data program: annual summary, calendar year 2008. Agricultural Marketing Service. https://www.ams.usda.gov/sites/ default/files/media/2008%20PDP%20Annual%20Summary.pdf.

78. Organophosphate pesticides break down in the body into 6 different kinds of chemicals, otherwise known as DAP metabolites. These metabolites can be converted into a common unit, nanomoles per liter, and added up to get a total. Based on data from NHANES, which includes a urine test for pesticides (Barr, D. B., Wong, L. Y., Bravo, R., Weerasekera, G., Odetokun, M., Restrepo, P., Kim, D. G., Fernandez, C., Whitehead Jr, R. D., Perez, J., Gallegos, M., Williams, B. L., & Needham, L. L. [2011]. Urinary concentrations of dialkylphosphate metabolites of organophosphorus pesticides: national health and nutrition examination survey 1999–2004. *International Journal of Environmental Research and Public Health, 2011* [8], 3063–3098. www.ncbi.nlm.nih.gov/pmc/articles/ PMC3166728/pdf/ijerph-08-03063.pdf), the average American female has about 13 units of DAP metabolites in her urine; the 90th percentile, 306 units, or the 95th percentile, 492 units (conversion factors utilized: DMP 0.126 mg/nmol; DMTP 0.142 mg/nmol; DMDTP 0.158 mg/nmol; DEP 0.154 mg/nmol; DETP 0.170 mg/nmol; DEDTP 0.186 mg/nmol (Arcury, T. A., Grzywacz, J. G., Davis, S. W., Barr, D. B., & Quandt, S. A. [2006]. Organophosphorus pesticide urinary metabolite levels of children in farmworker households in eastern North Carolina. *American Journal of Industrial Medicine, 49* [9], 751–760. http://onlinelibrary.wiley.com/doi/10.1002/ajim.20354/full). These are figures published in 2011 based on data from 2003–2004, a few years after the ban on residential

organophosphates was put in place. A study from the University of California–Berkeley measured women's DAP levels during pregnancy and then tested their children's IQ at 7 years of age. They found "a 7 IQ point-difference between children in the highest quintile of prenatal DAP levels and those in the lowest quintile" (Bouchard, M. F., Chevrier, J., Harley, K. G., Kogut, K., Vedar, M., Calderon, N., Trujillo, C., Johnson, C., Bradman, A., Barr, D. B., & Eskenazi, B. [2011, August]. Prenatal exposure to organophosphate pesticides and IQ in 7-year-old children. *Environmental Health Perspectives, 119* [8], 1189–1195. https://www.ncbi.nlm.nih.gov/pmc/articles/PMC3237357/). The highest quintile had a median level of 508 units, which is similar to the 492 above.

79. Food does appear to be the primary source of exposure. One group of researchers studied a group of pregnant Latina women in the Salinas Valley, a large agricultural region of California where thousands of tons of pesticides are sprayed each year. They created an elaborate model of potential exposure routes and compared the exposure of the Latina population with the average American population from NHANES. They concluded that "in both populations diet is the common and dominant exposure pathway" (McKone, T. E., Castorina, R., Harnly, M. E., Kuwabara, Y., Eskenazi, B., & Bradman, A. [2007]. Merging models and biomonitoring data to characterize sources and pathways of human exposure to organophosphorus pesticides in the Salinas Valley of California. *Environmental Science & Technology, 41* [9], 3233–3240. http://escholarship.org/uc/item/65f8n1th;jsessionid=B20C481862C98AEC35EECBF72CAEA029). Another study similarly stated: "Our findings suggest that most maternal pesticide exposure probably occurs through the diet, as is the case for the general U.S. population" (Bouchard, M. F., et al., Prenatal exposure to organophosphate pesticides and IQ in 7-year-old children).

That's not to say that it's healthy to live near fields being sprayed—quite the contrary. If a crop is sprayed with pesticides within two miles of your house between your third and eighth week of pregnancy, you may have up to double the chance of a fetal death due to birth defects (Bell, E. M., Hertz-Picciotto, I., & Beaumont, J. J. [2001]. A case-control study of pesticides and fetal death due to congenital anomalies. *Epidemiology, 12* [2], 148–156. http://journals.lww.com/epidem/Abstract/2001/03000/A_Case_Control_Study_of_Pesticides_and_Fetal_Death.5.aspx). Keep in mind such defects are very rare, so even with double the odds, you still are very unlikely to lose the baby; on the other hand, the pesticides nearby clearly have some effect. And the Latina women in the above study all had elevated levels of DAP metabolites vs. the average American group. But the majority of their exposure still came from elsewhere—namely, food.

80. US Department of Agriculture. (2015, September). The Pesticide Data Program: Helping monitor the safety of America's food supply. Agricultural Marketing Service. https://www.ams.usda.gov/sites/default/files/media/PDP%20factsheet.pdf.

81. All of the pesticides have been converted to a single scale of equivalence based on their various potency levels vs. a single reference pesticide, methamidophos; summaries of PDP data downloaded from www.whatsonmyfood.org.

82. The Environmental Working Group produces a list called the "Dirty Dozen" that doesn't completely match the findings here, although there is plenty of overlap. That's because their ranking is a combined figure based on measuring contamination in 6 different ways, 5 of which are about the number of pesticides (percent of samples tested with detectable pesticides, percent of samples with two or more pesticides, average number of pesticides found on a single sample, maximum number of pesticides found on a single sample, and total number of pesticides found on the commodity) and only one of which is about the total amount of pesticides (average amount in parts per million of all pesticides found), which is the statistic shown above (Frequently asked questions about produce & pesticides. [n.d.]. Environmental Working Group. https://www.ewg.org/foodnews/faq.php#.WipB1rbMzBJ).

83. Lu, C., Toepel, K., Irish, R., Fenske, R. A., Barr, D. B., & Bravo, R. (2006). Organic diets significantly lower children's dietary exposure to organophosphorus pesticides. *Environmental Health Perspectives, 114* (2), 260. www.ncbi.nlm.nih.gov/pmc/articles/PMC1367841/pdf/ehp0114-000260.pdf.

84. Lairon, D. (2010). Nutritional quality and safety of organic food: a review. *Agronomy for sustainable development, 30* (1), 33–41. http://hal.archives-ouvertes.fr/docs/00/88/65/13/PDF/hal-00886513.pdf.

85. Sagoo, S. K., Little, C. L., & Mitchell, R. T. (2001). The microbiological examination of ready-to-eat organic vegetables from retail establishments in the United Kingdom. *Letters in Applied Microbiology, 33* (6), 434–439. http://onlinelibrary.wiley.com/doi/10.1046/j.1472-765X.2001.01026.x/full.

86. Let's say on a typical day, you eat a couple of servings of fruit and a couple of servings of vegetables. As of this writing, a Granny Smith apple costs $0.79 while an organic one is $1.19 on the Stop&Shop website. Ordinary frozen green beans cost $1.67 for a 16-oz bag, while organic cost $2.69. So if we round up and say $2.00 a day extra to go organic and multiply that figure by 280 days (40 weeks) of being pregnant, that works out to $560.

87. Threat score: 5% (probability, based on my conclusion that almost 5% of American women have exposure levels high enough to dock 7 points off the IQ of their offspring) x 100 (impact: statistically detectable impairment) x 1 (certainty: well proven) = 5.

88. Brucker-Davis, F., Wagner-Mahler, K., Delattre, I., Ducot, B., Ferrari, P., Bongain, A., Kurzenne, J. Y., Mas, J. C., Fénichel, P, & Cryptorchidism Study Group from Nice Area. (2008). Cryptorchidism at birth in Nice area (France) is associated with higher prenatal exposure to PCBs and DDE, as assessed by colostrum concentrations. *Human Reproduction, 23* (8), 1708–1718. http://humrep.oxfordjournals.org/content/23/8/1708.full.

89. Environmental Working Group. (2004). Exposures add up—survey results. Environmental Working Group's Skin Deep Cosmetics Database. http://www.ewg.org/skindeep/2004/06/15/exposures-add-up-survey-results/#.Wc4FUcIm7jY.

90. Lorente, C., Cordier, S., Bergeret, A., De Walle, H. E. K., Goujard, J., Aymé, S., Knill-Jones, R., Calzolari, E., & Bianchi, F. (2000). Maternal occupational risk factors for oral clefts. *Scandinavian Journal of Work, Environment & Health, 26* (2), 137–145. https://www.ncbi.nlm.nih.gov/pubmed/10817379.

91. Nguyen, R. H., Wilcox, A. J., Moen, B. E., McConnaughey, D. R., & Lie, R. T. (2007). Parent's occupation and isolated orofacial clefts in Norway: a population-based case-control study. *Annals of Epidemiology, 17* (10), 763–771. www.sciencedirect.com/science/article/pii/S1047279707002153.

92. Organization of Teratology Information Specialists. (2016, December). Hair treatments and pregnancy. MotherToBaby. www.mothertobaby.org/files/hairtreatments.pdf.

93. Chua-Gocheco, A., Bozzo, P., & Einarson, A. (2008). Safety of hair products during pregnancy: personal use and occupational exposure. *Canadian Family Physician, 54* (10), 1386–1388. http://www.cfp.ca/content/54/10/1386.short.

94. Calafat, A. M., Wong, L. Y., Ye, X., Reidy, J. A., & Needham, L. L. (2008). Concentrations of the sunscreen agent benzophenone-3 in residents of the United States: National Health and Nutrition Examination Survey 2003-2004. *Environmental Health Perspectives, 116* (7), 893–897. www.ncbi.nlm.nih.gov/pmc/articles/PMC2453157/pdf/ehp0116-000893.pdf.

95. Why does this chemical seem to affect only baby girls and not boys? The hypothesis is that oxybenzone is a hormone disruptor, but how this works is still not clear. (Wolff, M. S., Engel, S. M., Berkowitz, G. S., Ye, X., Silva, M. J., Zhu, C., Wetmur, J., & Calafat, A. M. [2008]. Prenatal phenol and phthalate exposures and birth outcomes. *Environmental Health Perspectives, 116* [8], 1092–1097. www.ncbi.nlm.nih.gov/pmc/articles/PMC2516577/pdf/ehp0116-001092.pdf.)

96. EWG's 11th annual guide to sunscreens. (n.d.). Environmental Working Group. http://www.ewg.org/sunscreen/#.WcnPj3aGPIU.

97. Threat score is 1 (if you choose to use hair dye) x 100 (impact: statistically detectable impairment) x 1/1,000 (certainty: unproven) = 0.1.

98. Threat score is 1/2 (just girls) x 1/3 (top third) (probability, based on the CDC suggestion that the top tercile of BP3 exposure is associated with lower birth weight among female infants) x 100 (impact: statistically detectable impairment) x 1/100 (certainty: ambiguous) = 0.167.

99. Threat score is 1 (probability you're exposed to chemicals in personal care products, unless you're Amish and use nothing but unadulterated bar soap) x 100 (impact: statistically detectable impairment) x 1/1,000 (certainty: unproven) = 0.1.

100. Herz, R. (2007). *The scent of desire: discovering our enigmatic sense of smell.* New York: William Morrow.

101. De Vader, C. (2010). Fragrance in the workplace: what managers need to know. *Journal of Management and Marketing Research*, 1–17. http://www.national-toxic-encephalopathy-foundation.org/wp-content/uploads/2012/01/fragInworkplace1.pdf.

102. Sarantis, H., Naidenko, O. V., Gray, S., Houlihan, J., & Malkan, M. (2010). Not so sexy: the health risks of secret chemicals in fragrance. Campaign for Safe Cosmetics and Environmental Working Group. https://www.ewg.org/sites/default/files/report/SafeCosmetics_FragranceRpt.pdf.

103. The EWG perfume report makes a number of scary claims about the various chemicals in some perfumes, including hormone disruptors. The problem is that the testing of these chemicals is still in the early stages. For example, I followed one of their citations to a report by the Endocrine Society (Diamanti-Kandarakis, E., Bourguignon, J. P., Giudice, L. C., Hauser, R., Prins, G. S., Soto, A. M., Zoeller, T., & Gore, A. C. [2009]. Endocrine-disrupting chemicals: an endocrine society scientific statement. *Endocrine Reviews, 30* [4], 293–342. http://edrv.endojournals.org/content/30/4/293.full.pdf+html), which made the following claim: "There are several properties of endocrine-disrupting chemicals that have caused controversy. First, even infinitesimally low levels of exposure—indeed, any level of exposure at all—may cause endocrine or reproductive abnormalities, particularly if exposure occurs during a critical developmental window." This sounds bad, but the citation for this statement is a study involving turtles, not humans. I'm not saying that what applies to turtles will never apply to humans; it very well might. I'm just making the point that thus far, very few studies of these chemicals have been done on humans.

104. Sheehan, D. M., Willingham, E., Gaylor, D., Bergeron, J. M., & Crews, D. (1999). No threshold dose for estradiol-induced sex reversal of turtle embryos: how little is too much? *Environmental Health Perspectives, 107* (2), 155. www.ncbi.nlm.nih.gov/pmc/articles/PMC1566346/pdf/envhper00507-0101.pdf.

105. Schlumpf, M., Schmid, P., Durrer, S., Conscience, M., Maerkel, K., Henseler, M., Gruetter, M., Herzog, I., Reolon, S., Ceccatelli, R., Faass, O., Stutz, E., Jarry, H., Wuttke, W., & Lichtensteiger, W. (2004). Endocrine activity and developmental toxicity of cosmetic UV filters—an update. *Toxicology, 205* (1), 113–122. http://www.sciencedirect.com/science/article/pii/S0300483X04003713.

106. Threat score is 1 (probability you're exposed to perfume in your daily life) x 100 (impact: statistically detectable impairment) x 1/1,000 (certainty: unproven) = 0.1.

107. Dottinga, R. (2009, November 18). Could plastics feminize boys' play? ABCNews.com. http://abcnews.go.com/Health/Healthday/plastics-chemicals-feminize-boys-play/story?id=9109200.

108. Swan, S. H., Main, K. M., Liu, F., Stewart, S. L., Kruse, R. L., Calafat, A. M., Mao, C., Redmon, J. B., Ternand, C., Sullivan, S., Teague, J. L., & the Study for Future Families

Research Team. (2005). Decrease in anogenital distance among male infants with prenatal phthalate exposure. *Environmental Health Perspectives, 113* (8), 1056. https://www.ncbi.nlm.nih.gov/pmc/articles/PMC1280349/.

109. Ibid.

110. Swan, S. (2006, January 9). Parents needn't wait for legislation to shield kids from toxins in products. SFGate.com. www.sfgate.com/cgi-bin/article.cgi?f=/c/a/2006/01/09/EDGMKGJGL61.DTL&hw=Swan&sn=009&sc=152.

111. Study links plastics to small genitals. (2005, May 27). FoxNews.com. www.foxnews.com/story/0,2933,157882,00.html.

112. Sample, I. (2005, May 27). Chemicals in plastics harming unborn boys: scientists say chemicals have gender bending effect. *The Guardian.* www.guardian.co.uk/uk/2005/may/27/health.gender.

113. The original Swan study hadn't actually linked phthalates to any negative outcomes in humans; it had simply raised the hypothesis that there could be a link and encouraged further study. In the words of a critique published by STATS, a nonprofit focused on uncovering the use and abuse of science and statistics in the media, "the media was in part led astray by Dr. Shanna Swan, the lead author of the study. She has publicly taken the position that the correlation between phthalate exposure in utero and anogenital index proves that phthalates are causing reproductive harm, even though the study found neither actual genital defects nor fertility problems" (Goldin, R. [2006, January 30]. Toy tantrums—the debate over the safety of phthalates. STATS, George Mason University). Risks of developmental effects have been extrapolated based on animal studies, but these effects have not yet been demonstrated in humans.

114. Kamrin, M. A. (2009). Phthalate risks, phthalate regulation, and public health: a review. *Journal of Toxicology and Environmental Health, Part B, 12* (2), 157–174. www.tandfonline.com/doi/pdf/10.1080/10937400902729226.

115. Witorsch, R. J., & Thomas, J. A. (2010). Personal care products and endocrine disruption: a critical review of the literature. *Critical Reviews in Toxicology, 40* (S3), 1–30. http://www.tandfonline.com/doi/abs/10.3109/10408444.2010.515563.

116. Overview of phthalates toxicity. (2002, April 12). United States Consumer Product Safety Commission. Bethesda, MD. https://www.cpsc.gov/s3fs-public/phthalover.pdf. Dibutyl Phthalate (DBP) posed "some risk of developmental effects in the offspring of some highly exposed women of reproductive age," and Bis(2-ethylhexyl)phthalate (DEHP) posed "some risk to males exposed during pregnancy." There was serious concern about the phthalate exposure of critically ill male infants undergoing certain medical treatments, but this is a book about pregnancy, so we won't cover that here.

117. Zhang, Y., Lin, L., Cao, Y., Chen, B., Zheng, L., & Ge, R. S. (2009). Phthalate levels and low birth weight: a nested case-control study of Chinese newborns. *The Journal of Pediatrics, 155* (4), 500–504. http://download.journals.elsevierhealth.com/pdfs/journals/0022-3476/PIIS0022347609003679.pdf.

According to this study, infants with the highest quartile of phthalate exposure had a maximum odds ratio of 4.67 for having low birth weight. The baseline incidence of LBW in the population as of 2010 was 8.15% according to the CDC (Martin, J. A., Hamilton, B. E., Ventura, S. J., Osterman, M. J., Wilson, E.C., & Mathews, T. J. [2012, August 28]. Births: final data for 2010. *National Vital Statistics Report 61* [1], 1–90. www.cdc.gov/nchs/data/nvsr/nvsr61/nvsr61_01.pdf), so applying the appropriate conversion formula (Higgins, J. P. T., et al., Computing absolute risk reduction or NNT from an odds ratio [OR]), that equates to a 21% absolute increase in LBW attributable to phthalate exposure for the top quartile exposed, or an absolute increase of 5.3% for the full population.

118. Latini, G., De Felice, C., Presta, G., Del Vecchio, A., Paris, I., Ruggieri, F., & Mazzeo, P. (2003). In utero exposure to di-(2-ethylhexyl) phthalate and duration of human pregnancy. *Environmental Health Perspectives, 111* (14), 1783. https://www.ncbi.nlm.nih.gov/pmc/articles/PMC1241724/.

119. Whyatt, R. M., Adibi, J. J., Calafat, A. M., Camann, D. E., Rauh, V., Bhat, H. K., Perera, F. P., Andrews, H., Just, A. C., Hoepner, L., Tang, D., & Hauser, R. (2009). Prenatal di(2-ethylhexyl) phthalate exposure and length of gestation among an inner-city cohort. *Pediatrics, 124* (6), e1213–e1220. http://pediatrics.aappublications.org/content/124/6/e1213.short.

120. Meeker, J. D., Hu, H., Cantonwine, D. E., Lamadrid-Figueroa, H., Calafat, A. M., Loch-Caruso, R., Hernandez-Avila, M., Loch-Caruso, R., & Téllez-Rojo, M. M. (2009). Urinary phthalate metabolites in relation to preterm birth in Mexico City. *Environmental Health Perspectives, 110* (10), 1587–1592. www.ncbi.nlm.nih.gov/pmc/articles/PMC2790514/pdf/ehp-117-1587.pdf.

121. Wigle, D. T., Arbuckle, T. E., Turner, M. C., Berube, A., Yang, Q., Liu, S., & Krewski, D. (2008). Epidemiologic evidence of relationships between reproductive and child health outcomes and environmental chemical contaminants. *Journal of Toxicology and Environmental Health, Part B, 11* (5–6), 373–517. www.tandfonline.com/doi/pdf/10.1080/10937400801921320.

122. US Centers for Disease Control and Prevention. (2009). Fourth national report on human exposure to environmental chemicals. US Department of Health and Human Services. www.cdc.gov/exposurereport/pdf/FourthReport.pdf.

123. NTP-CERHR. (2003). NTP-CERHR monograph on the potential human reproductive and developmental effects of di-*n*-butyl phthalate (DBP). 4: i-III90. US Department of Health and Human Services. http://ntp.niehs.nih.gov/ntp/ohat/phthalates/dbp/dbp_monograph_final.pdf.

124. McDonald, L. (2007). *The toxic sandbox: the truth about environmental toxins and our children's health.* New York: Perigree Books.

125. Clark, K., Cousins, I. T., & Mackay, D. (2003). Assessment of critical exposure pathways. In *Series anthropogenic compounds.* Berlin, Heidelberg: Springer, 227–262. www.springer-link.com/content/23488863232214q9/fulltext.pdf.

126. Fromme, H., Gruber, L., Schlummer, M., Wolz, G., Böhmer, S., Angerer, J., Mayer, R., Liebl, B., & Bolte, G. (2007). Intake of phthalates and di(2-ethylhexyl)adipate: results of the integrated exposure assessment survey based on duplicate diet samples and biomonitoring data. *Environment International, 33* (8), 1012–1020. www.sciencedirect.com/science/article/pii/S016041200700102X.

127. Rudel, R. A., Gray, J. M., Engel, C. L., Rawsthorne, T. W., Dodson, R. E., Ackerman, J. M., Rizzo, J., Nudelman, J. L., & Brody, J. G. (2011). Food packaging and bisphenol A and bis(2-ethyhexyl) phthalate exposure: findings from a dietary intervention. *Environmental Health Perspectives, 119* (7), 914–920. www.ncbi.nlm.nih.gov/pmc/articles/PMC3223004/.

128. Blount, B. C., Silva, M. J., Caudill, S. P., Needham, L. L., Pirkle, J. L., Sampson, E. J., Lucier, G. W., Jackson, R. J., & Brock, J. W. (2000). Levels of seven urinary phthalate metabolites in a human reference population. *Environmental Health Perspectives, 108* (10), 979. www.ncbi.nlm.nih.gov/pmc/articles/PMC1240132/pdf/ehp108-000979.pdf.

129. Threat score is 5.3% (probability of an increase in low birth weight, as calculated in a previous footnote) x 10 (impact: statistically detectable impairment) x 1/10 (certainty: preliminary) = 0.82.

130. Urbina, I. (2013, April 13). Think those chemicals have been tested? NYTimes.com. www.nytimes.com/2013/04/14/sunday-review/think-those-chemicals-have-been-tested.html?_r=0.

131. EWG's guide to healthy cleaning. (Updated 2017). Environmental Working Group. http://www.ewg.org/guides/cleaners#.WcpmUXaGPIU.

132. Alcohol ethoxysulfates, alcohol ethoxylates (C10-C16) sodium salt, polyethyleneimine ethoxylates, PEG-75, laureth-9, alcohol ethoxylates (C16-18, 25EO), and diethylene glycol.

133. Helmenstine, A. M. (2017, September 3). The chemistry of how borax works as a cleaner (sodium borate). About.com. http://chemistry.about.com/od/howthingsworkfaqs/a/how-boraxworks.htm.

134. **Rats:** Price, C. J., Strong, P. L., Marr, M. C., Myers, C. B., & Murray, F. J. (1996). Developmental toxicity NOAEL and postnatal recovery in rats fed boric acid during gestation. *Toxicological Sciences, 32* (2), 179–193. http://toxsci.oxfordjournals.org/content/32/2/179.full.pdf.

   Rabbits: Price, C. J., Marr, M. C., Myers, C., Seely, J. C., Heindel, J. J., & Schwetz, B. A. (1996). The developmental toxicity of boric acid in rabbits. *Toxicological Sciences, 34* (2), 176–187. http://toxsci.oxfordjournals.org/content/34/2/176.full.pdf.

   Mice: Heindel, J. J., Price, C. J., Field, E. A., Marr, M. C., Myers, C. B., Morrissey, R. E., & Schwetz, B. A. (1992). Developmental toxicity of boric acid in mice and rats. *Fundamental and Applied Toxicology, 18* (2), 266–277. www.sciencedirect.com/science/article/pii/027205909290055M.

135. Member state committee draft support document for identification of boric acid as a substance of very high concern because of its CMR properties. (2010). ECHA (European Chemicals Agency). https://echa.europa.eu/documents/10162/13638/svhc_supdoc_boric_acid_publication_3576_en.pdf/d51fd473-40ec-4831-bc2d-6f53bdf9cbbe.

136. Munn, S. J., Aschberger, K., Cosgrove, O., De Coen, W., Lund, B. O., Pakalin, S. Paya-Perez, A., & S. Vegro (eds.). (2007). European Union risk assessment report: perboric acid, sodium salt. Including addendum 2007. European Chemicals Bureau, Institute for Health and Consumer Protection. http://echa.europa.eu/documents/10162/6434698/orats_summary_perboricacid_sodiumsalt_en.pdf.

137. National Teratology Information Service (NTIS). (2005). Sodium hypochlorite (bleach) exposure in pregnancy. Regional Drug and Therapeutics Centre. Newcastle.

138. Cyclotetrasiloxane (otherwise known as D4), suspected to be an endocrine disruptor based on results from animal studies (Vier, R. L., Bennett, D. R., & Hunter, M. J. [1975]. Effects of oral 2,6-*cis*-diphenylhexamethyl-cyclotetrasiloxane on the reproductive system of the male *macaca mulatta*. *Acta Pharmacologica et Toxicologica, 36* [s3], 68–80. http://onlinelibrary.wiley.com/doi/10.1111/j.1600-0773.1975.tb03085.x/abstract), is on the "EU Priority list of substances for further evaluation of their role in endocrine disruption" (List of undesirable substances). (2009). Danish Environmental Protection Agency. http://eng.mst.dk/chemicals/chemicals-in-products/assessment-of-chemicals/list-of-undesirable-substances/) and is being evaluated by the Canadian National Health Department and the Californian Office of Environmental Health Hazard Assessment for its potential effects in humans as an endocrine (hormone) disruptor.

139. Otherwise known as diethylene glycol monomethyl ether or 2-(2-methoxyethoxy)ethanol. 2-(2-methoxyethoxy)ethanol. (n.d.). PubChem Open Chemistry Database. http://pubchem.ncbi.nlm.nih.gov/summary/summary.cgi?cid=8134.

140. Hardin, B. D., Goad, P. T., & Burg, J. R. (1986). Developmental toxicity of diethylene glycol monomethyl ether (diEGME). *Toxicological Sciences, 6* (3), 430–439. www.sciencedirect.com/science/article/pii/0272059086902162.

141. Scortichini, B. H., John-Greene, J. A., Quast, J. F., & Rao, K. S. (1984). Teratologic evaluation of dermally applied dietykene glycol monomethyl ether in rabbits.

Fundamental and Applied Toxicology, 7, 68–75. www.sciencedirect.com/science/article/pii/0272059086901983.

142. European Union. (2008, December 24). Decision No 1348/2008/EC of the European Parliament and of the Council of 16 December 2008 amending Council Directive 76/769/EEC as regards restrictions on the marketing and use of 2-(2- methoxyethoxy)ethanol, 2-(2-butoxyethoxy)ethanol, methylenediphenyl diisocyanate, cyclohexane and ammonium nitrate. Published in the *Official Journal of the European Union*, L 348. http://eur-lex.europa.eu/LexUriServ/LexUriServ.do?uri=OJ:L:2008:348:0108:0112:EN:PDF.

143. Lorente, C., et al., Maternal occupational risk factors for oral clefts.

144. Herdt-Losavio, M. L., Lin, S., Chapman, B. R., Hooiveld, M., Olshan, A., Liu, X., DePersis, R. D., Zhu, J., & Druschel, C. M. (2010). Maternal occupation and the risk of birth defects: an overview from the National Birth Defects Prevention Study. *Occupational and Environmental Medicine, 67* (1), 58–66. www.processcleaningsolutions.com/pdf/5_Job%20related%20birth%20deffects.pdf.

145. Blatter, B. M., Roeleveld, N., Zielhuis, G. A., Gabreels, F. J., & Verbeek, A. L. (1996). Maternal occupational exposure during pregnancy and the risk of spina bifida. *Occupational and Environmental Medicine, 53* (2), 80–86. http://oem.bmj.com/content/53/2/80.full.pdf.

146. Sherriff, A., Farrow, A., Golding, J., & Henderson, J. (2005). Frequent use of chemical household products is associated with persistent wheezing in pre-school age children. *Thorax, 60* (1), 45–49. http://thorax.bmj.com/content/60/1/45.full.pdf+html.

    Another study has suggested that frequent use of chemical household products during pregnancy may be linked to a higher likelihood of future asthma in children, but the authors rightly point out that this could actually be due to exposure after birth, since the same mothers who use lots of chemicals during pregnancy may continue to do so after their children are born.

147. McCarthy, J. P. (Updated 2016, May). Toxic matters: protecting our families from toxic substances. University of California, San Francisco Program on Reproductive Health and the Environment From Advancing Science To Ensuring Prevention (FASTEP). https://prhe.ucsf.edu/sites/prhe.ucsf.edu/files/TM_Brochure_en_1.pdf. At www.cdc.gov/preconception/planning.html.

148. One of their detergents, Arm & Hammer Plus OxiClean Liquid Detergent HE, Cool Breeze, even has sodium borate in it.

149. Threat score of spina bifida is 0.7 (elevation in risk) x 3.66 /10,000 (incidence of spina bifida from the Metropolitan Atlanta Congenital Defects Program) x 10,000 (impact: significant impairment) x 1/10 (certainty: preliminary) = 0.26.

    Threat score of cleft palate is 0.4 (elevation in risk) x 12.2 /10,000 (incidence of oral clefts from the Metropolitan Atlanta Congenital Defects Program) x 10,000 (impact: significant impairment) x 1/10 (certainty: preliminary) = 0.49. Total: 0.74.

150. Threat score is 1 (probability) x 100 (impact: statistically detectable impairment) x 1/1000 (certainty: unproven) = 0.1.

151. Nesting instinct. (n.d.). Wikipedia. http://en.wikipedia.org/wiki/Nesting_instinct.

152. Sørensen, M., Andersen, A. M. N., & Raaschou-Nielsen, O. (2010). Non-occupational exposure to paint fumes during pregnancy and fetal growth in a general population. *Environmental Research, 110* (4), 383–387. www.sciencedirect.com/science/article/pii/S0013935110000423.

153. Windham, G. C., Shusterman, D., Swan, S. H., Fenster, L., & Eskenazi, B. (1991). Exposure to organic solvents and adverse pregnancy outcome. *American Journal of Industrial Medicine, 20* (2), 241–259. http://onlinelibrary.wiley.com/doi/10.1002/ajim.4700200210/full.

154. According to the CDC, "solvents are substances that are capable of dissolving or dispersing one or more other substances. Organic solvents are carbon-based solvents (i.e., they contain carbon in their molecular structure). Millions of US workers are exposed to organic solvents that are used in such products as paints, varnishes, lacquers, adhesives, glues, and degreasing/cleaning agents, and in the production of dyes, polymers, plastics, textiles, printing inks, agricultural products, and pharmaceuticals" (Centers for Disease Control and Prevention. [Last updated 2017, October 10]. Workplace safety & health topics: organic solvents. The National Institute for Occupational Safety and Health. www.cdc.gov/niosh/topics/organsolv/).

155. Windham, et al., Exposure to organic solvents and adverse pregnancy outcome.

156. Correa, A., Gray, R. H., Cohen, R., Rothman, N., Shah, F., Seacat, H., & Com, M. (1996). Ethylene glycol ethers and risks of spontaneous abortion and subfertility. *American Journal of Epidemiology, 143* (7), 707–717. http://aje.oxfordjournals.org/content/143/7/707.full.pdf.

157. Khattak, S., Guiti, K., McMartin, K., Barrera, M., Kennedy, D., & Koren, G. (1999). Pregnancy outcome following gestational exposure to organic solvents: a prospective controlled study. *JAMA, 281* (12), 1106–1109. http://jama.jamanetwork.com/article.aspx?articleid=189189.

158. Cordier, S., Bergeret, A., Goujard, J., Ha, M. C., Aymé, S., Bianchi, F., Calzolari, E., De Walle, H. E. K., Knill-Jones, R., Candela, S. Dale, I., Dananché, B., De Vigan, C., Fevotte, J., Kiel, G., & Mandereau, L. (1997). Congenital malformations and maternal occupational exposure to glycol ethers. *Epidemiology, 8* (4), 355–363. http://www.jstor.org/stable/3702574?seq=1#page_scan_tab_contents.

159. Laumon, B., Martin, J. L., Bertucat, I., Verney, M. P., & Robert, E. (1996). Exposure to organic solvents during pregnancy and oral clefts: a case-control study. *Reproductive Toxicology, 10* (1), 15–19. www.sciencedirect.com/science/article/pii/0890623895020136.

160. Jenkins, K. J., Correa, A., Feinstein, J. A., Botto, L., Britt, A. E., Daniels, S. R., Elixson, M., Warnes, C. A., & Webb, C. L. (2007). Noninherited risk factors and congenital cardiovascular defects: current knowledge: a scientific statement from the American Heart Association Council on Cardiovascular Disease in the Young. *Circulation, 115* (23), 2995–3014. https://circ.ahajournals.org/content/115/23/2995.full.

161. Till, C., Koren,. G, & Rovet, J. F. (2001). Prenatal exposure to organic solvents and child neurobehavioral performance. *Neurotoxicology and Teratology 23* (3), 235–245. http://www.sciencedirect.com/science/article/pii/S0892036201001416.

162. Laslo-Baker, D., Barrera, M., Knittel-Keren, D., Kozer, E., Wolpin, J., Khattak, S., Hackman, R., Rovet, J., & Koren, G. (2004). Child neurodevelopmental outcome and maternal occupational exposure to solvents. *Archives of Pediatrics & Adolescent Medicine, 158* (10), 956–961. http://archpedi.ama-assn.org/cgi/reprint/158/10/956.pdf.

163. Pelé, F., Muckle, G., Costet, N., Garlantézec, R., Monfort, C., Multigner, L., Rouget, F., & Cordier, S. (2013). Occupational solvent exposure during pregnancy and child behaviour at age 2. *Occupational and Environmental Medicine, 70* (2), 114–119. http://hal.archives-ouvertes.fr/docs/00/79/50/43/PDF/Occupationnal_solvent_exposure_child_behavior_HAL.pdf.

164. Janulewicz, P. A., White, R. F., Martin, B. M., Winter, M. R., Weinberg, J. M., Vieira, V., & Aschengrau, A. (2012). Adult neuropsychological performance following prenatal and early postnatal exposure to tetrachloroethylene (PCE)-contaminated drinking water. *Neurotoxicology and Teratology, 34* (3), 350–359. www.ncbi.nlm.nih.gov/pmc/articles/PMC3553661/.

165. Wilkins-Haug, L., & Gabow, P. A. (1991). Toluene abuse during pregnancy: obstetric complications and perinatal outcomes. *Obstetrics and Gynecology, 77* (4), 504–509. http://europepmc.org/abstract/MED/2002970.

166. Holmberg, P. C., & Nurminen, M. (1980). Congenital defects of the central nervous system and occupational factors during pregnancy: a case-referent study. *American Journal of Industrial Medicine, 1* (2), 167–176. http://onlinelibrary.wiley.com/doi/10.1002/ajim.4700010207/abstract.

167. Holmberg, P. C., Hernberg, S., Kurppa, K., Rantala, K., & Riala, R. (1982). Oral clefts and organic solvent exposure during pregnancy. *International Archives of Occupational and Environmental Health, 50* (4), 371–376. www.springerlink.com/content/n620078v1p1m4142/.

168. Scélo, G., Metayer, C., Zhang, L., Wiemels, J. L., Aldrich, M. C., Selvin, S., Month, S., Smith, M. T., & Buffler, P. A. (2009). Household exposure to paint and petroleum solvents, chromosomal translocations, and the risk of childhood leukemia. *Environmental Health Perspectives, 117* (1), 133–139. www.ncbi.nlm.nih.gov/pmc/articles/PMC2627857/.

169. There are 2,600 total cases of childhood leukemia annually in the United States, of which 80% are acute lymphoblastic, or 2,080 (Parkin, D., Ferlay, J., Whelan, S. L., & Storm, H. H. [2005]. Cancer incidence in five continents [Vol. 1]. Diamond Pocket Books [P] Ltd.).

170. "Low-VOC" paints are becoming increasingly trendy and are probably better on average than normal paints. According to Consumer Reports, "In response to stricter federal and regional standards, manufacturers have reduced the levels of volatile organic compounds—some of the noxious chemicals that can make paint smell like paint—in their products. Earlier low-VOC paints lacked the durability of higher-VOC finishes, but now all the paints in our tests are claimed to have low or no VOCs, and many performed very well." (Paint buying guide. [Last updated 2017, February]. ConsumerReports.org. www.consumer reports.org/cro/paints/buying-guide.

171. Threat score is 21% x 2,080 / 4,112,000 (probability of leukemia, since there are 2,080 cases each year as calculated in a previous footnote, out of a total of 4,112,000 live births per year from Appendix I) x 10,000 (impact: significant impairment) x 1/10 (certainty: preliminary) = 0.11.

172. Fritz Haber and the nitrogen cycle. (2002, July 10). NPR.org. www.npr.org/templates/story/story.php?storyId=1146429.

173. Smil, V. (1999). Detonator of the population explosion. *Nature, 400* (6743), 415. http://vaclavsmil.com/wp-content/uploads/docs/smil-article-1999-nature7.pdf.

174. Wolfe, D. W. (2002). Tales from the underground: a natural history of subterranean life. Cambridge, MA: Basic Books.

175. Mueller, D. K. (1995). Nutrients in ground water and surface water of the United States: an analysis of data through 1992. *Water-Resources Investigations Report (USA)*. http://pubs.er.usgs.gov/publication/wri954031.

176. Nitrates and nitrites: TEACH chemical summary. (2007, May 22). Environmental Protection Agency. https://archive.epa.gov/region5/teach/web/pdf/nitrates_summary.pdf.

177. Mueller, Nutrients in ground water and surface water of the United States.

178. Centers for Disease Control and Prevention. (1996). Spontaneous abortions possibly related to ingestion of nitrate-contaminated well water—LaGrange County, Indiana, 1991–1994. *Morbidity and Mortality Weekly Report, 45* (26), 569–572. https://www.cdc.gov/mmwr/preview/mmwrhtml/00042839.htm.

179. Cedergren, M. I., Selbing, A. J., Löfman, O., & Källen, B. A. (2002). Chlorination byproducts and nitrate in drinking water and risk for congenital cardiac defects. *Environmental Research, 89* (2), 124–130. www.sciencedirect.com/science/article/pii/S0013935101943622.

180. Arbuckle, T. E., Sherman, G. J., Corey, P. N., Walters, D., & Lo, B. (1988). Water nitrates and CNS birth defects: a population-based case-control study. *Archives of Environmental Health: An International Journal, 43* (2), 162–167. www.tandfonline.com/doi/abs/10.1080/00039896.1988.9935846.

181. Dorsch, M. M., Scragg, R. K., McMichael, A. J., Baghurst, P. A., & Dyer, K. F. (1984). Congenital malformations and maternal drinking water supply in rural South Australia: a case-control study. *American Journal of Epidemiology, 119* (4), 473–486. http://aje.oxford-journals.org/content/119/4/473.short.

182. Croen, L. A., Todoroff, K., & Shaw, G. M. (2001). Maternal exposure to nitrate from drinking water and diet and risk for neural tube defects. *American Journal of Epidemiology, 153* (4), 325–331. http://aje.oxfordjournals.org/content/153/4/325.full.

183. Manassaram, D. M., Backer, L. C., & Moll, D. M. (2007). A review of nitrates in drinking water: maternal exposure and adverse reproductive and developmental outcomes. *Ciencia & Saude Coletiva, 12* (1), 153–163. http://www.scielo.br/scielo.php?pid=S1413-81232007000100018&script=sci_arttext.

184. Nitrate and nitrite in drinking-water: background for development of WHO guidelines for drinking-water quality. (2016). World Health Organization. www.who.int/water_sanitation_health/dwq/chemicals/nitrate-nitrite-background-jan17.pdf.

185. Preston-Martin, S., Pogoda, J. M., Mueller, B. A., Holly, E. A., Lijinsky, W., & Davis, R. L. (1996). Maternal consumption of cured meats and vitamins in relation to pediatric brain tumors. *Cancer Epidemiology Biomarkers & Prevention, 5* (8), 599–605. http://cebp.aacrjournals.org/content/5/8/599.full.pdf.

186. Pogoda, J. M., & Preston-Martin, S. (2001). Maternal cured meat consumption during pregnancy and risk of paediatric brain tumour in offspring: potentially harmful levels of intake. *Public Health Nutrition, 4* (02), 183–189. https://www.cambridge.org/core/journals/public-health-nutrition/article/maternal-cured-meat-consumption-during-pregnancy-and-risk-of-paediatric-brain-tumour-in-offspring-potentially-harmful-levels-of-intake/8BD-0F0BBDD4B52399DC7774ACBD1E21C.

187. Sarasua, M. S., & Savitz, D. A. (1994). Cured and broiled meat consumption in relation to childhood cancer: Denver, Colorado (United States). *Cancer Causes & Control, 5* (2), 141–148. https://link.springer.com/article/10.1007%2FBF01830260?LI=true.

188. McCredie, M., Maisonneuve, P., & Boyle, P. (1994). Antenatal risk factors for malignant brain tumours in New South Wales children. *International Journal of Cancer, 56* (1), 6–10. www.ncbi.nlm.nih.gov/pubmed/8262678.

189. Huncharek, M., & Kupelnick, B. (2004). A meta-analysis of maternal cured meat consumption during pregnancy and the risk of childhood brain tumors. *Neuroepidemiology, 23* (1–2), 78–84. www.karger.com/Article/Abstract/73979.

190. IARC Working Group on the Evaluation of Carcinogenic Risks to Humans. (2010). Ingested nitrate and nitrite, and cyanobacterial peptide toxins. *IARC Monographs on the Evaluation of Carcinogenic Risks in Humans, 94,* 1–412. http://monographs.iarc.fr/ENG/Monographs/vol94/index.php.

191. Nitrates and nitrites: TEACH chemical summary.

192. "Research over the past 15 years has led to a paradigm change in our ideas about health effects of both nitrite and nitrate. Whereas historically nitrite and nitrate were considered harmful food additives and listed as probable human carcinogens . . . they are now considered by some as indispensable nutrients essential for cardiovascular health by promoting nitric oxide (NO) production" (Bryan, N. S., Alexander, D. D., Coughlin, J. R., Milkowski, A. L., & Boffetta, P. [2012]. Ingested nitrate and nitrite and stomach cancer

risk: an updated review. *Food and Chemical Toxicology, 50* [10], 3646–3665. http://www. sciencedirect.com/science/article/pii/S0278691512005406).

193. Sindelar, J. J., & Milkowski, A. L. (2011). Sodium nitrite in processed meat and poultry meats: a review of curing and examining the risk/benefit of its use. *American Meat Science Association White Paper Series, (3)*, 1–14. www.themeatsite.com/articles/contents/nitrite_report.pdf.

194. Neuman, W. (2011, July 1). What's inside the bun? NYTimes.com. www.nytimes. com/2011/07/02/business/02hotdog.html?_r=0.

195. IARC Working Group on the Evaluation of Carcinogenic Risks to Humans, Ingested nitrate and nitrite, and cyanobacterial peptide toxins.

196. Milkowski, A. L. (2011). Sources of exposure to nitrogen oxides. Pages 49–65 in: Bryan, N. S., & Loscalzo, J. (2011). Nitrite and nitrate in human health and disease. New York: Humana Press.

197. IARC Working Group on the Evaluation of Carcinogenic Risks to Humans, Ingested nitrate and nitrite, and cyanobacterial peptide toxins.

198. Nitrate levels converted to nitrite equivalents based on the US EPA reference doses for nitrate (7.0 mg nitrate ion/kg body weight per day) and nitrite (0.33 mg nitrite ion/kg body weight per day). Agency for Toxic Substances and Disease Registry. (2011, January). ToxFAQs for nitrate and nitrite. Toxic substances portal: nitrate and nitrite. www.atsdr. cdc.gov/toxfaqs/tf.asp?id=1186&tid=258.

199. Threat score is 1% (probability you're exposed to elevated nitrate levels in drinking water) x 100 (impact: statistically detectable impairment) x 1/1,000 (certainty: unproven) = 0.001.

200. Lim, L. (2013, January 14). Beijing's 'Airpocalypse' spurs pollution controls, public pressure. NPR.org. www.npr.org/2013/01/14/169305324/ beijings-air-quality-reaches-hazardous-levels.

201. US Department of Transportation, Office of Planning, Environment & Realty. (2011, May 6). Census 2000 population statistics. DOT.gov. www.fhwa.dot.gov/planning/ census_issues/archives/metropolitan_planning/cps2k.cfm.

202. Wilhelm, M., & Ritz, B. (2003). Residential proximity to traffic and adverse birth outcomes in Los Angeles County, California, 1994–1996. *Environmental Health Perspectives, 111* (2), 207. www.ncbi.nlm.nih.gov/pmc/articles/PMC1241352/pdf/ehp0111-000207.pdf.

203. Wilhelm, M., & Ritz, B. (2005). Local variations in CO and particulate air pollution and adverse birth outcomes in Los Angeles County, California, USA. *Environmental Health Perspectives, 113* (9), 1212. www.ncbi.nlm.nih.gov/pmc/articles/PMC1280404/.

204. Volk, H. E., Lurmann, F., Penfold, B., Hertz-Picciotto, I., & McConnell, R. (2013). Traffic-related air pollution, particulate matter, and autism. *JAMA Psychiatry, 70* (1), 71–77. www. sesalmaul.org/userfiles/board/classroom/20130603935-Q232U2.pdf.

205. Perera, F. P., Rauh, V., Tsai, W. Y., Kinney, P., Camann, D., Barr, D., Bernert, T., Garfinkel, R., Tu, Y. H., Diaz, D., Dietrich, J., & Whyatt, R. M. (2003). Effects of transplacental exposure to environmental pollutants on birth outcomes in a multiethnic population. *Environmental Health Perspectives, 111* (2), 201. www.ncbi.nlm.nih.gov/pmc/articles/ PMC1241351/pdf/ehp0111-000201.pdf.

206. Perera, F. P., Li, Z., Whyatt, R., Hoepner, L., Wang, S., Camann, D., & Rauh, V. (2009). Prenatal airborne polycyclic aromatic hydrocarbon exposure and child IQ at age 5 years. *Pediatrics, 124* (2), e195–e202. http://pediatrics.aappublications.org/content/124/2/e195.

207. Perera, F. P., Tang, D., Wang, S., Vishnevetsky, J., Zhang, B., Diaz, D., Camann, D., & Rauh, V. (2012). Prenatal polycyclic aromatic hydrocarbon (PAH) exposure and child

behavior at age 6–7 years. *Environmental Health Perspectives, 120* (6), 921–926. www.ncbi. nlm.nih.gov/pmc/articles/PMC3385432/.

208. Perera, F. P., Whyatt, R. M., Jedrychowski, W., Rauh, V., Manchester, D., Santella, R. M., & Ottman, R. (1998). Recent developments in molecular epidemiology: a study of the effects of environmental polycyclic aromatic hydrocarbons on birth outcomes in Poland. *American Journal of Epidemiology, 147* (3), 309–314. http://aje.oxfordjournals.org/content/147/3/309.full.pdf.

209. Dejmek, J., Solanský, I., Benes, I., Lenícek, J., & Srám, R. J. (2000). The impact of polycyclic aromatic hydrocarbons and fine particles on pregnancy outcome. *Environmental Health Perspectives, 108* (12), 1159. www.ncbi.nlm.nih.gov/pmc/articles/PMC1240197/pdf/ehp0108-001159.pdf.

210. Choi, H., Jedrychowski, W., Spengler, J., Camann, D. E., Whyatt, R. M., Rauh, V., Tsai, W. Y., & Perera, F. P. (2006). International studies of prenatal exposure to polycyclic aromatic hydrocarbons and fetal growth. *Environmental Health Perspectives,* 1744–1750. www.ncbi. nlm.nih.gov/pmc/articles/PMC1665416/.

211. Tang, D., Li, T. Y., Liu, J. J., Chen, Y. H., Qu, L., & Perera, F. (2006). PAH–DNA adducts in cord blood and fetal and child development in a Chinese cohort. *Environmental Health Perspectives, 114* (8), 1297. www.ncbi.nlm.nih.gov/pmc/articles/PMC1552014/.

212. Tang, D., Li, T. Y., Liu, J. J., Zhou, Z. J., Tao, Y., Chen, Y. H., Rauh, V. A., Xie, J., & Perera, F. P. (2008). Effects of prenatal exposure to coal-burning pollutants on children's development in China. *Environmental Health Perspectives, 116* (5), 674–679. www.ncbi.nlm.nih. gov/pmc/articles/pmc2367664/.

213. Perera, F., Li, T. Y., Zhou, Z. J., Tao, Y, Chen, Y. H., Qu, L., Rauh, V. A., Zhang, Y., & Tang, D. Benefits of reducing prenatal exposure to coal-burning pollutants to children's neurodevelopment in China. *Environmental Health Perspectives, 116* (10), 1396–1400. www.ncbi.nlm.nih.gov/pmc/articles/PMC2569101/.

214. Shah, P. S., & Balkhair, T. (2011). Air pollution and birth outcomes: a systematic review. *Environment International, 37* (2), 498–516. www.sciencedirect.com/science/article/pii/S0160412010002254.

215. Parker, J., Rich, D. Q., Glinianaia, S. V., Leem, J. H., Wartenberg, D., Bell, M. L., Bonzini, M., Brauer, M., Darrow, L., Gehring, U., Gouveia, N., Grillo, P., Ha, E., Van Den Hooven, E. H., Jalaludin, B., Jesdale, B. M., Lepeule, J., Morello-Frosch, R., Morgan, G. G., Slama, R., Pierik, F. H., Pesatori, A. C., Sathyanarayana, S., Seo, J., Strickland, M., Tamburic, L., & Woodruff, T. J. (2011). The International Collaboration on Air Pollution and Pregnancy Outcomes: initial results. *Environmental Health Perspectives, 119* (7), 1023–1028. www. ncbi.nlm.nih.gov/pmc/articles/PMC3222970/.

216. Slama, R., Darrow, L., Parker, J., Woodruff, T. J., Strickland, M., Nieuwenhuijsen, M., Glinianaia, S., Hoggatt, K. J., Kannan, S., Hurley, F., Kalinka, J., Šrám, R., Brauer, M., Wilhelm, M., Heinrich, J., & Ritz, B. (2008). Meeting report: atmospheric pollution and human reproduction. *Environmental Health Perspectives, 116* (6), 791–8. www.ncbi.nlm. nih.gov/pmc/articles/pmc2430236/.

217. Barn, P. (2010). Residential air cleaner use to improve indoor air quality and health: a review of the evidence. National Collaborating Centre for Environmental Health. http:// www.ncceh.ca/sites/default/files/Air_Cleaners_Oct_2010.pdf.

218. Brauner, E. V., Forchhammer, L., Møller, P., Barregard, L., Gunnarsen, L., Afshari, A., Wåhlin, P., Glasius, M., Dragsted, L. O., Basu, S., Raaschou-Nielsen, O., & Loft, S. (2008). Indoor particles affect vascular function in the aged: an air filtration–based intervention study. *American Journal of Respiratory and Critical Care Medicine, 177* (4), 419–425. http:// www.atsjournals.org/doi/abs/10.1164/rccm.200704-632OC.

219. Sublett, J. L., Seltzer, J., Burkhead, R., Williams, P. B., Wedner, H. J., & Phipatanakul, W. (2010). Air filters and air cleaners: rostrum by the American Academy of Allergy, Asthma & Immunology Indoor Allergen Committee. *Journal of Allergy and Clinical Immunology, 125* (1), 32–38. www.ncbi.nlm.nih.gov/pmc/articles/PMC2824428/.

220. Agency for Toxic Substances and Disease Registry. (1993). Toxicological profile for polycyclic aromatic hydrocarbons (PAHs). US Department of Health and Human Services Public Health Service. www.atsdr.cdc.gov/ToxProfiles/tp69.pdf.

221. Smith, A.P. (2013, July 22). The kitchen as a pollution hazard. NYTimes.com. http://well. blogs.nytimes.com/2013/07/22/the-kitchen-as-a-pollution-hazard/.

222. Jedrychowski, W., Perera, F. P., Tang, D., Stigter, L., Mroz, E., Flak, E., Spengler, J., Budzyn-Mrozek, D., Kaim, I., & Jacek, R. (2012). Impact of barbecued meat consumed in pregnancy on birth outcomes accounting for personal prenatal exposure to airborne polycyclic aromatic hydrocarbons. Birth cohort study in Poland. *Nutrition, 28* (4), 372–377. www.ncbi.nlm.nih.gov/pmc/articles/PMC3288524/.

223. Park, A. (2011, August 2). Could microwaves be associated with children's asthma? Time.com. http://healthland.time.com/2011/08/02/microwaves-and-asthma-exposure-to-magnetic-fields-during-pregnancy-ups-asthma-risk-among-newborns/.

224. To address a popular misconception, ultrasound is not a form of radiation but rather a type of sound wave. Ultrasound appears to be totally harmless in pregnancy; for more detail, see Appendix VI.

225. World Health Organization. (n.d.). What are electromagnetic fields? Summary of health effects. Electromagnetic fields (EMF).www.who.int/peh-emf/about/WhatisEMF/en/index1. html.

226. The WHO has flagged two studies which indicate a possible link between magnetic field exposure and miscarriage (Lee, G. M., Neutra, R. R., Hristova, L., Yost, M., & Hiatt, R. A. [2002]. A nested case-control study of residential and personal magnetic field measures and miscarriages. *Epidemiology, 13* [1], 21–31. http://modx.buergerwelle.de/assets/files/ miscarriages_emf.pdf; Li, D. K., Odouli, R., Wi, S., Janevic, T., Golditch, I., Bracken, T. D., Senior, R., Rankin, R., & Iriye, R. [2002]. A population-based prospective cohort study of personal exposure to magnetic fields during pregnancy and the risk of miscarriage. *Epidemiology, 13* [1], 9–20. www.psicomag.com/biblioteca/2002/Li%20%2002. pdf) but caveats that it's too soon to draw firm conclusions (Kheifets, L., Repacholi, M., Saunders, R., & Van Deventer, E. [2005]. The sensitivity of children to electromagnetic fields. *Pediatrics, 116* [2], e303–e313. http://pediatrics.aappublications.org/content/116/2/e303.short.

227. Kheifets, L., et al., The sensitivity of children to electromagnetic fields.

228. World Health Organization, What are electromagnetic fields? Summary of health effects.

229. The International Labour Organization, the International Commission on Non-Ionizing Radiation Protection, and the World Health Organization. (2007). Environmental health critera 238: extremely low frequency fields. World Health Organization. www.who.int/ entity/peh-emf/publications/Complet_DEC_2007.pdf.

230. The National Institute of Health has concluded that your child may be at higher risk of developing childhood leukemia longer term (The National Institute of Environmental Health Sciences and the National Institutes of Health. [2002, June]. Electric and magnetic fields associated with the use of electric power. NIEHS/DOE EMF RAPID program. www. niehs.nih.gov/health/materials/electric_and_magnetic_fields_associated_with_the_use_ of_electric_power_questions_and_answers_english_508.pdf), although keep in mind this is a very rare disease—even if the risk is doubled, that's only 5–8 cases per 100,000 children per year (Kheifets, L., et al., The sensitivity of children to electromagnetic fields).

231. Electric and magnetic fields and health: personal exposure. [n.d.]. EMFs.info. www.emfs. info/Sources+of+EMFs/exposure/.

232. Mader, D. L., & Peralta, S. B. (1992). Residential exposure to 60-Hz magnetic fields from appliances. *Bioelectromagnetics, 13* (4), 287–301. http://onlinelibrary.wiley.com/ doi/10.1002/bem.2250130404/full.

233. World Health Organization, What are electromagnetic fields? Summary of health effects.

234. World Health Organization, What are electromagnetic fields? Summary of health effects.
    All measurements from a distance of 30 cm away, except TV and fluorescent light, which are from a distance of 1 meter.

235. Li, D. K., Chen, H., & Odouli, R. (2011). Maternal exposure to magnetic fields during pregnancy in relation to the risk of asthma in offspring. *Archives of Pediatrics & Adolescent Medicine, 165* (10), 945–950. http://jamanetwork.com/journals/jamapediatrics/ fullarticle/1107612..

236. Vecchia, P., Matthes, R., Ziegelberger, G., Lin, J., Saunders, R., & Swerdlow, A. (2009). Exposure to high frequency electromagnetic fields, biological effects and health consequences (100 kHz-300 GHz). International Commission on Non-Ionizing Radiation Protection. http://publicsde.regie-energie.qc.ca/projets/34/DocPrj/R-3770-2011-B-0136-AUDI-PIECE-2012_05_18.pdf.

237. International Programme on Chemical Safety. (1993). Environmental health criteria 137: electromagnetic fields (300 Hz to 300 GHz). World Health Organization. www.inchem.org/ documents/ehc/ehc/ehc137.htm.

238. Kheifets, L., et al., The sensitivity of children to electromagnetic fields.

239. World Health Organization, What are electromagnetic fields? Summary of health effects.

240. Ibid.

241. Friberg, L., & Elinder, C. G. (1985). Electric and magnetic fields and health outcomes. Encylopaedia of Occupational Health and Safety, Chapter 49–Radiation: Non-Ionizing. www.ilocis.org/documents/chpt49e.htm.

242. Committee on the Possible Effects of Electromagnetic Fields on Biologic Systems. (1997). Possible health effects of exposure to residential electric and magnetic fields. Washington, DC: National Academies Press. http://books.nap.edu/openbook/0309054478/html/index. html.

243. Ahlbom, I. C., Cardis, E., Green, A., Linet, M., Savitz, D., Swerdlow, A., & the International Commission for Non-Ionizing Radiation Protection Standing Committee on Epidemiology. (2001). Review of the epidemiologic literature on EMF and health. *Environmental Health Perspectives, 109* (Suppl 6), 911. www.ncbi.nlm.nih.gov/pmc/articles/ PMC1240626/pdf/ehp109s-000911.pdf.

244. **Threat score is 10th percentile x 13% (probability of a child developing asthma, as cited in the study postulating a link to magnetic fields—this is therefore a high upper bound, since 100% of cases of asthma are unlikely to be attributable to magnetic field exposure) x 100 (impact: statistically detectable impairment) x 1/10 (certainty: ambiguous) = 0.013.**

245. Brent, R. L. (1989). The effect of embryonic and fetal exposure to X-ray, microwaves, and ultrasound: counseling the pregnant and non-pregnant patient about these risks. *Seminars in Radiation Oncology, 16,* 347–368. www.ncbi.nlm.nih.gov/pubmed/2678486.

246. Radiation. (n.d.). Wikipedia. http://en.wikipedia.org/wiki/Radiation.

247. ACOG Committee on Obstetric Practice. (2017, October). Guidelines for diagnostic imaging during pregnancy and lactation: ACOG committee opinion number 273 (replaces number 656, February 2016). *Obstetrics and Gynecology 2017, 130,* e210–216. https://www.acog. org/Resources-And-Publications/Committee-Opinions/Committee-on-Obstetric-Practice/ Guidelines-for-Diagnostic-Imaging-During-Pregnancy-and-Lactation.

248. ACOG Committee on Obstetric Practice. (2004, September). Guidelines for diagnostic imaging during pregnancy: ACOG committee opinion number 299 (replaces number 158, September 1995). *Obstetrics and Gynecology, 104* (3), 647. https://www.acog.org/Resources-And-Publications/Committee-Opinions/Committee-on-Obstetric-Practice/Guidelines-for-Diagnostic-Imaging-During-Pregnancy-and-Lactation.

249. Brent, R. L., The effect of embryonic and fetal exposure to X-ray, microwaves, and ultrasound.

250. Friedberg, W., & Copeland, K. (2003). What aircrews should know about their occupational exposure to ionizing radiation (No. DOT/FAA/AM-03/16). Civil Aerospace Medical Institute, Federal Aviation Administration, Oklahoma City. www.dtic.mil/cgi-bin/GetTRDoc?AD=ADA423589.

251. Radon: molecular action and genetic effects. (n.d.). University of Minnesota School of Public Health. http://enhs.umn.edu/hazards/hazardssite/radon/radonmolaction.html.

252. Radiation protection: Radon. (2013, February 13). US Environmental Protection Agency.

253. The origins range from processes on the sun (and presumably other stars as well) to as-yet-unknown nonthermal mechanisms in the farthest reaches of the observable universe, although the exact sources are often difficult to pinpoint. Magnetic fields bend cosmic ray direction so that they arrive nearly randomly from all directions, hiding any clue of the direction of their initial sources (Cosmic ray. [n.d.]. Wikipedia. http://en.wikipedia.org/wiki/Cosmic_rays).

254. Friedberg, W., What aircrews should know about their occupational exposure to ionizing radiation.

255. The U.S. Transportation Security Administration (TSA) currently uses millimeter wave Advanced Imaging Technology (AIT) to screen passengers and states that these are safe for pregnant women (TSA travel tips for pregnant passengers. [2014, July 22]. Transportation Security Administration Blog. https://www.tsa.gov/blog/2014/07/22/tsa-travel-tips-pregnant-passengers), as they use radio frequency energy and the energy projected is thousands of times less than a cell phone transmission. Another technology called the backscatter X-ray was recently phased out in the United States for privacy reasons, but it's still in use elsewhere in the world. Although this technology uses ionizing radiation, the Department of Homeland Security states that "an airline passenger that has been screened receives an equivalent dose of radiation from less than two minutes of flight at altitude" (Fact sheet: advanced imaging technology (AIT) health & safety. (n.d.). Homeland Security: Office of Health Affairs. http://epic.org/foia/dhs/bodyscanner/appeal/TSA-AIT_ScannerFactSheet.pdf).

256. EPA 402-F-14-015: cosmic radiation. (2014, August). US Environmental Protection Agency Office of Radiation and Indoor Air. https://www3.epa.gov/radtown/docs/cosmic-radiation.pdf.

257. Friedberg, W., What aircrews should know about their occupational exposure to ionizing radiation.

258. There is a product being specifically marketed to pregnant women called "Belly Armor" that claims to provide protection for the fetus, but it doesn't protect against ionizing radiation, only the non-iodizing radiation discussed in the previous chapter (FAQs: do Belly Armor products shield against ionizing radiation? [n.d.]. BellyArmor.com. www.bellyarmor.com).

259. Threat score: 1/10,000 x 2.02 (probability of developing cancer later in life) x 10,000 (impact: significant impairment) x 1 (certainty: well proven) = 2.02.

260. Threat score: 1/10,000 x 0.028 x 2 (probability of developing cancer later in life) x 10,000 (impact: significant impairment) x 1 (certainty: well proven) = 0.06.

261. Threat score: 1/10,000 x 0.95 (probability of developing cancer later in life) x 10,000 (impact: significant impairment) x 1 (certainty: well proven) = 0.95.

262. Reynolds, C. (2012, November 30). Agatha Christie's methods of murder. *The home of Agatha Christie.* http://www.agathachristie.com/news/2012/ agatha-christies-methods-of-murder.

263. Gerald, M. C. (1993). *The poisonous pen of Agatha Christie.* Austin: University of Texas Press. www.nejm.org/doi/full/10.1056/NEJM199404143301522.

264. Arsenic in your food. (2012, November). ConsumerReports.org. http://consumerreports. org/cro/magazine/2012/11/arsenic-in-your-food/index.htm.

265. World Health Organization. (2010). Exposure to arsenic: a major public health concern. Geneva: WHO Public Health and Environment, 1–5. www.who.int/entity/ipcs/features/ arsenic.pdf.

266. Sepkowitz, K. (2012, September 20). Why rice contains detectable levels of arsenic. *The Daily Beast.* www.thedailybeast.com/articles/2012/09/20/why-rice-contains-detectable- levels-of-arsenic.html#url=/articles/2012/09/20/why-rice-contains-detectable-of- arsenic.html.

267. Agency for Toxic Substances and Disease Registry (ATSDR). (2007, August). Toxicological profile for arsenic. US Department of Health and Human Services Public Health Service. www.atsdr.cdc.gov/ToxProfiles/tp.asp?id=22&tid=3.

268. National Research Council Subcommittee on Arsenic in Drinking Water. (1999). *Arsenic in drinking water.* Washington, DC: The National Academies Press. https://www.nap.edu/ catalog/6444/arsenic-in-drinking-water.

269. Aschengrau, A., Zierler, S., & Cohen, A. (1989). Quality of community drinking water and the occurrence of spontaneous abortion. *Archives of Environmental Health: An International Journal, 44* (5), 283–290. www.tandfonline.com/doi/abs/10.1080/00039896.1 989.9935895.

270. Concha, G., Vogler, G., Lezcano, D., Nermell, B., & Vahter, M. (1998). Exposure to inorganic arsenic metabolites during early human development. *Toxicological Sciences, 44* (2), 185–190. https://academic.oup.com/toxsci/article/44/2/185/1611532/ Exposure-to-Inorganic-Arsenic-Metabolites-during.

271. World Health Organization, Exposure to arsenic: a major public health concern.

272. Ahmad, S. A., Salim Ullah Sayed, M. H., Barua, S., Khan, M. H., Faruquee, M. H., Jalil, A., Hadi, S. A., & Talukder, H. K. (2001). Arsenic in drinking water and pregnancy outcomes. *Environmental Health Perspectives, 109* (6), 629. www.ncbi.nlm.nih.gov/pmc/articles/ PMC1240346/pdf/ehp0109-000629.pdf.

273. World Health Organization. Exposure to arsenic: a major public health concern.

274. Agency for Toxic Substances and Disease Registry, Toxicological profile for arsenic.

275. DeSesso, J., Jacobson, C., Scialli, A., Farr, C., & Holson, J. (1998). An assessment of the developmental toxicity of inorganic arsenic. *Reproductive Toxicology, 12* (4), 385–433. http://europepmc.org/abstract/MED/9717692/ reload=0;jsessionid=JHgEUeF4AZWnOlUhVWM5.0.

276. DeSesso, J. M. (2001). Teratogen update: inorganic arsenic. *Teratology, 64* (3), 170–173. http://teratology.org/updates/64pg170.pdf.

277. Questions & answers: arsenic in rice and rice products. (2017, October 25). US Food and Drug Administration. www.fda.gov/Food/FoodborneIllnessContaminants/Metals/ ucm319948.htm.

278. Kay, J. (2012, December 10). Should doctors warn pregnant women about environmental risks? *Scientific American*. www.scientificamerican.com/article/should-doctors-warn-pregnant-women-about-environmental-risks/.

279. Committee opinion number 575: exposure to toxic environmental agents. (2013, October). *Obstetrics and Gynecology, 2013* (122), 931–935. www.acog.org/Resources_And_Publications/Committee_Opinions/Committee_on_Health_Care_for_Underserved_Women/Exposure_to_Toxic_Environmental_Agents.

280. Hamblin, J. (2014, March 18). The toxins that threaten our brains. *The Atlantic*. www.theatlantic.com/features/archive/2014/03/the-toxins-that-threaten-our-brains/284466/.

281. "Over the past decade, the federal government has invested substantially more money in looking at just how pregnant women and children have been affected by industrial chemicals. The EPA has awarded millions of dollars in related research grants, and the NIH started funding a network of what it calls Centers for Children's Environmental Health and Disease Prevention Research. There is one at Mount Sinai and another at Harvard, and there are others at Columbia, UC Berkeley, and elsewhere. Those centers have established strong research programs called prospective birth-cohort studies. Scientists enroll pregnant female subjects and carefully record objective measures of environmental exposure, using things like blood samples, urine samples, and maybe even dust and air samples from their homes. After the babies are born, the researchers follow up with them at various points in their childhoods" (Hamblin, J., The toxins that threaten our brains).

3

GUiLTY PLEASURES

Voluntary Poison

*I*f only it were the 1800s, when doctors prescribed iced champagne as a cure for morning sickness.[1, 2] If only we lived in the age of Camelot, when Jackie Kennedy could smoke with a bump and attract not a whiff of media scrutiny.[3, 4] If only we could still indulge in our decadent pleasures without a disapproving Cricket whispering words of warning from our shoulder.

We know it's wrong, perhaps even sinful, to continue some of our indulgences as we did pre-pregnancy, but many of us simply can't help ourselves. According to a National Institutes of Health survey, at least one in five pregnant women continue to smoke and drink.[5] Some even use marijuana and cocaine (see chart on following page).

Is some or all of this flagrantly irresponsible behavior doing irreparable damage to our unborn children? Or is our puritanical culture causing the indulgent (or addicted) among us unnecessary stress? Let's find out.

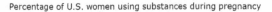

Percentage of U.S. women using substances during pregnancy

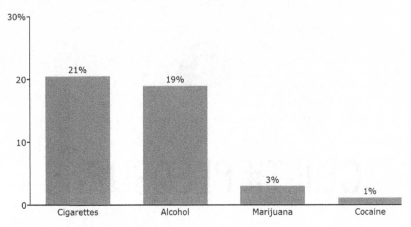

Stub It Out: Cigarettes

We've all seen the SURGEON GENERAL'S WARNING written in bold black lettering on the side of cigarette packages: "Smoking by Pregnant Women May Result in Fetal Injury, Premature Birth, and Low Birth Weight." If smoking still retains an element of glamour despite years of public education campaigns (think Audrey Hepburn with her cigarette holder, or the sirens from *Mad Men*), smoking while pregnant decidedly does not. Penelope Cruz, Kate Moss, Nicole Richie, and Uma Thurman have all been publicly skewered for supposedly lighting up while pregnant, and publicists have been always quick to point out their desire to stop.[6, 7, 8, 9]

There's no controversy anymore about the health effects of smoking. It not only harms you, it harms your chances of a successful pregnancy.[10] According to the surgeon general, the evidence is sufficient to infer a causal relationship between maternal active smoking and premature rupture of the membranes, placental problems, preterm delivery, shortened gestation, fetal growth restriction, and low birth weight, and the evidence is suggestive of a causal relationship between maternal active smoking and ectopic pregnancy and miscarriage.[11] According to the CDC, 11 percent of miscarriages, 5 to 8 percent of preterm deliveries, 13 to 19 percent of term low-birth-weight deliveries,[12, 13] and 5 to 7 percent of preterm-related deaths in the United States are attributable to prenatal smoking.[14] Even smoking fewer than ten cigarettes a day may increase the risk of miscarriage.[15]

The message is resonating. Almost half of smokers manage to stop while pregnant[16] (most pick up the habit again later, but that's another subject). It feels cruel to even cover smoking in a book like this. If you're still smoking, it's probably because you're finding it impossible to quit. And unfortunately, smoking-cessation strategies such as nicotine replacement patches,[17] electronic cigarettes,[18] cognitive behavioral therapy, and regular measurement of nicotine levels all have success rates well below 10 percent.[19]

There is one type of intervention that works noticeably better, however, helping up to a quarter of women stop. That intervention is "financial incentives," otherwise known as bribery.[20, 21] So if you really want to stop smoking while you're pregnant, here's my suggestion: buy some nicotine test kits (various brands are available at reasonable prices on Amazon). Then set up a regular direct debit into a good friend's bank account, involving a sum of money large enough to matter to you. Provide your friend with instructions to cancel each payment only after receiving a negative test from you (www.stickk. com, a site set up by Yale University economists, provides help with setting up such a contract).

Perhaps you're not a smoker yourself, but you're concerned about secondhand smoke. Now that smoking bans are spreading across the country like wildfire, any exposure you're getting is likely to be at home. According to the surgeon general, the evidence linking secondhand smoke to reproductive effects like miscarriage remains inadequate. Unfortunately, that's not the end of the story—there is sufficient evidence to infer a causal relationship between secondhand smoke and sudden infant death syndrome.[22] So if you need to convince your partner to quit, it might be worth starting before the baby is born. (If getting the smoker in the house to quit is impossible, you might consider buying a couple of HEPA air filters, which won't eliminate the effect of secondhand exposure but may reduce the impact somewhat.[23]) Keep in mind: a little bribery never hurts.

Threat level for heavy smoking (20+ cigarettes a day): Very high[24]

Threat level for moderate smoking (10 to 19 a day): Very high[25]

Threat level for light smoking (<10 a day): Very high[26]

The Religion of Drink: Alcohol

Kenora, Ontario, 1981: The young woman is in the final stages of labor, gritting her teeth and screaming through the contractions. Standing by her side is her physician, encouraging and coaching her as she pushes. But unbeknownst to the mother-to-be, another individual lurks in the back corner of the room, watching the labor with careful attention. The baby's head finally begins to emerge. The doctor frees the shoulders, and the baby slips out in a gush of fluid. The mouth and nose are cleared, the cord is cut, and the baby is wrapped in a swaddling blanket. But then, in one quick motion, the physician turns and delivers the bleating bundle into the arms of the stranger, who rushes from the room. The mother, still woozy from her ordeal, slowly props herself up on one elbow. A look of confusion and fear passes over her face. "Where's my baby?"

Little does she know she is about to fight a protracted legal battle over her rights to raise her own child. The baby has been confiscated into the protective care of the local Children's Aid Society on the grounds of prenatal child abuse.[27] The mother's crime? Consumption of alcohol during pregnancy.

New York, NY, 2010: The waiter pauses, the starched white cloth draped over his arm, the perspiring wine bottle hovering over the woman's glass. She gestures for him to proceed. He reluctantly pours a few drops in the bottom of the glass, enough for a tasting. She waves for him to continue. He pours a full glass and turns away, covertly shaking his head in disgust. "Don't worry, sir," she calls out after him, her close-to-full-term bump protruding against the table. "I asked my doctor, and he said it was OK—it will help me relax."

To which religious sect do you belong? Are you among the righteous abstainers, who wave away the tiniest sip during pregnancy? Or are you part of the persecuted minority, those who persist in drinking despite the opprobrium of those around you? Actually, your affiliation when it comes to alcohol can be predicted in large part by your nationality. According to recent surveys, only 12 percent of American women report drinking during pregnancy. This is unsurprising, given the US surgeon general's categorical warning that pregnant women should not drink alcohol.[28] But Americans are absurdly conservative teetotalers in the eyes of other parts of the world: the figure rises to 34 percent in Australia, and all the way up to 52 percent in France and 54 percent in the UK.[29, 30] That's right: more than half of mothers in Great Britain are actively willing to admit to a researcher that they consumed alcohol while pregnant, which means the true figure could well be much higher. Those poor, deluded Brits, dousing their unsuspecting fetuses in poisonous alcohol.

May 2007, England: "Women who are pregnant or trying for a baby should stop drinking alcohol altogether, the Government's leading doctors [at the UK Department of Health] give warning today. The new advice radically revises existing guidelines, which say that women can drink up to two units once or twice a week."[31]

May 2007, England: "It emerged yesterday that the Royal College of Obstetricians and Gynecologists intended to stick with its advice that moderate drinking was perfectly safe, which could leave many pregnant women confused. The college said that it would examine the new advice and decide whether to adopt it 'in due course.'"[32]

October 2007, England: "Confusion over whether women can safely drink during pregnancy deepened yesterday with new guidance stating that a small glass of wine a day is okay. The National Institute for Health and Clinical Excellence [an independent body that sets national treatment guidelines for the UK public health service] said that women can drink up to 1.5 units of alcohol a day without harming their unborn baby. This contradicts Department of Health advice that mothers-to-be should not drink at all, and will leave women wondering which set of 'official' guidelines to follow."[33]

How can three august bodies, presumably staffed with leading scientific minds in the field, have come to such inconsistent conclusions? The answer is that their differences of opinion are philosophical rather than factual. Should government agencies account for the human tendency to push boundaries or not? The speed limit says 65 miles per hour; surely that means you can safely drive at 75. The bottle of aspirin says "not to exceed 4 doses in 24 hours," but your headache is killing you. So you pop double that amount, knowing the lawsuit-wary manufacturers must have included a healthy margin of error.

The UK Department of Health has even admitted that this is the case with its revision of the alcohol policy down to a no-tolerance stance: "Fiona Adshead, the deputy chief medical officer, said that the change was meant to send 'a strong signal' to the thousands of women who drank more than the recommended limit that they were putting their babies at risk. But she admitted that it was not in response to any new medical evidence."[34] No tolerance is simply a national insurance policy.

The media have helped sow confusion around the effects of alcohol during pregnancy. In October 2008, the *Times*, a prominent British newspaper, ran the following headline: "Drinking alcohol occasionally when pregnant 'does no harm.'"[35] According to the article, "researchers at University College London (UCL) examined data on the behavior and mental skills of 12,495 three-year-olds . . . boys born to mothers who drank lightly were 40 percent *less* likely to have conduct problems than those whose mothers abstained, and were 30 percent less likely to be hyperactive. They also had higher scores on tests of vocabulary . . . Girls born to light drinkers were 30 percent less likely to have emotional symptoms and peer problems compared with those born to abstainers, although these differences could partially be explained by family and social backgrounds, the researchers said."[36]

The *Times* was not the only paper to carry the story. "Light drinking during pregnancy may benefit baby,"[37] crowed Fox News, among others. Could this result be true? Does alcohol possess some mysterious property that causes babies to thrive? Was your great-grandmother onto something when she plied her children with brandy to put them to sleep? The idea doesn't make much intuitive sense.

It wasn't long before the scientific community responded. By February 2009, a group of researchers in Toronto had written a response entitled "Does Light Drinking During Pregnancy Improve Pregnancy Outcome? A Critical Commentary." In four brief pages, the authors did their best to rip this study to shreds, pointing out a variety of reasons why the methodology was flawed.[38] Did the mainstream media take note, splashing further headlines across the front pages? Of course not. Critical commentaries don't make for sensational stories that sell newspapers. Instead, women across the UK and the US were left with the erroneous perception that not only had they been given carte blanche to drink moderately during pregnancy, but they might actually be benefiting their fetus by doing so.

It's only natural for the government to interpret, the media to hype, and the academics to scrutinize the evidence about prenatal drinking. So let's examine the evidence directly ourselves. How compelling is the case against alcohol in pregnancy?

There's no doubt whatsoever that when alcohol is consumed in excessive amounts, it passes through the placenta, reaches the fetus, and causes irreversible damage. You may have seen such a photo: the baby's eyes are small and beady, the upper lip looks abnormally thin, and the skin between the nose and mouth is strangely smooth rather than grooved. These are the classic features of fetal alcohol syndrome (FAS), a term coined in 1973 when doctors noticed that women who drank throughout pregnancy typically gave birth prematurely, and their infants frequently suffered from noticeable facial defects and intellectual disability. FAS has since been recognized as the leading known cause of mental disability in the Western world, affecting about 1 in 500 children globally.[39] In the first trimester, when the brain is still forming, alcohol can cause major structural brain deformities. If you drank before realizing you were pregnant, you're in good company. According to the CDC, one in twenty pregnant women consumes alcohol prior to pregnancy recognition.[40, 41] Unfortunately, there is no "safe" window in early pregnancy (e.g., prior to implantation) when the fetus is protected from exposure to alcohol. Research in both animals[42, 43] and humans[44, 45] has shown the potential for harmful effects from high levels of exposure ("binge drinking") even in very early pregnancy. Later in pregnancy, alcohol can damage the hippocampus and cause problems with areas such as learning, memory, and emotion. Women who drink heavily throughout pregnancy have a rate of fetal alcohol syndrome somewhere between 2.5 and 4 percent.[46]

Evidence on the impact of drinking small amounts of alcohol is far less definitive. There are a variety of troubles plaguing these types of studies (which also apply to some of the other guilty pleasures covered later in this chapter). One problem is that small effects tend to get lost in random noise. If you're evaluating a new baby formula that claims to make children grow one millimeter taller, you're going to have a difficult time proving your claim if one of the children getting the placebo has a professional basketball player for a parent. The only way around this problem is a very large sample size, which means a costly study.

Another problem is that it's hard to isolate the effects of small amounts of alcohol from other influential factors. People who drink alcohol aren't necessarily the same as people who abstain. For example, drinkers are more likely to smoke and do drugs, both of which may negatively impact their children. On the flip side, people who drink may be more sociable and outgoing by nature, and those who drink only in moderation may have more self-control than those who binge drink or have to abstain altogether. A randomized, controlled study could adjust for these effects, but it's not exactly ethical to urge a random group of women to drink more than they would have while pregnant. This means researchers are left to compare self-selected drinkers with teetotalers and do their best to statistically adjust for the fact that these two populations are likely different in many ways beyond just their inclination toward drinking alcohol. Add to this the fact that alcohol use during pregnancy is often underreported by mothers due to its social stigma, and you can see why the answer to this very important question remains wide open.

There is hope in sight: researchers are currently developing bio-markers, or objective tests of how much a mother has drunk during pregnancy.[47] And there are a number of studies recently published and more underway that are bound to shed further light on the subject.[48, 49] Many of these newer studies are "prospective": the researchers find a population of pregnant women, evaluate their drinking habits, and then follow the offspring over a number of years. This takes patience, but it eliminates the problem of mothers misrecalling their drinking habits, another problem with some of the existing studies.

In the meantime, some information would be better than none. One option is to look at animal studies, in which researchers have the freedom to, say, douse pregnant rats with alcohol and then dissect the brains of their fetuses to examine the effects. With high alcohol exposure in the womb, rat babies develop the rat equivalent of fetal alcohol syndrome. But even at low levels of alcohol exposure, researchers find evidence of brain cell loss in the fetuses[50]—although the fetal brains manage to recover functionality over time by reorganizing and bringing in cells from elsewhere to take over the required tasks.[51]

It's always difficult to know whether animal studies can be generalized to people. So let's turn to human studies, despite their imperfections. Let me introduce you to the Seattle socialites. In 1974, a group of researchers at the University of Washington, Seattle, chose 250 women who drank at "social drinking" levels and 250 infrequent drinkers and abstainers and interviewed them in their fifth month of pregnancy. The researchers then evaluated the children at birth, eight months, eighteen months, and four, seven, eleven, and fourteen years, publishing reports of their findings along the way.[52, 53]

This was a great study because the women were a homogeneous group at low risk for adverse pregnancy outcomes (primarily white, married, and middle class). The researchers asked women about their drinking habits while they were still pregnant (and did their best to ensure honest reports) rather than requiring them to recall their drinking habits later.[54] Finally, these women were very moderate social drinkers, consuming a median of one drink per day before realizing they were pregnant and less than one drink per day mid-pregnancy.

The researchers bided their time. By age seven, "the children's performance in general was very good, with mean IQ of 107.6." However, a closer look revealed subtle differences in performance between the children of drinkers versus abstainers: "The more alcohol use reported by the mother, the longer the time delay to attach to the nipple in the newborn, the longer the delay to self-correct errors on a fine motor maze task at age 4 years, and the longer the reaction time on vigilance tasks at 4 and 7 years . . . [By age 7], children exposed to more than 1 ounce of absolute alcohol per day mid-pregnancy [equivalent to 2 drinks per day] had a mean IQ 6.7 points lower than children exposed to less than this amount, even after adjustment [for other confounding factors]."

Two drinks per day is still rather a lot, you say. So what's the smallest amount of alcohol that has ever been shown to have an effect? One study of ~500 African-American women found that children exposed to even a single drink per week in the womb were more likely to demonstrate aggressive and delinquent behavior at age seven,[55] although the populations of drinkers versus non-drinkers were different on several dimensions and the effect was small. A group of researchers followed 580 Pittsburgh babies to age fourteen and concluded "prenatal alcohol exposure continues to affect size [weight, height, head circumference] at age 14 . . . at levels below one drink per day."[56] And finally, perhaps the largest study to consider this question analyzed ~32,000 pregnancies in the United States and concluded that drinking even less than one unit per day in the second half of pregnancy increased the chance of having a low-birth-weight infant.[57]

In contrast, plenty of studies have found no appreciable effect from small amounts of alcohol. For example, one study of 665 women in Australia found that moderate drinking had no effect on measurements of newborns at birth,[58] while another Australian study followed the children of 2,900 women for fourteen years and found no link between low and moderate levels of alcohol consumption in pregnancy and later behavior in children.[59] A study in Scotland concluded that drinking fewer than three drinks per week appeared to have no effect on mental and motor development at eighteen months of age.[60] And a series of studies in Denmark found that low to moderate drinking in early pregnancy had no significant effect on developmental outcomes in children.[61]

There has also been plenty of research examining a link between drinking and miscarriage, and again the results have been mixed. There's only one discernible pattern: studies from North America (where drinking during pregnancy is frowned upon) tend to show a link, while studies from Europe and Australia (where drinking during pregnancy is more socially acceptable) don't.[62] This strange fact suggests that maybe we are indeed measuring the impact of lifestyle choices that are correlated with willingness to flout public opinion on important health topics rather than just the effects of alcohol consumption.

In summary, we still have no idea whether small amounts of alcohol are harmful. According to one frequently cited review, "given the state of our knowledge, it is impossible to conclude whether low-level alcohol intake in pregnancy has clinically significant deleterious effects on the individual or not."[63] No wonder the governments of the world can't agree on a policy!

In the end, I'd probably call myself an agnostic when it comes to the religion of alcohol in pregnancy. I'm not the disapproving waiter, nor am I the pregnant woman freely drinking several glasses of wine with dinner. If I see you raising a celebratory glass of champagne to toast to the health of your bump, I'll smile and toast with you. But rather than downing my glass, I'll be taking a token sip.

Threat level for drinking heavily throughout pregnancy: Very high[64]

Threat level for drinking minimally (<1 drink per day): Very low[65]

A Need for Weed: Marijuana

When you're pregnant, sometimes even the thought of food is enough to bring on intractable waves of nausea. You're supposed to be gaining weight, but instead you're steadily losing it, spending much of the day huddled over the toilet. If you have the misfortune to fall in the 0.5 percent of women who experience *hyperemesis gravidarum*, otherwise known as severe, debilitating morning sickness during pregnancy, you're now in luck.[66] A drug proven to relieve nausea in chemotherapy patients[67] and effective at reducing symptoms of nausea in 92 percent of pregnant women[68] has recently been added to the arsenal available to your doctor. The downside? If you fill your doctor's prescription, there's a very real chance you could be arrested the day your baby is born.[69, 70]

We have recently reached an inflection point in our attitude toward cannabis in the United States. As various states experiment with legalizing medical marijuana, unintentional loopholes inevitably proliferate. At the moment, pregnant women are not explicitly banned from using marijuana, and physicians are not legally required to ask patients if they're pregnant before prescribing it. Yet hospitals can still report a pregnant woman to Child Protective Services if they suspect she's been using the substance.[71] For many women, this risk would be unacceptable. But for those debilitated by nausea, the upside can outweigh the downside.[72]

I seriously doubt you're planning to get high while pregnant. *Hyperemesis gravidarum* is hardly a common problem, and for those who don't suffer it, you no doubt have sufficient willpower to quit smoking pot. Actress Evan Rachel Wood, the former fiancée of Marilyn Manson, may have complained, but even she chose to swear off weed during her pregnancy.[73] Nevertheless, I am covering the topic, and here's why: if we're going to have societal taboos about pregnancy, let's at least make sure we've gotten our taboos right—particularly at a moment when our laws are being rewritten.

Yet again, research on marijuana use is difficult for all the obvious reasons. THC, the active ingredient in marijuana, does travel through the placenta to reach the baby.[74] But women who smoke weed while pregnant are also more likely to smoke cigarettes, drink, use other drugs, come from a lower socioeconomic background, eat a poorer diet, skip prenatal care,[75] and/or report their exposure inaccurately.[76] In the face of all these limitations, what can we conclude about the effects of smoking pot during pregnancy? It might reduce birth weight slightly. Some studies have observed this effect,[77, 78] although not others.[79, 80] The authors of one meta-analysis point out that the effect appears to be "weaker than has been observed for cigarette smoking."[81]

Researchers have also poured lots of energy into investigating longer-term effects in children. Have they managed to find the marijuana equivalent of fetal alcohol syndrome, without the facial defects? Here, it's even more difficult to say. One long-term study of low-risk, white, middle-class women from Canada concluded that by age four, children with prenatal marijuana exposure had more behavioral problems and more difficulty with "visual perceptual tasks, language comprehension, sustained attention, and memory."[82] Another long-term study of higher-risk women from Pittsburgh found subtle effects of marijuana on IQ at age three[83] and on hyperactivity and impulsiveness at age ten.[84] Heavy marijuana use (smoking at least once a day) had more noticeable effects.[85]

But women who cavalierly continue to smoke pot while pregnant are likely to be more negligent parents in general, so the effects become hard to separate. As a review from 2009 puts it, the "postnatal behavioral effects of prenatal cannabis exposure seem modest. The causal interpretation of any such effects is weakened by the inability of these studies to control for the confounding effects of other drug use during pregnancy, poor parenting, and genetic factors."[86]

There is one way to avoid this problem, and that's to travel outside the US. In Jamaica, "ganja" may technically be illegal,[87] but the law is widely ignored.[88] More important, marijuana is culturally integrated, playing "ritual and medicinal as well as recreational functions."[89] And unlike the United States and Canada, "marijuana use by women in Jamaica has been relatively uncontaminated by other drugs; even alcohol and tobacco are used only minimally by women."[90] In this environment, a small study of marijuana-exposed babies has shown no negative impact on these children at three days or one month old, or at ages four and five.[91, 92]

Should you give up smoking pot while pregnant? The evidence is hardly definitive. (There is also no good evidence yet on the effects of

edible marijuana during pregnancy, although this topic has been identified as an important research gap.[93]) Should you be arrested if you
don't? Here, we can be a bit more definitive: certainly not.

Threat level for smoking marijuana: Very low[94]

Conclusions: The Crack Babies That Weren't

1985: US Congressman George Miller (founding chairman of the
House Select Committee on Children, Youth, and Families), using
the newly minted term "crack babies," declares on national television
that "these children, who are the most expensive babies ever born in
America, are going to overwhelm every social service delivery system
that they come into contact with throughout the rest of their lives."[95]
Tom Brokaw, Peter Jennings, and Dan Rather all launch coverage of
the "crack baby" epidemic.[96]

1997: The charity C.R.A.C.K. (Children Requiring a Caring
Kommunity) is founded and begins to generate national press coverage for paying drug-addicted mothers $200 to accept long-acting
contraception or sterilization.[97, 98]

2000: The US Supreme Court hears a case in which mothers at the
Medical University of South Carolina were screened for cocaine then
arrested directly after giving birth.[99]

The movement to protect crack babies rode a wave of good inten-
tions. No one wanted an entire generation of American children
growing up stunted by the effects of burgeoning drug use. The only
problem was . . . they weren't. It's not that cocaine is harmless—it may
slightly increase the risk of miscarriage.[100] And the children of women
who used cocaine early in pregnancy appear to be more likely to be
born underweight or premature,[101, 102, 103, 104] to have a slightly higher
rate of certain birth defects,[105] and, later in life, to have slightly more
difficulty controlling their behavior and paying attention for long periods of time.[106] But the effects are subtle: newborns of cocaine-abusing
mothers show no dramatic symptoms of withdrawal,[107] and reviews
have concluded that longer-term, exposed children have "similar performance patterns to non-exposed children living in similar

low-income, urban settings . . . prenatal cocaine exposure does not seem to confer significant risk to school-aged children's performance on global measures of intellectual functioning."[108, 109]

If you're reading a book like this, I suspect you're unlikely to be among the one percent of women who use cocaine while pregnant. You're certainly not a crack addict, and even if you had a social cocaine habit, you've probably put that lifestyle on hold (which would be a very sensible choice, given the potential downsides described above). So why am I bothering to discuss this topic? Because the story about cocaine again highlights our skewed perspectives of relative risk.

Here's a comparison between cocaine and cigarettes: "When prenatal cocaine and tobacco exposure are compared dispassionately, it becomes clear how sociopolitical forces shape discrepant interpretations of similar scientific data. The mechanisms of nicotine and cocaine effects on the developing brain are similar . . . Prenatal tobacco exposure has been associated with infant mortality, moderate impairment of cognitive functioning, and a range of behavioral problems (which, unlike those associated with cocaine exposure, are detectable on relatively insensitive epidemiologic measures) . . . but there are no sterilization campaigns for mothers who use tobacco. No pregnant women have been charged with child abuse for tobacco use in pregnancy. Teachers do not dread having a 'tobacco kid' assigned to their class."[110]

Similarly, a number of experts have recently gone on record in the media to make another point that's obvious once you examine the data: alcohol is far more dangerous to a fetus than cocaine is.[111, 112] According to the Institute of Medicine, "Of all the substances of abuse, including heroin, cocaine, and marijuana, alcohol produces by far the most serious neurobehavioral effects in the fetus."[113] But women who would never even remotely consider taking an illicit drug during their pregnancy may be fairly casual about drinking alcohol.

Our taboos may be outdated, but they persist powerfully nevertheless. Your local cocaine dealer won't be achieving the social acceptance or prestige of a sommelier anytime soon.

Threat level for abusing cocaine: Medium[114, 115]

Notes

1. Inman, T. (1860). On morning sickness: its significance as a symptom. *British Medical Journal, 1* (169), 223. www.ncbi.nlm.nih.gov/pmc/articles/PMC2252653/pdf/ brmedjo6049-0005.pdf.

2. Kershaw, R. (1892). Special hospitals. *British medical journal, 2* (1644), 50. www.ncbi.nlm. nih.gov/pmc/articles/PMC2420633/pdf/brmedjo8854-0050d.pdf.

3. Jackie Kennedy, pregnant and smoking, Hyannis Port, 1963. (2012, August 25). PhotosOfWar.net. https://www.pinterest.co.uk/pin/226657793719744526/.

4. Smith, S. B. (2005). *Grace and power: the private world of the Kennedy White House*. New York: Random House.

5. National Institute on Drug Abuse Division of Epidemiology & Prevention Research. (1996). National Pregnancy & Health Survey: drug use among women delivering livebirths, 1992. Department of Health and Human Services, National Institutes of Health. https://babel. hathitrust.org/cgi/pt?id=pur1.32754066652243;view=1up;seq=2.

6. Penelope Cruz busted for smoking while pregnant; is her habit harming her unborn child? (2011, April 14). iNewsWire.com. www.i-newswire.com/ penelope-cruz-busted-for-smoking/102559.

7. Nicholl, K. (n.d.). Pregnancy? It's a drag for Kate. *The Daily Mail*. www.dailymail.co.uk/ health/article-111881/Pregnancy-Its-drag-Kate.html.

8. Adams, C. (2007, October 30). Pregnant Nichole Richie seen smoking cigarette. AceShowBiz. com. www.aceshowbiz.com/news/view/00012082.html.

9. Money to burn: Uma Thurman risks $250 fine as she lights up illegally in a public park. (2011, March 8). *The Daily Mail*. www.dailymail.co.uk/tvshowbiz/article-1364222/Uma-Thurman-risks-250-fine-lights-illegally-public-park.html.

10. DiFranza, J. R., Aligne, C. A., & Weitzman, M. (2004). Prenatal and postnatal environmental tobacco smoke exposure and children's health. *Pediatrics, 113* (Supplement 3), 1007–1015. http://pediatrics.aappublications.org/content/113/Supplement_3/1007.long.

    For a thorough review of the current knowledge on how the various chemicals in cigarettes contribute to problems in pregnancy, see the following publication: How tobacco smoke causes disease: the biology and behavioral basis for smoking-attributable disease—a report of the surgeon general. (2010). Centers for Disease Control and Prevention. www.ncbi.nlm.nih.gov/books/NBK53022/.

11. The health consequences of smoking: a report of the surgeon general. (2004). US Department of Health and Human Services. www.cdc.gov/tobacco/data_statistics/sgr/2004/ pdfs/chapter5.pdf.

12. PRAMS (the Pregnancy Risk Assessment Monitoring System) and smoking data tables. (2011, December 19). Centers for Disease Control and Prevention. https://www.cdc.gov/ prams/index.htm.

13. Centers for Disease Control. (2001). Women and smoking: a report of the surgeon general. CDC Office on Smoking and Health, Atlanta, GA. www.cdc.gov/tobacco/data_statistics/ sgr/2001/complete_report/pdfs/chp3.pdf.

14. Dietz, P. M., England, L. J., Shapiro-Mendoza, C. K., Tong, V. T., Farr, S. L., & Callaghan, W. M. (2010). Infant morbidity and mortality attributable to prenatal smoking in the US. *American Journal of Preventive Medicine, 39* (1), 45–52. http://www.sciencedirect.com/ science/article/pii/S0749379710002588.

15. According to a 2010 report from the Surgeon General (Centers for Disease Control and Prevention, How tobacco smoke causes disease). "The 2004 Surgeon General's report on

the health consequences of smoking found the evidence suggestive but not sufficient to infer a causal relationship between smoking and miscarriage (USDHHS 2004). However, numerous studies are available since the handful reviewed at that time, and most show positive associations. . . . In a meta-analysis of data from 13 studies [DiFranza, J. R., & Lew, R. A. (1995). Effect of maternal cigarette smoking on pregnancy complications and sudden infant death syndrome. *Journal of Family Practice, 40* (4), 385–394. www.ncbi.nlm.nih.gov/pubmed/7699353], the pooled ORs for miscarriage in smokers were 1.24 for cohort studies and 1.32 for case-control studies." An average of these two gives an odds ratio of 1.28. The baseline incidence of miscarriage in the population is 19.9% as calculated in a previous footnote on lead. So applying the appropriate conversion formula (Higgins, J. P. T., & Green, S. [eds.]. [2011, March]. Computing absolute risk reduction or NNT from an odds ratio [OR]. *Cochrane Handbook for Systematic Reviews of Interventions* 12.5.4.3. http://handbook.cochrane.org/chapter_12/12_5_4_3_computing_absolute_risk_reduction_or_nnt_from_an_odds.htm), that equates to a 4.23% absolute increase in miscarriage attributable to smoking in general. To break this down by number of cigarettes, according to one study (Armstrong, B. G., McDonald, A. D., & Sloan, M. [1992]. Cigarette, alcohol, and coffee consumption and spontaneous abortion. *American Journal of Public Health, 82* [1], 85–87. www.ncbi.nlm.nih.gov/pmc/articles/PMC1694397/pdf/amjph00538-0087.pdf), the odds ratios for miscarriage are 1.07 for 1–9 cigarettes a day, 1.22 for 10–19 per day, and 1.68 for 20+ per day. So that works out to absolute increases in miscarriage of 1.1%, 3.36%, and 9.55% respectively.

16. Centers for Disease Control and Prevention, PRAMS and smoking data tables.

17. Wisborg, K., Henriksen, T. B., Jespersen, L. B., & Secher, N. J. (2000). Nicotine patches for pregnant smokers: a randomized controlled study. *Obstetrics & Gynecology, 96* (6), 967–971. www.pi.nhs.uk/smoking/paper.pdf.

The jury remains out on using nicotine replacement products such as nicotine gum and the nicotine patch during pregnancy. These products can help people quit smoking and are recommended by the Agency of Health Care Policy and Research regardless of pregnancy status (Fiore, M. C., Wetter, D. W., Bailey, W. C., Bennett, G., Cohen, S. J., Dorfman, S. F., Goldstein, M. G., Gritz, E. R., Hasselblad, V., Henningfield, J. E., Heyman, R. B., Holbrook, J., Husten, C., Jaen, C. R., Kohler, C., Kottke, T. E., Lando, H. A., Manley, M., Mecklenburg, R., Melvin, C., Mullen, P. D., Nett, L. M., Piasecki, T. M., Robinson, L., Rothstein, D., Schriger, D. L., Stitzer, M. L., Stachenko, S., Tommasello, A., Villejo, L., Wewers, M. E., & Baker, T. B. [1996]. The Agency for Health Care Policy and Research smoking cessation clinical practice guideline. *JAMA, 275* [16], 1270–1280. http://jama.jamanetwork.com/article.aspx?articleid=401129). However, according to the United States Preventive Task Force, the safety and efficacy of these products during pregnancy has not been sufficiently well studied (US Preventive Services Task Force. [2009]. Counseling and interventions to prevent tobacco use and tobacco-caused disease in adults and pregnant women: US Preventive Services Task Force reaffirmation recommendation statement. *Annals of Internal Medicine, 150* [8], 551. http://annals.org/aim/article/2443060/).

18. Bullen, C., Howe, C., Laugesen, M., McRobbie, H., Parag, V., Williman, J., & Walker, N. (2013). Electronic cigarettes for smoking cessation: a randomised controlled trial. *The Lancet, 382* (9905), 1629–1637. http://www.sciencedirect.com/science/article/pii/S0140673613618425.

19. Lumley, J., Chamberlain, C., Dowswell, T., Oliver, S., Oakley, L., & Watson, L. (2009). Interventions for promoting smoking cessation during pregnancy. *Cochrane Database of Systematic Reviews, 3* (3). http://onlinelibrary.wiley.com/doi/10.1002/14651858.CD001055.pub3/full.

20. Ibid.

21. Higgins, S. T., Washio, Y., Heil, S. H., Solomon, L. J., Gaalema, D. E., Higgins, T. M., & Bernstein, I. M. (2012). Financial incentives for smoking cessation among pregnant and newly postpartum women. *Preventive Medicine, 55,* S33–S40. www.ncbi.nlm.nih.gov/pmc/articles/PMC3399924/.

22. US Department of Health and Human Services. (2006). The health consequences of involuntary exposure to tobacco smoke: a report of the surgeon general. US Department of Health and Human Services, Centers for Disease Control and Prevention, Coordinating Center for Health Promotion, National Center for Chronic Disease Prevention and Health Promotion, Office on Smoking and Health, 709. www.surgeongeneral.gov/library/reports/secondhandsmoke/chapter5.pdf.

23. Butz, A. M., Matsui, E. C., Breysse, P., Curtin-Brosnan, J., Eggleston, P., Diette, G., Williams, D., Yuan, J., Bernert, J. T., & Rand, C. (2011). A randomized trial of air cleaners and a health coach to improve indoor air quality for inner-city children with asthma and secondhand smoke exposure. *Archives of Pediatrics & Adolescent Medicine, 165* (8), 741. www.ncbi.nlm.nih.gov/pubmed/21810636.

24. Threat score is 9.55% (probability of miscarriage) x 100,000 (impact: death) x 1 (certainty: well proven) = 9,550.

25. Threat score is 3.36% (probability of miscarriage) x 100,000 (impact: death) x 1 (certainty: well proven) = 3,360.

26. Threat score is 1.1% (probability of miscarriage) x 100,000 (impact: death) x 1 (certainty: well proven) = 1,100.

27. *Children's Aid Society for the District of Kenora vs. J. L.* (1981) 134 D. I. R. (3d) 249 (Ont. Prov. Ct.).

28. General, U. S., & Carmona, V. A. R. H. (2004). Advisory on alcohol use in pregnancy. US Department of Health and Human Services. www.cdc.gov/ncbddd/fasd/documents/surgeongenbookmark.pdf.

29. Peadon, E., Payne, J., Bower, C., Elliott, E., Henley, N., O'Leary, C., D'Antoine, H., & Bartu, A. (2007). Alcohol and pregnancy: women's knowledge, attitudes and practice. *Journal of Paediatrics and Child Health, 43* (7–8), A12.

30. De Chazeron, I., Llorca, P. M., Ughetto, S., Vendittelli, F., Boussiron, D., Sapin, V., Coudore, F., & Lemery, D. (2008). Is pregnancy the time to change alcohol consumption habits in France? *Alcoholism: Clinical and Experimental Research, 32* (5), 868–873. https://www.ncbi.nlm.nih.gov/pubmed/18373726.

31. Bennett, R. (2007, May 25). Zero—the new alcohol limit in pregnancy. TheTimes.co.uk. www.thetimes.co.uk/tto/health/article1962101.ece.

32. Ibid.

33. MacRae, F. (2007, October 10). Now pregnant women are told: 'It IS safe to drink daily glass of wine.' *The Daily Mail.* www.dailymail.co.uk/health/article-486780/Now-pregnant-women-told-It-IS-safe-drink-daily-glass-wine.html.

34. Bennett, R., Zero—the new alcohol limit in pregnancy.

35. Drinking alcohol occasionally when pregnant 'does no harm'. (2008, October 31). TheTimes.co.uk. www.thetimes.co.uk/tto/health/article1962101.ece.

36. Kelly, Y., Sacker, A., Gray, R., Kelly, J., Wolke, D., & Quigley, M. A. (2009). Light drinking in pregnancy, a risk for behavioural problems and cognitive deficits at 3 years of age? *International Journal of Epidemiology, 38* (1), 129–140. http://ije.oxfordjournals.org/content/38/1/129.full?HITS=10&hits=10&andorexacttitle=&maxtoshow=&author1=kelly&RESULTFORMAT=1.

37. Light drinking during pregnancy may benefit baby. (2008, October 31). FoxNews.com. www.foxnews.com/story/2008/10/31/light-drinking-during-pregnancy-may-benefit-baby/.

38. What were the flaws in the UCL study? The authors of the response pointed out two major shortcomings. The first issue was that the mother's drinking levels were established based on asking the mothers themselves to recall their own drinking habits during pregnancy a full nine months after the birth of their babies, or fifteen to eighteen months since the first trimester. This is problematic on many levels. Mothers may no longer recall exactly how much they drank so long ago; their recall may be biased by their knowledge of how their baby has been behaving more recently; or, most importantly, they may knowingly underreport their drinking: "It has been well established that maternal self-reports of alcohol use are often unreliable due to fears of stigmatization, embarrassment, shame or guilt. . . . Combined use of the AUDIT questionnaire and samples for direct ethanol metabolites detect more potential alcohol consumers than any of these tests on its own" (Alvik, A., Haldorsen, T., Groholt, B., & Lindemann, R. [2006]. Alcohol consumption before and during pregnancy comparing concurrent and retrospective reports. *Alcoholism: Clinical and Experimental Research, 30* [3], 510–515. http://onlinelibrary.wiley.com/doi/10.1111/j.1530-0277.2006.00055.x/full; Ernhart, C. B., Morrow-Tlucak, M., Sokol, R. J., & Martier, S. [1988]. Underreporting of alcohol use in pregnancy. *Alcoholism: Clinical and Experimental Research, 12* [4], 506–511. http://onlinelibrary.wiley.com/doi/10.1111/j.1530-0277.1988.tb00233.x/full; Sayal, K. [2009]. Commentary: light drinking in pregnancy: can a glass or two hurt? *International Journal of Epidemiology, 38* [1], 140–142. http://ije.oxfordjournals.org/content/38/1/140.full.pdf). Women are understandably embarrassed to admit to a researcher that they drank during their pregnancy, and direct tests for alcohol levels reveal plenty of drinkers who claim not to be. The second problem with the study is the more important one, namely that the researchers likely picked up correlation rather than causation. As the typical example goes: on days when it rains, people tend to carry umbrellas; this doesn't mean that carrying umbrellas causes it to rain. Even the primary author of the study herself acknowledged that this might have been an issue: "The reasons behind these findings might in part be because light drinkers tend to be more socially advantaged than abstainers, rather than being due to the physical benefits of low level alcohol consumption seen, for example, in heart disease" (Parkinson, C. [2008, October 31]. Light drinking 'no risk to baby.' BBCNews.com. http://news.bbc.co.uk/1/hi/health/7699579.stm). Other researchers looking at the question of alcohol use in pregnancy have come to similar conclusions: "Substance-use research suggests that moderate drinkers are mentally healthier than both abstainers and addicts (Stranges, S., Notaro, J., Freudenheim, J. L., Calogero, R. M., Muti, P., Farinaro, E., Russell, M., Nochajski, T. H., & Trevisan, M. [2006]. Alcohol drinking pattern and subjective health in a population-based study. *Addiction, 101* [9], 1265–1276. http://onlinelibrary.wiley.com/doi/10.1111/j.1360-0443.2006.01517.x/full), which is attributed to the self-efficacy and behavioral self-management required for moderating substance intake (Peele, S., & Brodsky, A. [2000]. Exploring psychological benefits associated with moderate alcohol use: a necessary corrective to assessments of drinking outcomes? *Drug and Alcohol Dependence, 60* [3], 221–247. http://www.sciencdirect.com/science/article/pii/S0376871600001125; Vaillant, G. E. [2009]. *The natural history of alcoholism revisited.* Cambridge, MA: Harvard University Press). The self-control that allows light–moderate drinkers to contain and manage their drinking quite plausibly enables better parenting and positive child well-being" (Finkenauer, C., Engels, R. C., & Baumeister, R. F. [2005]. Parenting behaviour and adolescent behavioural and emotional problems: the role of self-control. *International Journal of Behavioral Development, 29* [1], 58–69. http://www.tandfonline.com/doi/abs/10.1080/01650250444000333; Robinson, M., Oddy, W. H., McLean, N. J., Jacoby, P., Pennell, C. E., De Klerk, N. H., Zubrick, S. R., Stanley, F. J., & Newnham, J. P. [2010]. Low–moderate prenatal alcohol exposure and risk to child behavioural development: a prospective cohort study. *BJOG:*

An International Journal of Obstetrics & Gynaecology, 117 [9], 1139–1152. http://onlineli-brary.wiley.com/doi/10.1111/j.1471-0528.2010.02596.x/full). People who drink socially may be the kind of people who make more relaxed, confident parents, or they may have simply passed along their social skills to their children genetically. Regardless, both of these are more plausible explanations than concluding the alcohol itself did the children good while in utero. As a final passing criticism, the authors of the critique point out that the study failed to find any negative effect of alcohol at all, even in heavy drinkers: "It is important to note that not only the light drinkers did not do worse than the abstinence group, the moderate and heavy drinkers did not do worse either. . . . This conclusion would go against a large body of evidence supporting a detrimental role of alcohol in pregnancy."

39. Abel, E., & Sokol, R. (1987). Incidence of fetal alcohol syndrome and economic impact of FAS-related anomalies: drug alcohol syndrome and economic impact of FAS-related anom-alies. *Drug and Alcohol Dependency, 19* (1), 51–70. http://www.sciencedirect.com/science/article/pii/0376871687900871.

40. Fact sheets—excessive alcohol use and risks to women's health. (Last reviewed 2016, March 7). Centers for Disease Control and Prevention: Alcohol and Public Health. www.cdc.gov/alcohol/fact-sheets/womens-health.htm.

41. Floyd, R. L., Decouflé, P., & Hungerford, D. W. (1999). Alcohol use prior to pregnancy recognition. *American Journal of Preventive Medicine, 17* (2), 101–107. www.sciencedirect.com/science/article/pii/S0749379799000598.

42. Mitchell, J. A. (1994). Effects of alcohol on blastocyst implantation and fecundity in the rat. *Alcoholism: Clinical and Experimental Research, 18* (1), 29–34. http://onlinelibrary.wiley.com/doi/10.1111/j.1530-0277.1994.tb00876.x/abstract.

43. Sandor, S., Checiu, M., Fazakas-Todea, I., & Garban, Z. (1979). The effect of ethanol upon early development in mice and rats. I. In vivo effect upon preimplantation and early post-implantation stages. *Morphologie et Embryologie, 26* (3), 265–274. http://europepmc.org/abstract/MED/6453289.

44. Floyd, R. L., et al., Alcohol use prior to pregnancy recognition.

45. Little, R. E., Asker, R. L., Sampson, P. D., & Renwick, J. H. (1986). Fetal growth and mod-erate drinking in early pregnancy. *American Journal of Epidemiology, 123* (2), 270–278. http://aje.oxfordjournals.org/content/123/2/270.short.

46. Sampson, P. D., Streissguth, A. P., Bookstein, F. L., Little, R. E., Clarren, S. K., Dehaene, P., Hanson, J. W., & Graham, J. M. (1997). Incidence of fetal alcohol syndrome and prevalence of alcohol-related neurodevelopmental disorder. *Teratology, 56* (5), 317–326. https://www.ncbi.nlm.nih.gov/pubmed/9451756.

   In one study referenced in the review, drinking consistently was defined as "either at least one ounce of absolute alcohol per day [in the United States, the standard drink contains 0.6 fluid ounces of alcohol (Standard drink. [n.d.]. Wikipedia. http://en.wiki-pedia.org/wiki/Standard_drink), so this is equivalent to about 2 drinks per day], or more than 17.5 drinks per month with ingestion of five or more drinks on at least one occasion." This study yielded two cases of FAS out of 80, or 2%. In another study, the rate of FAS among a population drinking an unspecified amount was 25/600, or 4%. Finally, according to another study, "determining the incidence of the fetal alcohol syndrome in only those infants whose mothers were alcoholic during their pregnancy is difficult, because obtaining a random or unselected sample of alcoholic women is virtually impos-sible. . . . Our own study of middle-class volunteers who recovered from alcoholism after the pregnancy yielded a rate of 4% of cases of the fetal alcohol syndrome" (Little, R. E., Streissguth, A. P., Barr, H. M., & Herman, C. S. [1980]. Decreased birth weight in infants of alcoholic women who abstained during pregnancy. *The Journal of Pediatrics, 96* (6), 974–977. www.sciencedirect.com/

science/article/pii/S0022347680806202, as cited in: Little, R. E., & Streissguth, A. P. [1981]. Effects of alcohol on the fetus: impact and prevention. *Canadian Medical Association Journal, 125* [2], 159. www.ncbi.nlm.nih.gov/pmc/articles/PMC1862275/pdf/ canmedaj01347-0039.pdf).

47. Littner, Yoav, & Cynthia F. Bearer. (2007). "Detection of alcohol consumption during pregnancy—current and future biomarkers." *Neuroscience & Biobehavioral Reviews, 31* (2), 261–269. www.researchgate.net/profile/Cynthia_Bearer/publication/6867925_Detection_ of_alcohol_consumption_during_pregnancy-Current_and_future_biomarkers/links/09e-4150954a154ef7f000000.pdf.

48. Sbrana, M., Grandi, C., Brazan, M., Junquera, N., Nascimento, M. S., Barbieri, M. A., Bettiol, H., & Cardoso, V. C. (2016). Alcohol consumption during pregnancy and perinatal results: a cohort study. *Sao Paulo Medical Journal, 134* (2), 146–152. www.scielo.br/ scielo.php?script=sci_arttext&pid=S1516-31802016000200146.

49. May, P. A., & Gossage. J. P. (2001). Estimating the prevalence of fetal alcohol syndrome: a summary. *Alcohol Research and Health, 25* (3), 159–167. https://pubs.niaaa.nih.gov/publi-cations/arh25-3/159-167.htm.

50. Young, C., & Olney, J. W. (2006). Neuroapoptosis in the infant mouse brain triggered by a transient small increase in blood alcohol concentration. *Neurobiology of Disease, 22* (3), 548–554. http://www.sciencedirect.com/science/article/pii/S0969996105003505.

51. Wozniak, D. F., Hartman, R. E., Boyle, M. P., Vogt, S. K., Brooks, A. R., Tenkova, T., Young, C., Olney, J. W., & Muglia, L. J. (2004). Apoptotic neurodegeneration induced by ethanol in neonatal mice is associated with profound learning/memory deficits in juveniles followed by progressive functional recovery in adults. *Neurobiology of Disease, 17* (3), 403–414. http://www.sciencedirect.com/science/article/pii/S0969996104001913.

52. Streissguth, A. P., Barr, H. M., & Sampson, P. D. (1990). Moderate prenatal alcohol exposure: effects on child IQ and learning problems at age 7 1/2 years. *Alcoholism: Clinical and Experimental Research, 14* (5), 662–669. http://onlinelibrary.wiley.com/ doi/10.1111/j.1530-0277.1990.tb01224.x/full.

53. Streissguth, A. P., Sampson, P. D., Olson, H. C., Bookstein, F. L., Barr, H. M., Scott, M., Fedlman, J., & Mirsky, A. F. (1994). Maternal drinking during pregnancy: attention and short-term memory in 14-year-old offspring—a longitudinal prospective study. *Alcoholism: Clinical and Experimental Research, 18* (1), 202–218. http://deepblue.lib.umich.edu/bit-stream/handle/2027.42/66151/j.1530-0277.1994.tb00904.x.pdf?sequence=1.

54. "(1) The study was conducted prior to general knowledge about the adverse effects of drinking during pregnancy, (2) the interview was conducted in the woman's own home without anyone else present, (3) the interview was conducted by a research assistant identified as not part of the hospital staff and (4) the mother was informed that the infor-mation would not become part of her medical record" (Streissguth, A. P., et al., Moderate prenatal alcohol exposure: effects on child IQ and learning problems at age 7 1/2 years).

55. Sood, B., Delaney-Black, V., Covington, C., Nordstrom-Klee, B., Ager, J., Templin, T., Janisse, J., Martier, S., & Sokol, R. J. (2001). Prenatal alcohol exposure and childhood behavior at age 6 to 7 years: I. dose-response effect. *Pediatrics, 108* (2), e34. http://pediatrics. aappublications.org/content/108/2/e34.short.

56. Day, N. L., Leech, S. L., Richardson, G. A., Cornelius, M. D., Robles, N., & Larkby, C. (2002). Prenatal alcohol exposure predicts continued deficits in offspring size at 14 years of age. *Alcoholism: Clinical and Experimental Research, 26* (10), 1584–1591. http://online library.wiley.com/doi/10.1111/j.1530-0277.2002.tb02459.x/abstract.

57. Mills, J. L., Graubard, B. I., Harley, E. E., Rhoads, G. G., & Berendes, H. W. (1984). Maternal alcohol consumption and birth weight: how much drinking during pregnancy is safe? *JAMA, 252* (14), 1875–1879. http://jama.jamanetwork.com/article.aspx?articleid=394673.

In this study, the probability of having a newborn below the 10th percentile in weight increased by an adjusted odds ratio of 1.11. The baseline incidence is by definition 10%, so applying the appropriate conversion formula (Higgins, J. P. T., et al., Computing absolute risk reduction or NNT from an odds ratio [OR]), that equates to a 0.98% absolute increase attributable to alcohol.

58. Walpole, I., Zubrick, S., & Pontre, J. (1990). Is there a fetal effect with low to moderate alcohol use before or during pregnancy? *Journal of Epidemiology and Community Health, 44* (4), 297–301. http://jech.bmj.com/content/44/4/297.full.pdf.

59. Robinson, M., et al., Low–moderate prenatal alcohol exposure and risk to child behavioral development.

60. 50 g, which is equivalent to ~6 units, or 3 standard glasses of wine, or 3 cans of beer (Forrest, F., Florey, C. D., Taylor, D., McPherson, F., & Young, J. A. [1991]. Reported social alcohol consumption during pregnancy and infants' development at 18 months. *British Medical Journal, 303* [6793], 22. www.ncbi.nlm.nih.gov/pmc/articles/PMC1670277/pdf/bmjo0134-0028.pdf).

61. As a caveat, these studies only evaluated children at age five, which may be too young to fully assess the impact of alcohol exposure, and they didn't evaluate memory or language capabilities, which can also be affected.

Astley, S., & Grant, T. (2012, July 5). Alcohol and pregnancy: Another perspective on the disputed Danish studies. Special to the Times, *Seattle Times.* http://depts.washington.edu/fasdpn/pdfs/astley-grant-Washington.pdf; Falgreen Eriksen, H. L., Mortensen, E. L., Kilburn, T., Underbjerg, M., Bertrand, J., Støvring, H., Wimberly, T., Grove, J., & Kesmodel, U. S. (2012). The effects of low to moderate prenatal alcohol exposure in early pregnancy on IQ in 5-year-old children. *BJOG: An International Journal of Obstetrics & Gynaecology, 119* (10), 1191–1200. http://onlinelibrary.wiley.com/doi/10.1111/j.1471-0528.2012.03394.x/abstract; Underbjerg, M., Kesmodel, U. S., Landrø, N. I., Bakketeig, L., Grove, J., Wimberley, T., Kilburn, T. R., Sværke, C., Thorsen, P., & Mortensen, E. L. (2012). The effects of low to moderate alcohol consumption and binge drinking in early pregnancy on selective and sustained attention in five-year-old children. *BJOG: An International Journal of Obstetrics & Gynaecology, 119* (10), 1211–1221. http://onlinelibrary.wiley.com/doi/10.1111/j.1471-0528.2012.03396.x/full; Skogerbø, Å., Kesmodel, U. S., Wimberley, T., Støvring, H., Bertrand, J., Landrø, N. I., & Mortensen, E. L. (2012). The effects of low to moderate alcohol consumption and binge drinking in early pregnancy on executive function in 5-year-old children. *BJOG: An International Journal of Obstetrics & Gynaecology, 119* (10), 1201–1210. http://onlinelibrary.wiley.com/doi/10.1111/j.1471-0528.2012.03397.x/full; Kesmodel, U. S., Bertrand, J., Støvring, H., Skarpness, B., Denny, C. H., & Mortensen, E. L. (2012). The effect of different alcohol drinking patterns in early to mid pregnancy on the child's intelligence, attention, and executive function. *BJOG: An International Journal of Obstetrics & Gynaecology, 119* (10), 1180–1190. http://onlinelibrary.wiley.com/doi/10.1111/j.1471-0528.2012.03393.x/full; Bay, B., Støvring, H., Wimberley, T., Denny, C. H., Mortensen, E. L., Eriksen, H. L. F., & Kesmodel, U. S. (2012). Low to moderate alcohol intake during pregnancy and risk of psychomotor deficits. *Alcoholism: Clinical and Experimental Research, 36* (5), 807–814. http://onlinelibrary.wiley.com/doi/10.1111/j.1530-0277.2011.01657.x/full; Skogerbø, Å., Kesmodel, U. S., Denny, C. H., Kjærsgaard, M. I. S., Wimberley, T., Landrø, N. I., & Mortensen, E. L. (2013). The effects of low to moderate alcohol consumption and binge drinking in early pregnancy on behaviour in five-year-old children: a prospective cohort study on 1628 children. *BJOG: An International Journal of Obstetrics & Gynaecology, 120* (9), 1042–1050. http://onlinelibrary.wiley.com/doi/10.1111/1471-0528.12208/full.

62. Abel, E. L. (1997). Maternal alcohol consumption and spontaneous abortion. *Alcohol and Alcoholism, 32* (3), 211–219. http://alcalc.oxfordjournals.org/content/32/3/211.full.pdf.

63. According to one frequently cited review, "given the current state of our knowledge it is impossible to conclude whether low-level alcohol intake in pregnancy has clinically significant deleterious effects on the individual or not" (Stratton, K. R., Howe, C. J., & Battaglia, F. C. [Eds.]. [1996]. *Fetal alcohol syndrome: diagnosis, epidemiology, prevention, and treatment.* Washington, DC: National Academies Press. https://books.google.com/books?id=SZcrAAAAYAAJ&printsec=frontcover#v=onepage&q&f=false). Other exhaustive reviews agree: Mattson, S. N., Crocker, N., & Nguyen, T. T. (2011). Fetal alcohol spectrum disorders: neuropsychological and behavioral features. *Neuropsychology Review, 21* (2), 81–101. www.ncbi.nlm.nih.gov/pmc/articles/pmc3410672/; Henderson, J., Gray, R., & Brocklehurst, P. (2007). Systematic review of effects of low-moderate prenatal alcohol exposure on pregnancy outcome. *BJOG: An International Journal of Obstetrics & Gynaecology, 114* (3), 243–252. http://onlinelibrary.wiley.com/doi/10.1111/j.1471-0528.2006.01163.x/full; Bay, B., & Kesmodel, U. S. (2011). Prenatal alcohol exposure—a systematic review of the effects on child motor function. *Acta Obstetricia et Gynecologica Scandinavica, 90* (3), 210–226. http://onlinelibrary.wiley.com/doi/10.1111/j.1600-0412.2010.01039.x/full.

64. Threat score is 4% (probability of the offspring of a heavy drinker being born with FAS as discussed in a previous footnote) x 10,000 (impact: significant impairment) x 1 (certainty: well proven) = 400.

65. Threat score is 0.98% (probability of having a low-birth weight infant, according to the largest study, as discussed in a previous footnote) x 100 (impact: statistically detectable impairment) x 1/100 (certainty: ambiguous) = 0.01.

66. Källén, B. (1987). Hyperemesis during pregnancy and delivery outcome: a registry study. *European Journal of Obstetrics & Gynecology and Reproductive Biology, 26* (4), 291–302. www.sciencedirect.com/science/article/pii/0028224387901274.

67. Tramèr, M. R., Carroll, D., Campbell, F. A., Reynolds, D. J. M., Moore, R. A., & McQuay, H. J. (2001). Cannabinoids for control of chemotherapy induced nausea and vomiting: quantitative systematic review. *BMJ, 323* (7303), 16. www.ncbi.nlm.nih.gov/pmc/articles/PMC34325/.

68. Westfall, R. E., Janssen, P. A., Lucas, P., & Capler, R. (2006). Survey of medicinal cannabis use among childbearing women: patterns of its use in pregnancy and retroactive self-assessment of its efficacy against 'morning sickness.' *Complementary Therapies in Clinical Practice, 12* (1), 27–33. http://www.sciencedirect.com/science/article/pii/S1744388105000939.

69. Estes, L. (2013, August 2). Mother arrested after infant tested positive for marijuana. CullmanTimes.com. www.cullmantimes.com/community/mother-arrested-after-infant-tested-positive-for-marijuana/article_fc5a81e3-859c-5d24-8e32-40b1fba6edc3.html.

70. Smith, T. (2013, May 2). Mother arrested after baby tests positive for marijuana. TimesDaily.com. www.timesdaily.com/archives/article_d9523ce9-72f3-50be-a72c-0817529cc415.html.

71. Sanchez, Y. W. (2012, November 13). New fear: medical marijuana, pregnancy. Azcentral.com. www.azcentral.com/news/politics/articles/20121102medical-marijuana-pregnancy-new-fear.html.

72. Using marijuana for morning sickness: miracle cure or criminal act? (2010, December 20). Nwmca.com. http://www.opposingviews.com/i/when-getting-baked-doesn-t-refer-only-to-the-bun-in-the-oven.

73. Johnson, Z. (2013, July 17). Evan Rachel Wood misses smoking weed now that she's pregnant. USWeekly.com. www.usmagazine.com/celebrity-moms/news/evan-rachel-wood-misses-smoking-pot-now-that-shes-pregnant-2013177.

74. What you need to know about marijuana use and pregnancy. (2017). Centers for Disease Control and Prevention. https://www.cdc.gov/marijuana/pdf/marijuana-pregnancy-508. pdf.

75. Cannabis: a short review. (n.d.). United Nations Office on Drugs and Crime. http://www. unodc.org/documents/drug-prevention-and-treatment/cannabis_review.pdf.

76. Day, N. L., Wagener, D. K., & Taylor, P. M. (1985). Measurement of substance use during pregnancy: methodologic issues. In: Pinkert, T. (Ed.). Current research on the consequences of maternal drug abuse. (1985). *NIDA Research Monograph, 1985* (59), 36–47. https://archives.drugabuse.gov/sites/default/files/monograph59_0.pdf.

77. Zuckerman, B., Frank, D. A., Hingson, R., Amaro, H., Levenson, S. M., Kayne, H., Parker, S., Vinci, R., Aboagye, K., Fried, L. E., Cabral, H., Timperi, R., & Bauchner, H. (1989). Effects of maternal marijuana and cocaine use on fetal growth. *New England Journal of Medicine, 320* (12), 762–768. www.nejm.org/doi/pdf/10.1056/NEJM198903233201203.

78. Fergusson, D. M., Horwood, L. J., & Northstone, K. (2002). Maternal use of cannabis and pregnancy outcome. *BJOG: An International Journal of Obstetrics & Gynaecology, 109* (1), 21–27. http://onlinelibrary.wiley.com/doi/10.1111/j.1471-0528.2002.01020.x/full.

79. Balle, J., Olofsson, M. J., & Hilden, J. (1999). Cannabis and pregnancy. *Ugeskr Laeger, 161* (36), 5024–8. www.ukcia.org/research/CannabisAndPregnancy.html.

80. Fried, P. A., Watkinson, B., & Gray, R. (1999). Growth from birth to early adolescence in offspring prenatally exposed to cigarettes and marijuana. *Neurotoxicology and Teratology, 21* (5), 513–525. www.sciencedirect.com/science/article/pii/S0892036299000094.

81. English, D. R., Hulse, G. K., Milne, E., Holman, C. D. J., & Bower, C. I. (1997). Maternal cannabis use and birth weight: a meta-analysis. *Addiction, 92* (11), 1553–1560. http:// addictioneducation.co.uk/out1.pdf.

   According to this study, the probability of low birth weight is increased by an odds ratio of 1.09. The baseline incidence of LBW in the population as of 2010 was 8.15% according to the CDC (Martin, J. A., Hamilton, B. E., Ventura, S. J., Osterman, M. J., Wilson, E. C., & Mathews, T. J. [2012, August 28]. Births: final data for 2010. *National Vital Statistics Report, 61* [1], 1–90. www.cdc.gov/nchs/data/nvsr/nvsr61/nvsr61_01.pdf), so applying the appropriate conversion formula (Higgins, J. P. T., et al., Computing absolute risk reduction or NNT from an odds ratio [OR]), that equates to a 0.67% absolute increase in LBW attributable to marijuana.

82. Fried, P. A. (1995). The Ottawa prenatal prospective study (OPPS): methodological issues and findings—it's easy to throw the baby out with the bath water. *Life Sciences, 56* (23), 2159–2168. www.sciencedirect.com/science/article/pii/002432059500203I.

83. Day, N. L., Richardson, G. A., Goldschmidt, L., Robles, N., Taylor, P. M., Stoffer, D. S., Cornelius, M. D., & Geva, D. (1994). Effect of prenatal marijuana exposure on the cognitive development of offspring at age three. *Neurotoxicology and Teratology, 16* (2), 169–175. www.sciencedirect.com/science/article/pii/0892036294901147.

84. Goldschmidt, L., Day, N. L., & Richardson, G. A. (2000). Effects of prenatal marijuana exposure on child behavior problems at age 10. *Neurotoxicology and Teratology, 22* (3), 325–336. www.sciencedirect.com/science/article/pii/S0892036200000660.

85. Goldschmidt, L., Richardson, G. A., Willford, J., & Day, N. L. (2008). Prenatal marijuana exposure and intelligence test performance at age 6. *Journal of the American Academy of Child & Adolescent Psychiatry, 47* (3), 254–263. www.sciencedirect.com/science/article/pii/ S089085670962308X.

86. Hall, W., & Degenhardt, L. (2009). Adverse health effects of non-medical cannabis use. *The Lancet, 374* (9698), 1383–1391. http://www.sciencedirect.com/science/article/pii/ S0140673609610370.

87. The Dangerous Drugs Act. (1987). Ministry of Justice, Government of Jamaica. www.moj. gov.jm/laws/dangerous-drugs-act.

88. Jamaican farmers offer illegal "pothead paradise" cannabis tours to tourists. (2013, September 9). Dailymail.co.uk. www.dailymail.co.uk/travel/article-2416031/Jamaican-farmers-offer-illegal-pothead-paradise-cannabis-tours-tourists.html.

89. Dreher, M. C., Nugent, K., & Hudgins, R. (1994). Prenatal marijuana exposure and neonatal outcomes in Jamaica: an ethnographic study. *Pediatrics, 93* (2), 254–260. http://pediatrics. aappublications.org/content/93/2/254.short.

90. Ibid.

91. Ibid.

92. Hayes, J. S., Lampart, R., Dreher, M. C., & Morgan, L. (1991). Five-year follow-up of rural Jamaican children whose mothers used marijuana during pregnancy. *The West Indian Medical Journal, 40* (3), 120–123. www.ncbi.nlm.nih.gov/pubmed/1957518.

93. Metz, T. D., & Stickrath, E. H. (2015). Marijuana use in pregnancy and lactation: a review of the evidence. *American Journal of Obstetrics and Gynecology, 213* (6), 761–778. www. shastahealth.org/sites/default/files/residency/learning-resources/not-your-mothers-marijuana.pdf.

94. Threat level is 0.67% (probability of low birth weight, as discussed in a previous footnote) x 100 (impact: statistically detectable impairment) x 1/100 (certainty: ambiguous) = .0067.

95. Torres, S. (Ed.). (1998). Living color: face and television in the United States. Durham, NC: Duke University Press, 111.

96. Winerip, M. (2013, May 20). Revisiting the 'crack babies' epidemic that was not. NYTimes. com. www.nytimes.com/2013/05/20/booming/revisiting-the-crack-babies-epidemic-that-was-not.html?_r=0.

97. Project prevention. (n.d.). Wikipedia. http://en.wikipedia.org/wiki/Project_Prevention.

98. O'Neill, A. M., & Carter, K. (1999, September 27). Desperate measure. People.com. http:// people.com/archive/desperate-measure-vol-52-no-12/.

99. Greenhouse, L. (2000, October 5). Justices consider limits of the legal response to risky behavior by pregnant women. NYTimes.com. www.nytimes.com/2000/10/05/us/justices-consider-limits-legal-response-risky-behavior-pregnant-women.html.

100. Ness, R. B., Grisso, J. A., Hirschinger, N., Markovic, N., Shaw, L. M., Day, N. L., & Kline, J. (1999). Cocaine and tobacco use and the risk of spontaneous abortion. *New England Journal of Medicine, 340* (5), 333–339. http://192.38.117.59/~kach/gammelex/Ness%20 et%20al.pdf.

101. Gouin, K., Murphy, K., & Shah, P. S. (2011). Effects of cocaine use during pregnancy on low birthweight and preterm birth: systematic review and metaanalyses. *American Journal of Obstetrics and Gynecology, 2011* (204), 1.e1–1.e12. www.issues4life.org/pdfs/201101000a-jog.pdf.

102. Bada, H. S., Das, A., Bauer, C. R., Shankaran, S., Lester, B., Wright, L. L., Verter, J., Smeriglio, V. L., Finnegan, L. P. & Maza, P. L. (2002). Gestational cocaine exposure and intrauterine growth: maternal lifestyle study. *Obstetrics & Gynecology, 100* (5, Part 1), 916–924. http://journals.lww.com/greenjournal/Abstract/2002/11000/Gestational_Cocaine_Exposure_and_Intrauterine.16.aspx.

103. Richardson, G. A., Hamel, S. C., Goldschmidt, L., & Day, N. L. (1999). Growth of infants prenatally exposed to cocaine/crack: comparison of a prenatal care and a no prenatal care sample. *Pediatrics, 104* (2), e18. http://pediatrics.aappublications.org/content/104/2/e18. short.

104. Bandstra, E. S., Morrow, C. E., Anthony, J. C., Churchill, S. S., Chitwood, D. C., Steele, B. W., Ofir, A. Y., & Xue, L. (2001). Intrauterine growth of full-term infants: impact of prenatal cocaine exposure. *Pediatrics, 108* (6), 1309–1319. http://pediatrics.aappublications.org/content/108/6/1309.short.

105. According to a CDC report based on data from Atlanta, women who reported using cocaine any time from one month before pregnancy through the first three months of pregnancy had a risk of urinary tract defects of 7.2 per 1,000 births vs. 1.5 per 1,000 births for the rest of the population; this held even after adjusting the data for factors known to be associated with cocaine use and birth defects, such as maternal age, alcohol use, and use of illicit drugs other than cocaine (Centers for Disease Control. [1989]. Urogenital anomalies in the offspring of women using cocaine during early pregnancy—Atlanta, 1968–1980. *Morbidity and Mortality Weekly Report, 38* [31], 536–541. www.cdc.gov/mmwr/preview/mmwrhtml/00001437.htm).

106. Ackerman, J. P., Riggins, T., & Black, M. M. (2010). A review of the effects of prenatal cocaine exposure among school-aged children. *Pediatrics, 125* (3), 554–565. http://pediatrics.aappublications.org/content/early/2010/02/08/peds.2009-0637.short.

107. Hadeed, A. J., & Siegel, S. R. (1989). Maternal cocaine use during pregnancy: effect on the newborn infant. *Pediatrics, 84* (2), 205–210. http://fullcircleadoptions.org/wp-content/uploads/2017/08/Maternal-Cocaine-Use-During-Pregnancy-Effect-on-the-Newborn-Infant.pdf.

108. Ackerman, J. P., et al., A review of the effects of prenatal cocaine exposure among school-aged children.

109. Frank, D. A., Augustyn, M., Knight, W. G., Pell, T., & Zuckerman, B. (2001). Growth, development, and behavior in early childhood following prenatal cocaine exposure: a systematic review. *JAMA, 285* (12), 1613–1625. http://jama.ama-assn.org/content/285/12/1613.full.

110. Frank, D. A., et al., Growth, development, and behavior in early childhood following prenatal cocaine exposure.

111. Martin, M. (2010, May 3). Crack babies: twenty years later. NPR.org. www.npr.org/templates/story/story.php?storyId=126478643.

112. Lavoie, D. (2007, December 25). Crack-vs.-powder disparity is questioned. USAToday.com. http://usatoday30.usatoday.com/news/nation/2007-12-24-2050621119_x.htm?csp=34.

113. Stratton, K. R., et al., Fetal alcohol syndrome: diagnosis, epidemiology, prevention, and treatment.

114. Threat score is (7.2-1.5)/1000 = .0057 (increased probability of a urogenital birth defect, based on numbers from the previous footnote) x 1,000 (minor impairment) x (certainty: well proven) = 5.7.

4

A DAY IN THE LIFE

Lifestyle

*I*t's a humdrum day, despite your growing belly. Your alarm goes off. You roll out of bed and grab a cup of coffee. Then you jump in the car to head to work, perhaps feeling slightly nauseous. By the end of the long and stressful afternoon, you're too tired to face the gym, so you head home to figure out dinner and then collapse into bed, exhausted.

Or perhaps your day is the opposite of humdrum. Maybe you have to fly cross country for an unavoidable business trip or stay out late celebrating a friend's engagement. Either way, according to the conventional wisdom, every twenty-four hours is filled with a minefield of potential threats to your baby. You're apparently not even off the hook from your maternal responsibilities when you're fast asleep. So let's figure out which of your daily activities are truly risky versus which are utterly harmless.

Sinister Slumber: Sleeping on the Left

LEFT. LEFT. SLEEP on your LEFT. The mantra is everywhere, from websites to popular pregnancy bibles.[1, 2, 3] If you don't sleep on your left side in the later stages of pregnancy, you risk cutting off the blood flow to the vena cava, which could harm your baby. Heeding this advice, I dutifully drifted off to sleep curled up in the correct position. Yet every morning I'd awake to find myself lying on my back, thwarted by my unconscious self, who was clearly not taking this important pregnancy advice seriously.

The inclusion of the anatomical term *vena cava* gives the "left side" recommendation an air of medical credibility. Whatever the vena cava might be, it definitely sounds like something that shouldn't be obstructed by a ponderous belly. But the evidence supporting this piece of advice is scant at best. A handful of studies have observed slightly decreased blood flow from lying on your back rather than your side during pregnancy. One of these studies makes no recommendation,[4] another concludes the implications are for operating positions for women undergoing surgery while pregnant,[5] and the last points out that standing reduces blood flow by twice as much as lying on the back, so the implications are primarily for women whose jobs require them to be on their feet.[6]

Only one study has attempted to link sleeping positions to birth outcomes. A group of researchers from New Zealand recently generated press coverage in the UK when they published a study suggesting that the wrong sleeping position could increase your risk of stillbirth.[7] But the authors themselves have pointed out several caveats, which have been echoed by the UK National Health Service:[8] This was a relatively small study, and the findings have yet to be replicated. The women who ultimately gave birth to stillborn babies weren't observed sleeping but were simply asked to recall their sleeping position after the fact. Correlation doesn't prove causation: perhaps women are more likely to sleep on their back because of the conditions leading to stillbirth rather than the other way around. And finally, failing to get up in the middle of the night to go to the bathroom was equally correlated with stillbirth, and we don't see anyone recommending that you start setting your alarm clock to schedule a 3 a.m. bathroom break.

We all move around frequently in our sleep, and without even thinking about it, you're likely to spontaneously move into positions that reduce artery compression.[9] I'll leave you with the words of two amusingly incredulous doctors:

> Recently, many of our patients have asked whether it is better for a pregnant woman to sleep on her left side. Finding that this relatively unimportant topic was increasingly encroaching upon our time with patients, we did some research. . . . Neither the Society of Obstetricians and Gynaecologists of Canada nor the American College of Obstetricians and Gynecologists recommends any pattern or position for sleep. Neither the Cochrane database nor the major obstetrics textbooks address this issue. . . . Advising women to sleep or lie exclusively on the left side is not practical and is irrelevant to the vast majority of patients. . . . First, we tell [our patients] that remaining in one position throughout the night results in pressure sores but that we all move naturally in our sleep to prevent this. Then we point out that if lying prone had been detrimental to a normal pregnancy, the species would long ago have ceased to exist.[10]

Threat level for sleeping in the wrong position: Very low

Wired: Caffeine

This psychotropic drug grew popular in the fifteenth century in the hidden alleyways of a port city in Yemen.[11] Nowadays, it can be procured on most major street corners in the United States. It's addictive and causes a host of withdrawal symptoms, including headache, depressed mood, difficulty concentrating, irritability, and, at times, nausea, vomiting, and muscle pain.[12] Exposure during pregnancy causes immediate changes in fetal heart rate, and the drug has been accused of causing permanent heart damage.[13] Nevertheless, a vast number of American women choose to abuse this drug during pregnancy. If you assume you're not among them, I'll give you a hint: that port in Yemen is the city of Mocha. Yes, the drug I'm discussing is caffeine.

Nowadays, caffeine addiction is almost universal: ~90 percent of women are caffeine drinkers.[14] But almost equally universal is the instinct to cut down on coffee while pregnant. A quarter of women virtuously stop drinking caffeine altogether.[15] The rest of us cut down from about one and a half cups to one (or, for those in the top 10 percent, from about three and a half cups down to two and a half).[16]

Why exactly are we forgoing the delightful pleasures of our habitual morning mochaccino? Perhaps it's simply maternal intuition that caffeine can't be good for a fetus. Or maybe we've been influenced by the scaremongering headlines. For example, here's a statement from Dr. Joseph Mercola: "The equivalent of just two cups of coffee during the entire pregnancy may affect your child's heart function and, if your baby is male, could also lead to a weight problem."[17] Turns out, Dr. Mercola is extrapolating from a study done in mice, not humans, but it certainly sounds ominous. Or how about this headline from *The New York Times* in 2008: "Pregnancy Problems Tied to Caffeine." The headline sounds dramatic, but the article goes on to acknowledge that "too much caffeine during pregnancy may increase the risk of miscarriage ... the subject has long been contentious, with conflicting studies, fuzzy data, and various recommendations given over the years."[18]

The conflicting results about the effects of caffeine during pregnancy have also puzzled public health authorities, so our official institutions aren't providing much further clarity.[19] Both the FDA and the National Institutes of Health are wishy-washy, saying you should simply ask your healthcare provider to advise you on how much caffeine you can drink.[20, 21] The Academy of Nutrition and Dietetics says to keep below 300 mg caffeine per day,[22] while the March of Dimes and the UK government both say the limit is 200 mg.[23, 24] Why all this uncertainty?

There are a number of undisputed facts about caffeine. First, with each passing month of pregnancy, your body metabolizes caffeine more slowly. By the time you reach your third trimester, it mysteriously takes you three times longer than normal to clear the caffeine out of your system.[25] That means there's still caffeine lingering in your system up to eighteen hours after you've finished your café latte.[26] So even though women tend to drink less caffeine later in pregnancy, the level of caffeine in the baby's cord blood actually tends to rise over the course of pregnancy.[27] Second, there's no doubt that caffeine crosses the placenta. Your fetus ends up with the same blood caffeine level as you, with a noticeable effect on its breathing and heart rate.[28, 29] A fetus can even develop a tolerance for caffeine, just as an adult can.[30]

But the long-term effects of caffeine on the baby are more difficult to study. For one thing, the majority of studies have asked pregnant women to simply report the number of caffeinated beverages they drink, but this is a very inaccurate way of estimating true caffeine exposure (cup sizes vary, caffeine content varies, and people may estimate incorrectly).[31] As one review of the field complains, "further studies utilizing 'cups' of tea, coffee, and colas will add little more to the understanding of caffeine toxicity."[32] Second, women who drink large amounts of caffeine are also more likely to smoke and drink. Although most studies attempt to control for this, it's hard to be completely sure the effects have been separated. Furthermore, given that drinking coffee while pregnant is socially acceptable, while drinking alcohol and smoking are less so, there's a risk that women accurately report their caffeine consumption but understate their other risky behaviors, so the caffeine appears to be at fault.[33] Finally, there's the fact that nausea is actually a positive sign of a healthy pregnancy, but women who feel nauseous may respond by cutting out coffee.[34] So this effect may also get entangled in studies that don't control for it.[35] That's why numerous major reviews of the field have all concluded that there's simply not enough evidence to conclude that caffeine does any harm, even at high levels of exposure.[36]

Only one major study has attempted to overcome these hurdles.[37] A research team in Denmark enlisted over 1,000 pregnant women who habitually drank at least three cups of coffee per day and randomly assigned half to receive a supply of normal instant coffee and the other half to receive decaf (all in unmarked boxes). The authors then followed each group from twenty weeks onward and ultimately concluded that switching the second group to decaf had no effect on birth weight or the incidence of preterm birth. Even this study wasn't perfect: it only studied the effects of caffeine in the second half of pregnancy, and the researchers didn't physically measure the women's caffeine levels to make sure no one in the decaf group felt a withdrawal headache coming on and started cheating. Nevertheless, the study provides some degree of comfort that the effects of caffeine can't be dramatic.

So the current guidelines for caffeine, like so many pregnancy dogmas, fall firmly into the category of "better safe than sorry." By all means, cut down if you wish to feel virtuous, but don't worry if you've already turned your fetus into a caffeine junkie. With Starbucks providing temptation on every corner, he or she is likely to become one soon enough anyway.

Threat level for caffeine: Very low

Don't Worry, Be Happy: Stress

Practice meditation. Book yourself a vacation, or at least a foot massage. But whatever you do, do not let yourself get stressed. Why not? According to various parenting books, maternal stress "conditions" the fetal brain, making a child more prone to impulsiveness and aggression.[38] Poor abstract reasoning and an inability to concentrate lead to academic failure and dropping out of school, which in turn often leads to a life of addiction and crime.[39] Exposure to prenatal maternal stress may ultimately put your child at risk of suffering from alcoholism, schizophrenia, or even suicide later in life.[40]

Do you buy this? Some women apparently do. A full three-quarters of the pregnant women who responded to a recent March of Dimes poll were concerned that stress in their life would harm their baby's health.[41] Mothers are stressed about being stressed. As the old adage goes, there's nothing to fear but fear itself.

So is there any truth to this? Major studies of stress during pregnancy have looked at mothers who experienced the death of a loved one, survived a natural disaster like Hurricane Katrina, or were forced to flee their homes as refugees. These studies suggest that, yes, women experiencing such "major life events" and "catastrophic disasters" are slightly more likely to deliver prematurely. Similarly, stress related to severe financial strain, homelessness, or living in a dangerous neighborhood can also contribute to premature birth.[42] But these circumstances may not be in one's control, so there's little point in dwelling on them here.

What about the types of women who responded to that March of Dimes poll, the ones who are anxious about pregnancy itself? An exhaustive review highlighted three recent large, well-designed studies from North America covering more than 8,500 women and concluded that stress does contribute to preterm birth.[43, 44, 45] Specifically, "the most consistent results are found for pregnancy-related stress and anxiety."[46] It's a classic self-fulfilling prophesy: if you're worried something will go wrong with your pregnancy, there's a small chance it might.

I'm not going to provide stress-relieving advice for the natural worrywarts out there, since the self-help section of any bookstore will be overflowing with suggestions. But I do hope that reading this book will help you put your sense of the risks of pregnancy into perspective. Most pregnancies turn out just fine. So all you really need to do, as the British say, is "keep calm and carry on."

Threat level for pregnancy anxiety: Medium[47]

Bringing Home the Bacon: Work

Wouldn't it be nice to trade in the daily commute for a leisurely morning lounging at home in your pajamas? You're nauseous and exhausted, your brain is fuzzy from the hormones, and all this hard work might even be bad for the baby. Not to mention there's that nursery to decorate . . .

Unfortunately for the two-thirds of women who work during pregnancy, you have no good excuse.[48] Your brain still works fine: "pregnancy brain" and "momnesia" are myths.[49, 50] Holding an ordinary job doesn't appear to pose any risk to the health of your baby.[51, 52, 53, 54, 55] And for those who might be self-conscious, even if you work right up until the very end, there's only about a one percent chance your water will break at work.[56] So the pajamas will just have to wait until after the baby is born (at which point I wish you luck getting back out of them).

That's not to say that all types of work get the green light. Your risk of complications may increase slightly if you work in certain occupations, including sales and service, manufacturing, mining, agriculture, cleaning, nursing, and childcare.[57, 58, 59] It's not particularly surprising that any job that involves long hours of standing,[60] physical fatigue,[61] lifting heavy weights,[62] or exposure to chemicals or germs might be suboptimal.[63] But keep in mind that the increases in risk are small, and the vast majority of women working in these sectors will go on to have successful pregnancies.[64]

There's also the question of stress at work. Full disclosure: this happens to be a topic close to my own heart. Less than a week after experiencing a stressful period at work, I gave birth to my first child five weeks prematurely. I couldn't help wondering if maybe, just maybe, the premature delivery was my fault. But mental stress at work is hard to measure objectively, so the evidence isn't conclusive. One study of female lawyers concluded that women working long hours during their first trimester had a higher rate of miscarriage.[65] In another study, those reporting that their job was "generally stressful and/or demanding" had higher odds of miscarriage,[66] although this could be recall bias or another case of the worrywart phenomenon. And a final study has suggested that working more than forty-two hours a week may increase the risk of preterm birth, although this could be related to physical rather than mental strain.[67]

I'll never know definitively whether I caused my baby to be born prematurely, and if I had to relive that phase of my life, I'd probably still choose to work. I'd never want to make women feel guilty for having to earn a living, encourage them to drop out of the workforce unnecessarily, or even suggest they should stop "leaning in," as per Sheryl Sandberg's advice. But if I'd realized there was even a small chance that my level of stress was affecting my baby, I like to think I would have convinced myself not to take the ups and downs at work so much to heart. On the other hand, maybe I would have gotten stressed about the stress and compounded the situation. Or maybe I simply would have carved out more time for that pregnancy yoga class I kept missing. *Ommm . . .*

Threat level for stress at work: Difficult to calculate without an objective measure of stress

Our Dangerous Machines: Driving

Driving a car is dangerous. I know this courtesy of my driver's education teacher, who showered our class with statistics and showed us gruesome pictures of car accidents in an attempt to scare us into driving carefully. Nevertheless, I feel completely blasé about getting in a car, and I suspect you do too.

That's because we drive all the time without incident. Our brains aren't wired to understand low-probability events. So if we've personally driven many times without anything bad happening, we naturally conclude that driving must be harmless (except for the unfortunate few who've experienced a crash firsthand). It's hard to be actively afraid of any activity that's a regular part of your daily life—you quickly become desensitized. Furthermore, we're rarely exposed to the dark side of driving. A car crash is too mundane a topic to elicit much media attention. Crashes happen all the time, but if they don't affect anyone you know, you're unlikely to hear about them. Finally, when driving, we have the illusion of control, so we assume our great skill will protect us. In fact, we have deeply unrealistic expectations of our abilities: 93 percent of Americans rate themselves as above-average drivers.[68]

The truth is, the average woman age 25–34 has a 6 in 100,000 chance of dying in a motor vehicle accident in any given year.[69] That's not a number that's likely to scare you, or even mean very much out of context, but it does put driving in a higher risk category than many of the other threats to pregnancy that we've discussed. And even if you survive a major crash, the impact could kill or seriously injure your fetus.[70] Getting in a car (as either a driver or passenger) really is dangerous. But pregnant women are rarely counseled about this threat.[71]

I'm not trying to imply that responsible women should never ride in a car while pregnant. I know this is unrealistic and totally impossible for the vast majority of women. But if you want to minimize a legitimate risk to your pregnancy, at least wear your seat belt religiously (with the lap belt below your bump).[72, 73, 74, 75] Seat belt use has been shown in many studies to reduce the risk of fetal as well as maternal trauma in the case of an accident,[76] but at the moment, more than 30 percent of pregnant women don't wear one or wear it improperly.[77] Driving slowly and cautiously also can't hurt. If you're worried about giving the drivers behind you road rage, all you'll need is a variant on the traditional bumper sticker: "Bump on Board."

Threat level for driving: Medium[78]

The Incredible Shrinking Seat: Deep Vein Thrombosis

October 2013: "American Airlines, United, and other carriers are wedging an extra seat into each coach row. . . . The solution . . . is to offer distractions like big meals, frequent snacks and lots of electronic entertainment."[79]

Irritating news for ordinary passengers. Life-threatening news for pregnant women stuck in economy? According to conventional wisdom, sitting still for long periods of time is a sure way to develop life-threatening deep vein thrombosis (DVT), a condition where a blood clot forms in a vein, most often in the leg, which can subsequently detach and travel to the lungs, causing a life-threatening blockage. So rather than sitting mesmerized by the TV on long-haul flights, pregnant women should be annoying the flight attendants by doing calisthenics in the aisles.

This view is not entirely unfounded. It's true that pregnant women are more likely to get blood clots. The risk of getting DVT is about 6 times higher when you're pregnant,[80] and the risk of death from a blood clot is 12 times higher (~1.4 per 100,000 pregnancies).[81] So DVT does represent a material threat to pregnancy. Fortunately, if you're diagnosed with a blood clot before any complications ensue, you can take heparin, a safe anticoagulant that doesn't cross the placenta. Your pregnancy will then carry minimal additional risk.[82]

When it comes to air travel, there's no data on the risk of deep vein thrombosis specifically from long-haul flights during pregnancy, so it's difficult to calculate a threat score. According to the UK Royal College of Obstetricians and Gynaecologists, "The true frequency of DVT during long-haul flights in pregnancy is unknown and difficult to determine, particularly as the condition may be asymptomatic."[83] On the other hand, in a study of thirty-one women who died of deep vein thrombosis during pregnancy, only two had taken a long-haul flight, which suggests that air travel isn't usually at fault.[84] And according to the American Congress of Obstetricians and Gynecologists, "recent studies suggest no increase in adverse pregnancy outcomes for occasional air travelers," so "pregnant women can observe the same precautions for air travel as the general population and can fly safely."[85] In other words, there's probably no reason to worry about flying specifically.[86]

Is it worth at least wearing those ugly compression stockings on the plane just in case? According to a review, compression stockings do reduce the risk of DVT in hospitalized surgical patients, but they haven't been tested in other settings.[87] And ACOG agrees that "no hard evidence exists" on the effectiveness of various preventive measures during pregnancy.[88] So wear the ugly stockings if you like, but don't feel guilty if you forget them at home. And by all means drink plenty of liquids, although it's unfortunately likely you'll become dehydrated regardless.[89]

A final note: deep vein thrombosis is actually two to five times more common soon after birth than it is during pregnancy. So try to remember that the nurse who insists you get up and walk around right after twelve hours of labor isn't as sadistic as she might appear.[90]

Overall threat level for deep vein thrombosis (not specific to air travel): Medium[91]

PB&J: Food Allergies

If you haven't heard yet, there's an epidemic of hypodermic syringes in schools across the country. I'm not implying our children are hooked on heroin. I'm referring to EpiPens. Over the last decade, the percentage of children suffering from food allergies has almost doubled from 3.4 percent to 5.1 percent,[92] and the number of children being admitted to the ER with severe allergic reactions has doubled over a similar time frame.[93] A sinister change in our environment is wreaking havoc on our children's immune systems, but we have no idea what it might be.

One intriguing theory holds that modern hygiene practices may be at fault. We could be unnaturally limiting our exposure to the common bacteria that ordinarily would have played a role in stimulating the development of a healthy immune system. Perhaps pregnant women should be visiting farms and wallowing in manure, although the research is too preliminary to reach any firm conclusions.[94, 95]

Researchers have also been investigating prenatal exposure to food allergens in the womb. Thus far, these studies have come up empty-handed—there's little evidence that excluding cow's milk, eggs, or fish from your diet while pregnant will have any effect on your child's likelihood of developing the corresponding allergies.[96, 97, 98, 99] As a result, neither the American Academy of Pediatrics[100] nor the equivalent European institutions currently recommend altering your diet dramatically during pregnancy for the sake of allergy avoidance.[101]

There was some controversy over that little legume from South America that used to be the standard snack on airlines until people started dying from it. For reasons unknown to anyone, peanuts (yes, they are technically legumes, not nuts) are the worst culprits when it comes to severe, life-threatening allergies. One small study suggested that mothers who scarfed down peanut products more than once a week during pregnancy were more likely to have children with peanut allergies.[102] Given that peanuts aren't considered an essential food in the American diet (PB&J notwithstanding), the American Academy of Pediatrics initially suggested caution was in order.[103] But these results have now been contradicted by one study that found no evidence of any effect[104] and another that suggested eating nuts during pregnancy may actually reduce the chance of having an allergic child.[105] The AAP has since reversed its position.[106]

So enjoy your peanut butter guilt-free while you can. Once your child emerges from the womb, there's at least a 1 percent chance that jar may need to be thrown out alongside the rat poison.[107]

Threat level for eating common allergens (e.g., nuts): Very low

Beached Whale: Weight Gain

March 2007: "April Branum went to her local emergency room complaining of stomach pain and emerged with the biggest shock of her life.[108] She was pregnant with a full-term fetus . . . at about 420 pounds, she was so large that no one—including herself—could tell she had carried a baby to term. The layers of fat padding her belly likely insulated the baby's movements, said her physician."

June 2009: "Today, the momlogic blog features the story of a woman with 'pregorexia.' . . . After the birth, her child developed seizures and attention deficit problems, which her doctor suggested may have been linked with poor fetal nutrition."[109]

In a country of 300 million people, it's never difficult to find examples of our species behaving weirdly. "Pregorexia" (anorexia during pregnancy) and pregnancies disguised by fat both make for sensational headlines, but they're fortunately not mainstream problems. On the other hand, our national obsession with our weight carries over into pregnancy. Pregnancy websites and books all contain the obligatory section on the topic of eating and weight gain, and your doctor will likely monitor your weight throughout your pregnancy and tell you if you fall outside the official parameters for pregnancy weight gain set by the Institute of Medicine.[110]

Why do we need to pay attention to the official parameters? Because otherwise, we risk putting on far too much weight, that's why! According to the IOM, underweight women typically gain within the guidelines, but "some normal weight women may exceed these guidelines and a majority of overweight or obese women will likely exceed them."[111] Yes, we are gluttons during pregnancy. A full 44 percent of us will gain more weight than we officially should.[112] And according to the IOM, "weight gains outside the recommended ranges are associated with twice as many poor pregnancy outcomes than are weight gains within the ranges."

Sounds alarming. But before you start panicking, renouncing your high-calorie pregnancy cravings, and stocking your refrigerator with lettuce and celery, I'd like to raise three objections, all based on conclusions from the very same IOM report that established the guidelines in the first place.[113]

First, despite all the hype about weight, there's not actually much evidence that excessive weight gain during pregnancy causes problems for the pregnancy itself. According to the IOM, the evidence for an association between maternal weight gain and stillbirth or preterm birth is "weak." There is "insufficient evidence" of long-term health consequences for the mother, and "limited data" regarding long-term health outcomes in children, making inferences "tenuous."

Second, in the cases where there is evidence of a link between weight gain and pregnancy outcomes, we can't separate correlation from causation. For example, there's a strong association between higher weight gain and needing a cesarean. But in the words of the IOM, "the literature does not allow inference of causality." In other words, merely observing that excessive weight gain and cesareans go together isn't enough. Perhaps there are underlying health factors that cause women to gain lots of weight and also cause them to need a cesarean. The weight gain could simply be a symptom. Similarly, weight gain in pregnancy is linked to later childhood obesity, but there's "insufficient evidence" that restricting the mother's weight gain while pregnant would solve the problem.

Finally, no one has shown that intervening and attempting to change a woman's eating behavior during pregnancy actually helps. Providing advice? "The influence of weight gain advice has not been conclusively demonstrated." Weighing women regularly? "Despite the widespread measurement of maternal weight gain during pregnancy, almost no data have been published assessing the usefulness or negative consequences of weighing women."[114] More elaborate interventions? "Approaches have included counseling on diet or exercise or both, provision of unique physical activity classes, dietary prescription, and even daily recording of dietary intake." But "these interventions have not had adequate statistical power to detect differences in obstetric outcomes."[115] As the IOM sums it all up, "we could identify no published experimental studies that examined whether it's possible to manipulate pregnancy weight gains and change pregnancy outcomes."[116] In other words, it's perfectly possible that regardless of what anyone tried to do to intervene, you'd still end up gaining the same amount of weight.

Let's be clear: pregnancy doesn't provide you carte blanche to start polishing off pints of Ben & Jerry's on a daily basis. But as long as you're not changing your diet radically, you might as well put your bathroom scale away, since there's little proof weighing that yourself regularly will help. There'll be plenty of time to obsess about that baby weight once your child is born. For now, you might as well enjoy eating (sensibly) for two.

Threat level for weight gain: Very low

Get Moving: Exercise and Recreation

1880s: Women are encouraged to remain confined indoors while pregnant[117] and often wear corsets to minimize the size of their bumps.[118]

1985: The American College of Obstetrics and Gynecology (ACOG) cautions that "the maximum heart rate during pregnancy should not exceed 140 beats per minute and women should not partake in strenuous exercise for more than 15 minutes."[119]

2002: ACOG reverses its position, admitting there's little evidence that exercise guidelines need be different for pregnant versus non-pregnant women.[120]

2010: Famed marathon runners Paula Radcliffe and Kara Goucher, discovering they're coincidentally due on the same day, pair up to train throughout their pregnancies.[121]

2010: Teresa Delfin, a keen rock climber from California, launches her Mountain Mama brand of apparel and sports gear, designed for active women who want to continue rock climbing, kayaking, and mountain biking throughout pregnancy.[122]

2011: Amber Danielle Miller, a sporty 27-year-old from Illinois, enters the Chicago marathon at thirty-nine weeks pregnant. She successfully crosses the finish line and then promptly heads to the hospital, giving birth to a healthy child four hours later.[123]

Women of the twenty-first century have been given the green light to exercise as much as we please. Previous fears that exercise might divert blood supply away from baby, cause dangerous fetal heart palpitations, raise temperatures to worrisome levels, or result in undersized babies have all proved to be unfounded.[124] The most recent report from the American College of Obstetrics and Gynecology points out that even intense training by athletes appears to carry very little risk.[125] What about the warnings that you shouldn't increase your activity beyond pre-pregnancy levels or try anything new? Nonsense: a review from 2011 concludes that previously inactive women can take up exercising during pregnancy without any problems.[126] Women who exercise may even have a lower risk of preterm birth, according to a recent study of 87,000 women in Denmark, although it's unclear if that's correlation or causation.[127]

Unfortunately, those of us with bumps have a tendency to do the opposite and become increasingly slothful. A quarter of non-pregnant women get the recommended level of physical activity, but that drops to only 16 percent of pregnant women.[128] Over half of those sitting around with their bumps say they feel too nauseous, and a quarter say they're too tired, which is fair enough.[129] But another 10 percent are worried about hurting themselves or the baby. This isn't surprising, given that doctors themselves tend to be misinformed about the effects of exercise. In a survey of ~400 obstetricians, 26 percent thought moderate exercise was ill advised, 38 percent thought that a woman shouldn't start a new exercise program during pregnancy, and a full 94 percent were against vigorous exercise.[130] Nowadays, concerns about exercise tend to revolve around five themes:

1. Abdominal trauma.

This concern is legitimate, but we hardly need doctors to advise us on the topic. Here are some words of wisdom from the American College of Obstetricians and Gynecologists: "Those activities with a high risk of falling or for abdominal trauma should be avoided during pregnancy, [including] ice hockey, soccer, basketball, gymnastics, horseback riding, downhill skiing, and vigorous racquet sports."[131] Sensible advice, surely, but also unnecessary. Here are the activities pregnant women are actually doing, according to a recent survey of ~2,000 women:[132]

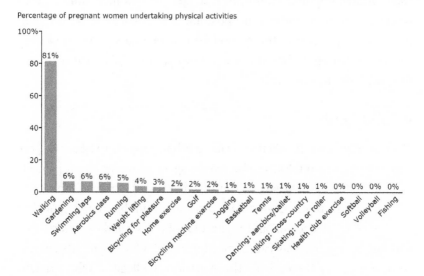

Percentage of pregnant women undertaking physical activities

That's right: pregnant women are going for walks. Perhaps they're also puttering in their gardens or going swimming, but they're certainly not playing ice hockey or vigorous racquet sports in large numbers. Besides, anyone with common sense is aware that these types of activities are risky for the baby as well as the mother. A die-hard rock climber like Teresa Delfin is clearly aware of the risk she's taking and is comfortable with it.[133]

2. High impact activities involving bouncing.

According to the Society of Obstetricians and Gynecologists of Canada, women should choose activities like walking and swimming that involve "less bouncing up and down of the center of gravity than running or jogging."[134] But there's very little evidence to suggest that bouncing up and down does any harm; for example, a study of ~90,000 pregnant women in Denmark looked at the effect of jogging on miscarriage and concluded that any potential increase in risk was statistically insignificant.[135]

3. Exercising in the supine position.

Lots of official bodies, including the Canadian government and the International Olympic Committee, suggest that women should avoid doing exercises in the supine position[136, 137, 138]—i.e., lying on their backs face up—during the second half of pregnancy. As we've seen from the sleeping studies, this is a purely hypothetical concern. There's little evidence to support it.

4. Joint laxity.

During pregnancy, the ligaments in your body appear to become more elastic.[139] As a result, lots of risk-averse agencies worry about protecting joints during pregnancy. The International Olympic Committee warns against rapid changes in direction and bouncing, and the Society of Obstetricians and Gynecologists of Canada cautions that running or jogging may cause knee injuries.[140] Once again, these concerns are purely theoretical. The American College of Obstetricians and Gynecologists sums it up nicely: "Despite a lack of clear evidence that musculoskeletal injuries are increased during pregnancy, these possibilities should nevertheless be considered when prescribing exercise in pregnancy."[141] That's right—there isn't any evidence. They're extrapolating about the risks of jogging from the fact that pregnant women have slightly more flexible fingers. Perhaps someone should study this topic directly someday. In the meantime, I'd argue the huge benefits of exercise should overrule any purely theoretical concerns. Just to clarify, the concern is about ligaments rather than muscles, so stretching is fine. Two studies have even examined the beneficial effects of stretching exercises during pregnancy.[142]

5. Exercising the abdominal muscles.

There's a common misconception that sit-ups during pregnancy are taboo. That's nonsense. In fact, according to one study, abdominal exercises help "improve muscle performance during labor, correct poor posture, and prevent rectus abdominus muscle separation."[143] Muscle separation sounds dire, but it's actually quite common. The rectus abdominus, otherwise known as the six pack for those in good shape, is actually two parallel muscles separated by a middle band of connective tissue. This connective tissue can tear during pregnancy from the pressure of the expanding belly, resulting in a very common and usually temporary condition called *diastasis recti*, which affects up to two-thirds of women by the third trimester.[144] Fortunately, it appears that regular sit-ups can help prevent this condition. For example, in a study in India, 14 out of 15 women who did no abdominal exercises developed *diastasis recti* versus only 8 out of 15 among those who did.[145]

It's easy to tell if you have *diastasis recti*: you'll see a vertical ridge forming when you strain your stomach muscles. If you do develop the condition, some suggest skipping the sit-ups,[146, 147] while others say sit-ups will simply become more difficult.[148] Probably the best answer is to only raise your head: "This activates just the superficial abdominal muscles that have separated. If the shoulders are raised off the floor, the deeper abdominal muscles will contract, causing an increase in the separation."[149] By the third trimester, sit-ups may slightly increase your risk of developing lower back pain, but who wants to be doing crunches with a huge belly anyway?[150]

So most mainstream exercise appears to be perfectly safe. What about trendy activities like Pilates and yoga? According to a review, there's "little evidence-based literature concerning these practices, so it should be recommended to be careful."[151] But preliminary studies would suggest both are fine. One study claims that "light muscle strengthening performed during the second and third trimesters of pregnancy has minimal effect on newborn body size and overall health."[152] And according to a review of yoga in pregnancy, preliminary evidence suggests that it's safe and may even improve birth outcomes: "While awaiting an appropriately designed trial . . . it remains a viable exercise option."[153]

In conclusion, you have no excuse. It's time to get off the couch and head to the gym or go for a jog. Don't expect it to be easy. Even marathon runner Paula Radcliffe, discussing her training regime with Kara Goucher, admitted that the two couldn't keep up the intensity of their normal routine: "No matter how hard we train, and no matter how many marathons we've run, nothing compares to pregnancy." But keep in mind that now's your chance. No matter how challenging, it's still easier to jog with a bump than a baby carriage.

Threat level for exercise: Very low

It's Getting Hot in Here: Hot Tubs and Saunas

The hosts of a ski resort bed and breakfast led my husband and me across a vast snowy lawn to the outdoor hot tub, positioned well away from the house to ensure privacy. After settling us in, they left, carrying our bathrobes and snow boots with them, promising to return with them "toasty warm." Half an hour later, they returned to find us miserably draped in awkward positions along the rim of the tub, trying to simultaneously avoid frostbite in our extremities while preventing our core body from overheating. So much for our romantic interlude.

Extreme weather aside, most of us are sensible enough to climb out of a hot tub when we feel our temperature rising. Our face flushes, we feel uncomfortable, and it's obvious that it's time to cool off. Nevertheless, warnings about the dangers of slipping into a hot tub while pregnant abound—it's a pregnancy taboo. And these warnings are not unfounded. There's evidence that getting overheated during pregnancy can cause neural tube defects in animals and in the children of women who have the misfortune to contract high fevers in early pregnancy.[154] The question is, when it comes to a voluntary activity like sitting in a hot tub or sauna, are we sensitive enough to our own body temperature to instinctively get out before causing harm to our babies?

The answer is: probably. One study that measured women's temperatures in hot tubs concluded you're unlikely to raise your body temperature to worrisome levels.[155] The women spontaneously took their arms out of the water to cool off and eventually climbed out completely before getting too hot. There will always be cases of extreme behavior (one woman whose baby had a neural tube defect reportedly sat in a 106°F hot tub for nearly an hour early in her pregnancy).[156] A couple of studies have also linked using a hot tub early in pregnancy with miscarriage,[157, 158] but both studies have been criticized for relying on the women to self-report their behavior, frequently after they'd already miscarried.[159]

Concerned about the possibility that hot tubs could be causing harm, the Consumer Product Safety Commission finally commissioned a study in 2005 to review all the evidence. What did this study conclude? "The potential for effects of maternal hyperthermia [overheating] due to hot tub/spa use cannot be discounted."[160] In other words, it's possible that soaking in a hot tub could cause problems, but there isn't any definitive proof. The study also points out that "approximately 50 percent of pregnancies in the US are unplanned, and the majority of these pregnancies are not recognized until the period of neural tube closure has already passed." So by the time you pick up a book like this, you're probably past the point where it matters. But if you want to be well-behaved and follow all the rules, the American College of Obstetricians and Gynecologists says to soak no more than ten minutes.[161]

Happen to enjoy sweating profusely in small, confined spaces? In that case, you're in luck: the evidence on saunas is even less definitive. Let's travel for a moment across the ocean to the small Nordic country of Finland. Finland is a country of five million people and two million saunas, purportedly the only nation in the world with more saunas than cars.[164, 165] In Finland, the typical sauna has no warning sign hanging outside mentioning any health risks, and more than 95 percent of pregnant women continue to go to the sauna at least once a week.[166] Yet the rate of neural tube defects in Finland is one of the lowest in the world.[167, 168] Pregnant women in Finland do appear to modify their behavior slightly—for example, staying in for a shorter time and lowering the temperature.[169, 170] Whether this is a cultural norm or whether women behave this way spontaneously is unclear. But a Finnish study comparing babies with and without birth defects concluded that "the relatively mild, temporal hyperthermia caused by the sauna should not be considered hazardous for the developing embryo,"[171] and another review from 2001 has concluded that "sauna is not harmful in moderation for healthy women with uncomplicated pregnancies."[172] If you want to be rule-abiding, fine: the American College of Obstetricians and Gynecologists recommends staying in the sauna for no more than fifteen minutes.[173]

So if you're lucky enough to have a hot tub in your backyard or a spa hotel on your travel itinerary, go for it. If you happen to be shy about showing off your bump, just be happy you're not in Finland. There may not be a sign to warn you outside the door, but you'll discover pretty quickly that Finnish saunas do have rules. It's just that it's clothing, not pregnancy, that's prohibited.[174]

Threat level for hot tubs and saunas: Very low

A Night on the Town: Loud Noise

The dance floor was heaving with jubilant wedding guests, young and old. My heavily pregnant friend was perched on a stool at one of the bordering tables, bopping her head in time with the music and probably regretting her choice of heels. I could barely hear her voice above the music, but she managed to shout into my ear, "My baby totally loves the music! I can feel him kicking and dancing around!"

Retreating to the bar in the adjoining room, I found another pregnant friend ensconced in a comfortable sofa. "Aren't you going to come dance?" I asked her.

"Oh no," she replied. "I need to stay here, where it's quieter. I could tell my baby was really disturbed by the loud music—he kept kicking and squirming around."

No one can read the mind of a fetus, these mothers included, so we'll never know whether those babies were kicking because they loved the music, hated it, or were merely reacting instinctively to a stimulus. I, too, did my fair share of dancing to loud music while pregnant and hoped my baby liked the music as much as I did. But I did feel a vague sense of guilt standing near the reverberating speakers. Was there a chance I could be damaging those tiny, sensitive eardrums?

There's no doubt babies can hear sounds well before they emerge from the womb, even prior to five months.[175] But no one has yet proven that loud sounds do a fetus any harm. A variety of studies have looked at women living next to airports,[176, 177, 178, 179] working in manufacturing,[180] working in a nut-shelling factory,[181] or in other loud environments.[182, 183] But according to a review of the field, none of these studies are definitive, because they didn't take factors like socioeconomic status and smoking into account, didn't actually measure the levels of noise, etc. The review concludes, "because of the paucity of information on the effects of prenatal noise exposure, our knowledge is incomplete."[184] Similarly, another in-depth discussion of the topic also concludes the jury is still out on whether loud noise affects hearing or is linked to other outcomes like premature birth.[185]

There's not even consensus on whether the occasional nightclub/rock concert/wedding band will do your *own* hearing any harm. One study has suggested that exposure to loud music doesn't appear to be linked to permanent hearing impairment.[186] On the other hand, the National Institutes of Health claims that ~15 percent of Americans age twenty to sixty-nine have hearing loss that may have been caused by exposure to loud sounds.[187]

So feel free to attempt to protect your little one from loud noise while you still can. But keep in mind that by age eighteen, he or she is unlikely to accept your proffered earplugs before heading out into the night. If your child ultimately ends up with hearing loss later in life, you can rest assured that it's far more likely to be his or her own fault, not yours.

Threat level for loud noise: Very low

Humping the Bump: Sexual Activity

Pregnancy is very sexy. If you don't believe me, check out Claudia Schiffer and Demi Moore posing on the covers of German *Vogue* and *Vanity Fair*, respectively. Or ask your partner. But up to half of mothers and a quarter of fathers worry that sexual activity will harm their baby, which is a bit of a libido killer.[188]

This one sits firmly in the category of myth. An exhaustive review of fifty-nine studies has concluded that as long as there are no obvious complications (like bleeding), sexual activity in pregnancy won't do any harm whatsoever.[189] And couples who maintain a healthy, enjoyable sex life during pregnancy are more likely to have a harmonious marriage both four months and three years after the birth (although, of course, this may be correlation rather than causation).

So if you're in the mood, go for it. If you're not feeling very glamorous, there's an absurdly named brand of lingerie called Hotmilk designed specifically for pregnant women.[190] If you've got it, flaunt it.

Threat level for sexual activity: Very low[191]

Conclusions: Strive Not to Drive

I suspect you've spent your first few pregnant months cutting down on your coffee consumption, avoiding miscellaneous threats like blue cheese and hot tubs, curtailing your activity in the sack, and perhaps stressing about stress at work. Your doctor has been carefully monitoring your weight gain. But neither of you have been obsessing about the length of your commute, despite the fact that driving is significantly more dangerous to your fetus than any of these other factors. This comparison is not meant to trivialize the impact or danger of contracting food poisoning during pregnancy. Given that foodborne infections can potentially be avoided through greater maternal awareness and vigilance, even a single fetal death is one too many. But the same mothers who religiously give up caffeine don't think twice about hopping in the car to pick up a decaf at Starbucks. And mothers who occasionally indulge in forbidden foods often feel guilty, while virtually no one feels guilt about getting into the car.

Let's say you're invited to a dinner party. It's the drive that should make you think twice, not the blue cheese or even the undercooked hamburgers offered by your host.

Notes

1. Babycenter.com Editorial Team. (Last updated 2015, August). What's the best sleeping position during pregnancy? BabyCenter.com. https://www.babycenter.com/404_whats-the-best-sleeping-position-during-pregnancy_7608.bc.

2. Downs, M. (2002, September 2). Sleep soundly during pregnancy. WebMD.com. www.webmd.com/baby/features/sleep-soundly-during-pregnancy.

3. Murkoff, H., & Mazel, S. (2008). *What to expect when you're expecting* (4th ed.). New York: Workman Publishing Company.

4. Kauppila, A., Koskinen, M., Puolakka, J., Tuimala, R., Kuikka, J. (1980). Decreased intervillous and unchanged myometrial blood flow in supine recumbency. *Obstetrics & Gynecology, 55* (2), 203–205. http://journals.lww.com/greenjournal/Abstract/1980/02000/Decreased_Intervillous_and_Unchanged_Myometrial.15.aspx.

5. Ellington, C., Katz, V. L., Watson, W. J., & Spielman, F. J. (1991). The effect of lateral tilt on maternal and fetal hemodynamic variables. *Obstetrics & Gynecology, 77* (2), 201–203. http://journals.lww.com/greenjournal/abstract/1991/02000/the_effect_of_lateral_tilt_on_maternal_and_fetal.7.aspx.

6. Clark, S. L., Cotton, D. B., Pivarnik, J. M., Lee, W., Hankins, G. D., Benedetti, T. J., & Phelan, J. P. (1991). Position change and central hemodynamic profile during normal third-trimester pregnancy and post partum. *American Journal of Obstetrics and Gynecology, 164* (3), 883–887. http://www.sciencedirect.com/science/article/pii/S0002937811905341.

7. Stacey, T., Thompson, J., Mitchell, E. A., Ekeroma, A. J., Zuccollo, J. M., & McCowan, L. M. (2011). Association between maternal sleep practices and risk of late stillbirth: a case-control study. *BMJ, 2011* (342), d3403. www.bmj.com/content/342/bmj.d3403.

8. Bazian (author), & the UK National Health Service (eds.). (2011, June 15). Mother's sleeping position and risk of stillbirth. NHS Choices. www.nhs.uk/news/2011/06June/Pages/mothers-sleeping-position-and-risk-of-stillbirth.aspx.

9. Mills, G. H., & Chaffe, A. G. (1994). Sleeping positions adopted by pregnant women of more than 30 weeks gestation. *Anaesthesia, 49* (3), 249–250. http://europepmc.org/abstract/med/8147522.

10. Farine, D., & Seaward, P. G. (2007). When it comes to pregnant women sleeping, is left right? *Journal of Obstetrics and Gynaecology Canada, 29* (10), 841–842. http://www.sciencedirect.com/science/article/pii/S1701216316326330.

11. Tengkuputeh. (2017, May 18). History of coffee. *Tengkuputeh*. https://tengkuputeh.com/2017/05/18/history-of-coffee/.

12. Juliano, L. M., & Griffiths, R. R. (2004). A critical review of caffeine withdrawal: empirical validation of symptoms and signs, incidence, severity, and associated features. *Psychopharmacology, 176* (1), 1–29. https://link.springer.com/article/10.1007/s00213-004-2000-x.

13. Mercola, J. (2009, January 3). How caffeine during pregnancy can damage your baby. Mercola.com. http://articles.mercola.com/sites/articles/archive/2009/01/03/how-caffeine-during-pregnancy-can-damage-your-baby.aspx.

14. Frary, C. D., Johnson, R. K., & Wang, M. Q. (2005). Food sources and intakes of caffeine in the diets of persons in the United States. *Journal of the American Dietetic Association, 105* (1), 110–113. http://www.sciencedirect.com/science/article/pii/S0002822304017302X.

15. Ibid.

16. A short Americano at Starbucks has ~75 mg of caffeine (Caffè Americano. [n.d.]. Starbucks.com. www.starbucks.com/menu/drinks/espresso/caffe-americano#size=93), and the average Nespresso capsule has ~60 mg (FAQs: How much caffeine is in each *Nespresso* Capsule?. [n.d.]. Nespresso.com. https://www.nespresso.com/us/en/grands-crus-coffee-range). The average female coffee drinker age 18–34 gets ~75% of her daily caffeine intake from coffee. When pregnant, the average woman 18–34 who continues to drink caffeine reduces her intake from ~100 mg to 58 mg; the 90th percentile reduces from 238 mg to 157 mg (Frary, C. D., Food sources and intakes of caffeine in the diets of persons in the United States).

17. Mercola, J., How caffeine during pregnancy can damage your baby.

18. Grady, D. (2008, January 21). Pregnancy problems tied to caffeine. NYTimes.com. www.nytimes.com/2008/01/21/health/21caffeine.html?_r=0.

19. Bech, B. H., Obel, C., Henriksen, T. B., & Olsen, J. (2007). Effect of reducing caffeine intake on birth weight and length of gestation: randomised controlled trial. *BMJ, 334* (7590), 409. www.ncbi.nlm.nih.gov/pmc/articles/PMC1804137/.

20. Medicines in my home: caffeine and your body. (2007). US Food and Drug Administration. https://www.fda.gov/Drugs/ResourcesForYou/Consumers/BuyingUsingMedicineSafely/UnderstandingOver-the-CounterMedicines/ucm092139.htm.

21. National Institute of Child Health and Human Development. (2013, July 15). What can I do to promote a healthy pregnancy? National Institutes of Health. www.nichd.nih.gov/health/topics/preconceptioncare/conditioninfo/pages/healthy-pregnancy.aspx.

22. Should I give up caffeine now that I'm pregnant? (n.d.). Academy of Nutrition and Dietetics.

23. March of Dimes. (2012, June). Eating and nutrition: caffeine in pregnancy. www.marchofdimes.com/pregnancy/caffeine-in-pregnancy.aspx.

24. UK National Health Service. (2013, May 6). Should I limit caffeine during pregnancy? NHS Choices. www.nhs.uk/chq/Pages/limit-caffeine-during-pregnancy. aspx?CategoryID=54&SubCategoryID=216.

25. Grosso, L. M., & Bracken, M. B. (2005). Caffeine metabolism, genetics, and perinatal outcomes: a review of exposure assessment considerations during pregnancy. *Annals of Epidemiology, 15* (6), 460–466. www.annalsofepidemiology.org/article/ S1047-2797(05)00014-1/abstract.

26. Aldridge, A., Bailey, J., & Neims, A. H. (1981, October). The disposition of caffeine during and after pregnancy. *Seminars in Perinatology, 5* (4), 310–314.

27. Grosso, L. M., Triche, E., Benowitz, N. L., & Bracken, M. B. (2008). Prenatal caffeine assessment: fetal and maternal biomarkers or self-reported intake? *Annals of Epidemiology, 18* (3), 172–178. www.ncbi.nlm.nih.gov/pmc/articles/PMC2275917/.

28. Goldstein, A., & Warren, R. (1962). Passage of caffeine into human gonadal and fetal tissue. *Biochemical Pharmacology, 11* (2), 166–168.

29. Salvador, H. S., & Koos, B. J. (1989). Effects of regular and decaffeinated coffee on fetal breathing and heart rate. *American Journal of Obstetrics and Gynecology, 160* (5), 1043–1047. www.sciencedirect.com/science/article/pii/0002937889901579.

30. Mulder, E. J. H., Tegaldo, L., Bruschettini, P., & Visser, G. H. A. (2009). Foetal response to maternal coffee intake: role of habitual versus non-habitual caffeine consumption. *Journal of Psychopharmacology, 24* (11), 1641–1648. http://jop.sagepub.com/content/24/11/1641. short.

31. Grosso, L. M., Prenatal caffeine assessment: fetal and maternal biomarkers or self-reported intake?

32. Brent, R. L., Christian, M. S., & Diener, R. M. (2011). Evaluation of the reproductive and developmental risks of caffeine. *Birth Defects Research Part B: Developmental and Reproductive Toxicology, 92* (2), 152–187. www.ncbi.nlm.nih.gov/pmc/articles/ PMC3121964/.

33. Higdon, J. V., & Frei, B. (2006). Coffee and health: a review of recent human research. *Critical Reviews in Food Science and Nutrition, 46* (2), 101–123. http://www.tandfonline. com/doi/abs/10.1080/10408390500400009.

34. Furneaux, E. C., Langley-Evans, A. J., & Langley-Evans, S. C. (2001). Nausea and vomiting of pregnancy: endocrine basis and contribution to pregnancy outcome. *Obstetrical & Gynecological Survey, 56* (12), 775–782. http://journals.lww.com/obgynsurvey/ Abstract/2001/12000/Nausea_and_Vomiting_of_Pregnancy__Endocrine_Basis.4.aspx.

35. Higdon, J. V., Coffee and health: a review of recent human research.

36. According to a review from 2002, "An association between caffeine consumption and a reproductive hazard is more likely to be seen in lower-quality studies than in studies that come closer to approximating the ideal. This is especially evident for 'lower' birth weight and congenital anomalies . . . it seems reasonable to conclude that no convincing evidence has been presented to show that caffeine consumption increases the risk of any reproductive adversity" (Leviton, A., & Cowan, L. [2002]. A review of the literature relating caffeine consumption by women to their risk of reproductive hazards. *Food and Chemical Toxicology, 40* [9], 1271–1310. www.sciencedirect.com/science/article/pii/ S0278691502000923). According to a review from 2004 addressing the potential link between caffeine and spontaneous abortion, "All of the studies reviewed suffer from important methodologic limitations that hinder both the interpretation of each study individually and the comparison of results across studies. . . . Until studies can overcome these limitations, evidence for a causal link between caffeine and spontaneous abortion

will remain inconclusive" (Signorello, L. B., & McLaughlin, J. K. [2004]. Maternal caffeine consumption and spontaneous abortion: a review of the epidemiologic evidence. *Epidemiology, 15* (2), 229–239. http://journals.lww.com/epidem/Abstract/2004/03000/Maternal_Caffeine_Consumption_and_Spontaneous.17.aspx). According to a review from 2006 addressing the link between caffeine and low birth weight, "A number of the available epidemiological studies have been criticized for inadequately controlling for important risk factors for low birth weight and fetal growth retardation, particularly smoking . . . it appears unlikely that caffeine intakes less than 300 mg/[day] will adversely affect fetal growth in nonsmoking women" (Higdon, J. V., Coffee and health: a review of recent human research.) According to a Cochrane review from 2009, "There is insufficient evidence to confirm or refute the effectiveness of caffeine avoidance on birth weight or other pregnancy outcomes" (Jahanfar, S., & Jaafar, S. H. [2013]. Effects of restricted caffeine intake by mother on fetal, neonatal and pregnancy outcome. *Cochrane Database of Systematic Reviews, 2015* (6). http://onlinelibrary.wiley.com/doi/10.1002/14651858.CD006965.pub4/full). The American College of Obstetricians and Gynecologists concluded in 2010 that "moderate caffeine consumption (less than 200 mg per day) does not appear to be a major contributing factor in miscarriage or preterm birth. The relationship of caffeine to growth restriction remains undetermined. A final conclusion cannot be made at this time as to whether there is a correlation between high caffeine intake and miscarriage" (ACOG Committee on Obstetric Practice. [2010, August]. ACOG committee opinion no. 462: moderate caffeine consumption during pregnancy. *Obstetrics and Gynecology, 2010* [116], 467–468. www.acog.org/Resources_And_Publications/Committee_Opinions/Committee_on_Obstetric_Practice/Moderate_Caffeine_Consumption_During_Pregnancy). The International Life Sciences Institute, a "nonprofit, worldwide organization whose mission is to provide science that improves public health and well-being," concluded in 2011 that "dietary exposures of caffeine are not teratogenic or are directly responsible for an increased risk of spontaneous abortion or fetal growth retardation. Studies that involve very high exposures to caffeine are difficult to evaluate because of the many confounding factors that contribute to the risks that are not adequately evaluated; however, the animal studies indicate that even the highest human exposures in the epidemiological studies are unlikely to have reproductive and developmental effects" (Brent, R. L., et al., Evaluation of the reproductive and developmental risks of caffeine).

37. Bech, B. H., Obel, C., Henriksen, T. B., & Olsen, J. (2007). Effect of reducing caffeine intake on birth weight and length of gestation: randomised controlled trial. *BMJ, 334* (7590), 409. www.ncbi.nlm.nih.gov/pmc/articles/PMC1804137/.

38. Wirth, F. (2001). *Prenatal parenting: the complete psychological and spiritual guide to loving your unborn child.* New York: Harper Collins, 32–33. As described in: Story, L. (2003). A head start in life? Prenatal parenting and the discourse of fetal stimulation. *Critical Studies in Gender, Culture & Social Justice, 27* (2), 41–48. http://forms.msvu.ca/atlantis/vol/272all/272story.PDF.

39. Verny, T. R., & Weintraub, P. (2002). *Tomorrow's baby: the art and science of parenting from conception through infancy.* New York: Simon and Schuster. As described in: Story, L., A head start in life?

40. Janov, A. (2000). *The biology of love.* New York: Prometheus Books. As described in: Story, L., A head start in life?

41. March of Dimes. (2009, December 9). Sushi and breastfeeding join birth defects and preterm birth as leading concerns of moms. MarchofDimes.com. www.marchofdimes.com/news/sushi-and-breastfeeding-join-birth-defects-and-preterm-birth-as-leading-concerns-of-moms.aspx.

42. Dunkel Schetter, C. (2011). Psychological science on pregnancy: stress processes, biopsychosocial models, and emerging research issues. *Annual Review of Psychology, 62*, 531–558. http://www.annualreviews.org/doi/abs/10.1146/annurev.psych.031809.130727.

43. Dole, N., Savitz, D. A., Hertz-Picciotto, I., Siega-Riz, A. M., McMahon, M. J., & Buekens, P. (2003). Maternal stress and preterm birth. *American Journal of Epidemiology, 157* (1), 14–24. https://academic.oup.com/aje/article/157/1/14/66374/Maternal-Stress-and-Preterm-Birth.

44. Orr, S. T., Reiter, J. P., Blazer, D. G., & James, S. A. (2007). Maternal prenatal pregnancy-related anxiety and spontaneous preterm birth in Baltimore, Maryland. *Psychosomatic Medicine, 69* (6), 566–570. http://journals.lww.com/psychosomaticmedicine/Abstract/2007/07000/Maternal_Prenatal_Pregnancy_Related_Anxiety_and.13.aspx.

45. Kramer, M. S., Lydon, J., Séguin, L., Goulet, L., Kahn, S. R., McNamara, H., Genest, J., Dassa, C., Chen, M. F., Sharma, S., Meaney, M. J., Thomson, S., Van Uum, S., Koren, G., Dahhou, M., Lamoureux, J., & Platt, R. W. (2009). Stress pathways to spontaneous preterm birth: the role of stressors, psychological distress, and stress hormones. *American Journal of Epidemiology, 169* (11), 1319–1326. https://academic.oup.com/aje/article/169/11/1319/159683/Stress-Pathways-to-Spontaneous-Preterm-Birth-The.

46. According to one study (Kramer, M. S., et al., Stress pathways to spontaneous preterm birth), mothers with the highest quartile of pregnancy-related anxiety had an odds ratio of 2.4 for preterm birth. The baseline incidence of preterm birth in the population as of 2010 was 12% according to the CDC (Martin, J. A., Hamilton, B. E., Ventura, S. J., Osterman, M. J., Wilson, E.C., & Mathews, T. J. [2012, August 28]. Births: final data for 2010. *National Vital Statistics Report 61* [1], 1–90. www.cdc.gov/nchs/data/nvsr/nvsr61/nvsr61_01.pdf), so applying the appropriate conversion formula (Higgins, J. P. T., & Green, S. [2011, March]. Computing absolute risk reduction or NNT from an odds ratio [OR]. *Cochrane Handbook for Systematic Reviews of Interventions*, 12.5.4.3. http://handbook.cochrane.org/chapter_12/12_5_4_3_computing_absolute_risk_reduction_or_nnt_from_an_odds.htm), that equates to a 12.7% absolute increase in preterm birth attributable to pregnancy-related anxiety for the top quartile or an absolute increase of 3% for the full population. (In case you were wondering, the researchers took into account the possibility that the women with poor birth outcomes could have known they were at higher statistical risk for pregnancy complications during pregnancy and were therefore rationally worried beforehand: "The association persisted after adjustment for perception of pregnancy risk, including perceived risk of preterm birth.")

47. Threat score is 3% (probability of preterm birth, as calculated in the previous footnote) x 100 (impact: statistically detectable impairment) x 1 (certainty: well proven) = 3.

48. Laughlin, L. L. (2011). Maternity leave and employment patterns of first-time mothers: 1961–2008. US Department of Commerce, Economics and Statistics Administration, US Census Bureau. www.census.gov/prod/2011pubs/p70-128.pdf.

49. Christensen, H., Leach, L. S., & Mackinnon, A. (2010). Cognition in pregnancy and motherhood: prospective cohort study. *The British Journal of Psychiatry, 196* (2), 126–132. http://bjp.rcpsych.org/content/196/2/126.short.

50. Crawley, R., Grant, S., & Hinshaw, K. (2008). Cognitive changes in pregnancy: mild decline or societal stereotype? *Applied Cognitive Psychology, 22* (8), 1142–1162. http://onlinelibrary.wiley.com/doi/10.1002/acp.1427/abstract.

51. Saurel-Cubizolles, M. J., Zeitlin, J., Lelong, N., Papiernik, E., Di Renzo, G. C., & Bréart, G. (2004). Employment, working conditions, and preterm birth: results from the Europop case-control survey. *Journal of Epidemiology and Community Health, 58* (5), 395–401. http://jech.bmj.com/content/58/5/395.full.

52. Maconochie, N., Doyle, P., Prior, S., & Simmons, R. (2007). Risk factors for first trimester miscarriage—results from a UK-population-based case-control study. *BJOG: An International Journal of Obstetrics & Gynaecology, 114* (2), 170–186. www.issues4life.org/pdfs/iariskptbo27.pdf.

53. McDonald, A. D. (1988). Work and pregnancy. *British Journal of Industrial Medicine, 45* (9), 577. www.ncbi.nlm.nih.gov/pmc/articles/PMC1009658/pdf/brjindmedoo149-0001.pdf.

54. Shi, L., & Chia, S. E. (2001). A review of studies on maternal occupational exposures and birth defects, and the limitations associated with these studies. *Occupational Medicine, 51* (4), 230–244. http://occmed.oxfordjournals.org/content/51/4/230.full.pdf.

55. Salihu, H. M., Myers, J., & August, E. M. (2012). Pregnancy in the workplace. *Occupational Medicine, 62* (2), 88–97. http://occmed.oxfordjournals.org/content/62/2/88.full.

56. According to the American College of Obstetricians and Gynecologists, there is a 9–11 percent chance your water will break before the onset of labor (Mercer, B. [1998]. ACOG Practice Bulletin #1: premature rupture of membranes. Washington, DC: ACOG.). According to an informal online poll (Surrogate Mothers Online. (n.d.). View poll results: What time of day did your water break? [used in the absence of any formal research on this topic]), 10 out of 54 women had their water break between 9 a.m. and 6 p.m., or 18.5%, and only 5/7 days are working days. So ~10% * 18.5% * 5/7 = 1.3%.

57. McDonald, A. D., McDonald, J. C., Armstrong, B., Cherry, N., Delorme, C., D-Nolin, A., & Robert, D. (1987). Occupation and pregnancy outcome. *British Journal of Industrial Medicine, 44* (8), 521–526. www.ncbi.nlm.nih.gov/pmc/articles/PMC1007870/pdf/brjindmedoo160-0017.pdf.

58. McDonald, A. D., Work and pregnancy.

59. Ahmed, P., & Jaakkola, J. J. (2007). Maternal occupation and adverse pregnancy outcomes: a Finnish population-based study. *Occupational Medicine, 57* (6), 417–423. http://occmed.oxfordjournals.org/content/57/6/417.full.pdf.

60. Henriksen, T. B., Hedegaard, M., Secher, N. J., & Wilcox, A. J. (1995). Standing at work and preterm delivery. *BJOG: An International Journal of Obstetrics & Gynaecology, 102* (3), 198–206. http://onlinelibrary.wiley.com/doi/10.1111/j.1471-0528.1995.tb09094.x/abstract?deniedAccessCustomisedMessage=&userIsAuthenticated=false.

61. Mozurkewich, E. L., Luke, B., Avni, M., & Wolf, F. M. (2000). Working conditions and adverse pregnancy outcome: a meta-analysis. *Obstetrics & Gynecology, 95* (4), 623–635. http://journals.lww.com/greenjournal/Abstract/2000/04000/Working_Conditions_and_Adverse_Pregnancy_Outcome_.29.aspx.

62. Juhl, M., Strandberg-Larsen, K., Stemann Larsen, P., Kragh Andersen, P., Wulff Svendsen, S., Peter Bonde, J., & Nybo Andersen, A. M. (2013). Occupational lifting during pregnancy and risk of fetal death in a large national cohort study. *Scandinavian Journal of Work, Environment & Health, 39* (4). http://www.jstor.org/stable/23558332.

63. According to one review, current advisories about occupational exposure to chemicals may not be sufficiently risk-averse: "The 201 chemicals already recognized as human neurotoxicants should be considered potentially hazardous to pregnant workers. Despite the lack of occupational epidemiology studies in this field, exposures that are not considered to be toxic in adults may still be harmful to fetal neurodevelopment." (Julvez, J., & Grandjean, P. [2009]. Neurodevelopmental toxicity risks due to occupational exposure to industrial chemicals during pregnancy. *Industrial Health, 47* [5], 459–468. https://www.jstage.jst.go.jp/article/indhealth/47/5/47_5_459/_article).

64. Palmer, K. T., Bonzini, M., & Bonde, J. P. (2013). Concise guidance: pregnancy—occupational aspects of management. *Clinical Medicine, 13* (1), 75. www.ncbi.nlm.nih.gov/pmc/articles/PMC3653071/.

There have also been no randomized trials studying the impact of reducing occupational fatigue on pregnancy outcomes.

65. Schenker, M. B., Eaton, M., Green, R., & Samuels, S. (1997). Self-reported stress and reproductive health of female lawyers. *Journal of Occupational and Environmental Medicine, 39* (6), 556–568. http://journals.lww.com/joem/Abstract/1997/06000/Self_Reported_Stress_and_Reproductive_Health_of.11.aspx.

66. Maconochie, N., Risk factors for first trimester miscarriage.

67. Saurel-Cubizolles, M. J., et al., Employment, working conditions, and preterm birth: results from the Europop case-control survey.

68. Svenson, O. (1981). Are we all less risky and more skillful than our fellow drivers? *Acta Psychologica, 47* (2), 143–148. http://heatherlench.com/wp-content/uploads/2008/07/svenson.pdf.

69. Centers for Disease Control and Prevention. (n.d.). CDC Wonder: About compressed mortality, 1999–2012. http://wonder.cdc.gov/cmf-icd10.html.

70. Klinich, K. D., Flannagan, C. A., Rupp, J. D., Sochor, M., Schneider, L. W., & Pearlman, M. D. (2008). Fetal outcome in motor-vehicle crashes: effects of crash characteristics and maternal restraint. *American Journal of Obstetrics and Gynecology, 198* (4), 450.e1–450.e9. http://www.sciencedirect.com/science/article/pii/S0002937808001452.

71. Sirin, H., Weiss, H. B., Sauber-Schatz, E. K., & Dunning, K. (2007). Seat belt use, counseling and motor-vehicle injury during pregnancy: results from a multi-state population-based survey. *Maternal and Child Health Journal, 11* (5), 505–510. http://citeseerx.ist.psu.edu/viewdoc/download?doi=10.1.1.579.7699&rep=rep1&type=pdf www.injurycontrol.com/Hank/reprints/pramsbelt.pdf.

72. Frequently asked questions: car safety for you and your baby. (2011) American College of Obstetricians & Gynecologists. www.acog.org/~/media/For%20Patients/faq018.pdf?dmc=1&ts=20120726T0948556730.

73. Should pregnant women wear seat belts? (2002, September). National Highway Traffic Safety Administration.

59. Klinich, K. D., et al., Fetal outcome in motor-vehicle crashes.

74. Hyde, L. K., Cook, L. J., Olson, L. M., Weiss, H. B., & Dean, J. M. (2003). Effect of motor vehicle crashes on adverse fetal outcomes. *Obstetrics & Gynecology, 102* (2), 279–286. http://www.sciencedirect.com/science/article/pii/S0029784403005180.

75. Wolf, M. E., Alexander, B. H., Rivara, F. P., Hickok, D. E., Maier, R. V., & Starzyk, P. M. (1993). A retrospective cohort study of seatbelt use and pregnancy outcome after a motor vehicle crash. *Journal of Trauma and Acute Care Surgery, 34* (1), 116–119. http://journals.lww.com/jtrauma/Abstract/1993/01000/A_Retrospective_Cohort_Study_of_Seatbelt_Use_and.21.aspx.

76. Pearlman, M. D., & Phillips, M. E. (1996). Safety belt use during pregnancy. *Obstetrics & Gynecology, 88* (6), 1026–1029. http://journals.lww.com/greenjournal/Abstract/1996/12000/Safety_Belt_Use_During_Pregnancy.22.aspx.

77. **Maternal death:** 6/100,000 (probability of mother dying as a driver or passenger in a motor vehicle, as referenced in the main text) x 100,000 (impact: death) x 1 (certainty: well-proven) = 6.0.

   Fetal death: one study estimates the fetal loss rate as 2.3 deaths per 100,000 live births, excluding cases pertaining to maternal deaths where there was no delivery, e.g. not double-counting the maternal death figure (Weiss, H. B., Songer, T. J., & Fabio, A. [2001]. Fetal deaths related to maternal injury. *JAMA, 286* [15], 1863–1868. https://www.ncbi.nlm.nih.gov/pubmed/11597288); another estimates 81% of 6.5 deaths per

100,000 live births (Weiss, H. B. [2001]. The epidemiology of traumatic injury-related fetal mortality in Pennsylvania, 1995–1997: the role of motor vehicle crashes. *Accident Analysis & Prevention, 33* [4], 449–454. http://www.sciencedirect.com/science/article/pii/S0001457500000580). Taking the midpoint, that's 3.8 deaths per 100,000 live births (probability) x 100,000 (impact: death) x 1 (certainty: well-proven) = 3.8.

Fetal injury: In an analysis of 57 crashes involving pregnant women, there were 12 fetal deaths and 11 crashes in which "the fetus survived but experienced major complications" (Klinich, K. D., Fetal outcome in motor-vehicle crashes; National Highway Traffic Safety Administration. [2012]. Traffic safety facts 2010: a compilation of motor vehicle crash data from the Fatality Analysis Reporting System and the General Estimates System. Early edition. Washington, DC: US Department of Transportation. https://crash-stats.nhtsa.dot.gov/Api/Public/ViewPublication/811659), so the rates for deaths and complications are similar. So 3.8 *11/12 per 100,000 live births (probability) x 10,000 (impact: significant impairment) x 1 (certainty: well-proven) = 0.3.

Total threat score = 6.0 + 3.8 + 0.3 = 10.1.

78. Ostrower, J., & Michaels, D. (2013, October 23). The incredible shrinking plane seat. WSJ. com. http://online.wsj.com/news/articles/SB10001424052702304384104579141941949066648.

79. Simpson, E. L., Lawrenson, R. A., Nightingale, A. L., & Farmer, R. D. T. (2001). Venous thromboembolism in pregnancy and the puerperium: incidence and additional risk factors from a London perinatal database. *BJOG: An International Journal of Obstetrics & Gynaecology, 108* (1), 56–60. http://onlinelibrary.wiley.com/doi/10.1111/j.1471-0528.2001.00004.x/full.

80. Lewis, G., & Drife, J. (2001). Why mothers die, 1997–1999. Report of the confidential enquiry into maternal deaths in the UK. London: Royal College of Obstetricians and Gynaecologists Press. As cited in: Drife, J. (2003). Thromboembolism: reducing maternal death and disability during pregnancy. *British Medical Bulletin, 67* (1), 177–190. http://bmb.oxfordjournals.org/content/67/1/177.long.

81. Sanson, B. J., Lensing, A. W., Prins, M. H., Ginsberg, J. S., Barkagan, Z. S., Lavenne-Pardonge, E., Brenner, B., Dulitzky, M., Nielsen, J. D., Boda, Z., & Tu, S. (1999). Safety of low-molecular-weight heparin in pregnancy: a systematic review. *Thrombosis and Haemostasis, 81* (5), 668–72. www.schattauer.de/de/magazine/uebersicht/zeitschriften-a-z/thrombosis-and-haemostasis/contents/archive/issue/898/manuscript/4826/show.html.

82. Royal College of Obstetricians and Gynaecologists. (2008). Air travel and pregnancy: Scientific Advisory Committee Opinion Paper 1. https://www.rcog.org.uk/globalassets/documents/guidelines/scientific-impact-papers/sip_1.pdf.

83. Drife, J. 2003. Thromboembolism: reducing maternal death and disability during pregnancy. *British Medical Bulletin, 67* (1), 177–190. http://bmb.oxfordjournals.org/content/67/1/177.long.

84. American College of Obstetricians and Gynecologists Committee on Obstetric Practice. ACOG committee opinion no. 433: air travel during pregnancy. (2002). *Obstetrics and Gynecology 2009* (114), 954–955. www.acog.org/~/media/Committee%20Opinions/Committee%20on%20Obstetric%20Practice/co443.pdf?dmc=1&ts=20131007T1730280146.

85. Huch, R., Baumann, H., Fallenstein, F., Schneider, K., Holdener, F., & Huch, A. (1986). Physiologic changes in pregnant women and their fetuses during jet air travel. *American Journal of Obstetrics and Gynecology, 154* (5), 996–1000. www.sciencedirect.com/science/article/pii/0002937886907362; Freeman, M., Ghidini, A., Spong, C. Y., Tchabo, N., Bannon, P. Z., & Pezzullo, J. C. (2004). Does air travel affect pregnancy outcome? *Archives of Gynecology and Obstetrics, 269* (4), 274–277. https://www.ncbi.nlm.nih.gov/pubmed/15205979.

There is some very preliminary evidence that flight attendants may have slightly higher rates of miscarriage, but this could be due to other factors, such as long hours spent standing (Aspholm, R., Lindbohm, M. L., Paakkulainen, H., Taskinen, H., Nurminen, T., & Tiitinen, A. [1999]. Spontaneous abortions among Finnish flight attendants. *Journal of Occupational and Environmental Medicine, 41* [6], 486–491. http://journals.lww.com/joem/Abstract/1999/06000/Spontaneous_Abortions_Among_Finnish_Flight.15.aspx).

86. Sachdeva, A., Dalton, M., Amaragiri, S. V., & Lees, T. (2014). Graduated compression stockings for prevention of deep vein thrombosis. *Cochrane Database of Systematic Reviews, 2014* (12). http://onlinelibrary.wiley.com/doi/10.1002/14651858.CD001484.pub3/full.

87. American College of Obstetricians and Gynecologists Committee on Obstetric Practice, ACOG committee opinion no. 433: air travel during pregnancy.

88. Ferrari, E., Chevallier, T., Chapelier, A., & Baudouy, M. (1999). Travel as a risk factor for venous thromboembolic disease: a case-control study. *CHEST Journal, 115* (2), 440–444. http://www.daigonline.de/site-content/die-daig/fachorgan/2004/ejomr-2005-vol.9/146.pdf.

89. Heit, J. A., Kobbervig, C. E., James, A. H., Petterson, T. M., Bailey, K. R., & Melton, L. J. (2005). Trends in the incidence of venous thromboembolism during pregnancy or postpartum: a 30-year population-based study. *Annals of Internal Medicine, 143* (10), 697–706. www.copacamu.org/IMG/pdf/Heit-ann_int_med.pdf.

90. Simpson, E. L., Lawrenson, R. A., Nightingale, A. L., & Farmer, R. D. T. (2001). Venous thromboembolism in pregnancy and the puerperium: incidence and additional risk factors from a London perinatal database. *BJOG: An International Journal of Obstetrics & Gynaecology, 108* (1), 56–60. http://onlinelibrary.wiley.com/doi/10.1111/j.1471-0528.2001.00004.x/full.

91. Threat score is 1.4/100,000 (probability of death from a blood clot, as referenced in the main text) x 100,000 (impact: death) x 1 (certainty: well proven) = 1.4.

92. Jackson, K. D., Howie, L. D., & Akinbami, L. J. (2013). Trends in allergic conditions among children: United States, 1997–2011. NCHS data brief no. 121. Hyattsville, MD: National Center for Data Statistics, 1–8. https://pdfs.semanticscholar.org/2aea/9abd11f5e51bf-c3756f41e6d3cb894b8bb1d.pdf.

93. Rudders, S. A., Banerji, A., Vassallo, M. F., Clark, S., & Camargo Jr, C. A. (2010). Trends in pediatric emergency department visits for food-induced anaphylaxis. *Journal of Allergy and Clinical Immunology, 126* (2), 385–388. http://www.jacionline.org/article/S0091-6749(10)00819-5/pdf.

94. Schaub, B., Liu, J., Höppler, S., Schleich, I., Huehn, J., Olek, S., Wieczorek, G., Illi, S., & Von Mutius, E. (2009). Maternal farm exposure modulates neonatal immune mechanisms through regulatory T cells. *Journal of Allergy and Clinical Immunology, 123* (4), 774–782. http://hzi.openrepository.com/hzi/bitstream/10033/71118/1/Schaub%20et%20al_final.pdf.

95. Lieberman, J. (2014). Should we encourage allergen immunotherapy during pregnancy? *Expert Review of Clinical Immunology, 10*, (3), 317–319. http://informahealthcare.com/doi/abs/10.1586/1744666X.2014.881718.

96. Zeiger, R. S., Heller, S., Mellon, M. H., Halsey, J. F., Hamburger, R. N., & Sampson, H. A. (1992). Genetic and environmental factors affecting the development of atopy through age 4 in children of atopic parents: a prospective randomized study of food allergen avoidance. *Pediatric Allergy and Immunology, 3* (3), 110–127. http://onlinelibrary.wiley.com/doi/10.1111/j.1399-3038.1992.tb00035.x/abstract.

97. Fälth-Magnuesson, K., & Kjeltmann, N. I. (1987). Development of atopic disease in babies whose mothers were receiving exclusion diet during pregnancy—a randomized study.

Journal of Allergy and Clinical Immunology, 80 (6), 868–875. www.sciencedirect.com/
science/article/pii/S0091674987802798.

98. Fälth-Magnusson, K., & Max Kjeltman, N. I. (1992). Allergy prevention by maternal elimination diet during late pregnancy—a 5-year follow-up of a randomized study. *Journal of
Allergy and Clinical Immunology, 89* (3), 709–713. www.sciencedirect.com/science/article/
pii/009167499290378F.

99. Lilja, G., Dannaeus, A., Foucard, T., Graff-Lonnevig, V., Johansson, S. G. O., & Öman, H.
(1989). Effects of maternal diet during late pregnancy and lactation on the development of
atopic diseases in infants up to 18 months of age—*in-vivo* results. *Clinical & Experimental
Allergy, 19* (4), 473–479. http://onlinelibrary.wiley.com/doi/10.1111/j.1365-2222.1989.
tb02416.x/abstract.

100. Greer, F.R., Sicherer, S.H., Burks, W.A., and the Committee on Nutrition and Section on
Allergy and Immunology. (2008). Effects of early nutritional interventions on the development of atopic disease in infants and children: the role of maternal dietary restriction,
breastfeeding, timing of introduction of complementary foods, and hydrolyzed formulas.
Pediatrics, 121 (1), 183–91. http://pediatrics.aappublications.org/content/121/1/183.short.

101. Høst, A., Koletzko, B., Dreborg, S., Muraro, A., Wahn, U., Aggett, P., Bresson, J. L.,
Hernell, O., Lafeber, H., Michaelsen, K. F., Micheli, J. L., Rigo, J., Weaver, L., Heymans,
H., Strobel, S., & Vandenplas, Y. (1999). Dietary products used in infants for treatment
and prevention of food allergy: joint statement of the European Society for Paediatric
Allergology and Clinical Immunology (ESPACI) Committee on Hypoallergenic Formulas
and the European Society for Paediatric Gastroenterology, Hepatology and Nutrition
(ESPGHAN) Committee on Nutrition. *Archives of Disease in Childhood, 81* (1), 80–84.
www.ncbi.nlm.nih.gov/pmc/articles/PMC1717972/pdf/v081p00080.pdf.

102. Frank, L., Marian, A., Visser, M., Weinberg, E., & Potter, P. C. (1999). Exposure to
peanuts in utero and in infancy and the development of sensitization to peanut allergens in
young children. *Pediatric Allergy and Immunology, 10* (1), 27–32. www.ncbi.nlm.nih.gov/
pubmed/10410914.

103. Zeiger, R. S. (2003). Food allergen avoidance in the prevention of food allergy in infants
and children. *Pediatrics, 111* (Supplement 3), 1662–1671. http://pediatrics.aappublications.
org/content/111/Supplement_3/1662.short.

104. Lack, G., Fox, D., Northstone, K., & Golding, J. (2003). Factors associated with the
development of peanut allergy in childhood. *New England Journal of Medicine, 348* (11),
977–985. www.nejm.org/doi/full/10.1056/NEJMoa013536.

105. Frazier, A. L., Camargo, C. A., Malspeis, S., Willett, W. C., & Young, M. C. (2014).
Prospective study of peripregnancy consumption of peanuts or tree nuts by mothers and
the risk of peanut or tree nut allergy in their offspring. *JAMA Pediatrics, 168* (2), 156–162.
www.siaip.it/upload/1660_poi130073.pdf.

106. Greer, F.R., et al., Effects of early nutritional interventions on the development of atopic
disease in infants and children.

107. Sicherer, S. H., Muñoz-Furlong, A., & Sampson, H. A. (2003). Prevalence of peanut and
tree nut allergy in the United States determined by means of a random digit dial telephone
survey: a 5-year follow-up study. *Journal of Allergy and Clinical Immunology, 112* (6),
1203–1207. www.jacionline.org/article/S0091-6749(03)02026-8/abstract.

108. Geozone. (2007, March 2). Obese woman shocked to learn she was pregnant. *Digital
Journal.* http://www.digitaljournal.com/article/131069.

109. Parker-Pope, T. (2009, June 2). During pregnancy, starving for two. NYTimes.com. http://
well.blogs.nytimes.com/2009/06/02/starving-for-twoa/?_r=0.

110. Yaktine, A. L., & Rasmussen, K. M. (Eds.). (2009). Weight gain during pregnancy: reexamining the guidelines. Washington, DC: National Academies Press. https://www.ncbi.nlm.nih.gov/pubmed/20669500.

111. Ibid.

112. Schieve, L. A., Cogswell, M. E., & Scanlon, K. S. (1998). Trends in pregnancy weight gain within and outside ranges recommended by the Institute of Medicine in a WIC population. *Maternal and Child Health Journal, 2* (2), 111–116. https://www.ncbi.nlm.nih.gov/pubmed/10728266.

113. Yaktine, A. L., et al., Weight gain during pregnancy.

114. Abrams, B., Altman, S. L., & Pickett, K. E. (2000). Pregnancy weight gain: still controversial. *The American Journal of Clinical Nutrition, 71* (5), 1233s–1241s. http://ajcn.nutrition.org/content/71/5/1233s.full.

115. Rasmussen, K. M., Catalano, P. M., & Yaktine, A. L. (2009). New guidelines for weight gain during pregnancy: what obstetrician/gynecologists should know. *Current Opinion in Obstetrics & Gynecology, 21* (6), 521. www.ncbi.nlm.nih.gov/pmc/articles/PMC2847829/.

116. Abrams, B., Pregnancy weight gain: still controversial.

117. Williams M. (1969). Keeping fit for pregnancy and labour. London: National Childbirth Trust. www.glowm.com/resources/glowm/cd/pages/v2/v2c008.html.

118. Reshaping the body: clothing and cultural practice—the maternity corset. (2007). University of Virginia, Historical Collections at the Claude Moore Health Sciences Library. http://exhibits.hsl.virginia.edu/clothes/maternity_corset/.

119. American College of Obstetricians and Gynecologists. (2003). Exercise during pregnancy and the postpartum period: ACOG technical bulletin number 189—February 1994. *Clinical Obstetrics and Gynecology, 46* (2), 496. www.sciencedirect.com/science/article/pii/0020729294907730.

120. American College of Obstetricians and Gynecologists, Exercise during pregnancy and the postpartum period.; Artal, R., & O'Toole, M. (2003). Guidelines of the American College of Obstetricians and Gynecologists for exercise during pregnancy and the postpartum period. *British Journal of Sports Medicine, 37* (1), 6–12. http://bjsm.bmj.com/content/37/1/6.short.

121. Parker-Pope, T. (2010, August 19). Two running stars train while pregnant. NYTimes.com. http://well.blogs.nytimes.com/2010/08/19/two-running-stars-train-while-pregnant/?_r=0.

122. Rubin, R. (2012, January 9). Exercise during pregnancy? Yes, even some extreme sports. USAToday.com. http://usatoday30.usatoday.com/news/health/wellness/pregnancy/story/2012-01-09/Exercise-during-pregnancy-Yes-emdash-even-some-extreme-sports/52471860/1.

123. Filas, L. (2011, October 10). DuPage woman gives birth after running, walking marathon. DailyHerald.com. www.dailyherald.com/article/20111010/news/710109819/.

124. Artal, R., Guidelines of the American College of Obstetricians and Gynecologists for exercise during pregnancy and the postpartum period.

125. Ibid.

126. Charlesworth, S., Foulds, H. J. A., Burr, J. F., and Bredin, S. S. D.. (2011). Evidence-based risk assessment and recommendations for physical activity clearance: pregnancy. *Applied Physiology, Nutrition, and Metabolism, 36* (2011), S33–S48. www.nrcresearchpress.com/doi/abs/10.1139/h11-061.

127. Juhl, M., Andersen, P. K., Olsen, J., Madsen, M., Jørgensen, T., Nøhr, E. A., & Andersen, A. M. N. (2008). Physical exercise during pregnancy and the risk of preterm birth: a study

within the Danish National Birth Cohort. *American Journal of Epidemiology, 167* (7), 859–866. http://aje.oxfordjournals.org/content/167/7/859.full.

The green light does come with the usual long list of caveats. For example, ACOG lists these warning signs as reasons to stop exercising and contact a doctor: "vaginal bleeding, fluid leaking from the vagina, decreased fetal movement, uterine contractions, muscle weakness, calf swelling or pain, headache, chest pain, increased shortness of breath, dizziness, or feeling faint." This is a typical example of unnecessary pregnancy advice. It's hard to imagine a woman moronic enough to continue her strenuous workout after feeling chest pain or starting to bleed. Moreover, none of this advice is specific to exercise—you should probably contact your doctor if you start feeling unwell, regardless of whether or not you've just stepped off the treadmill.

128. Evenson, K. R., Savitz, A., & Huston, S. L. (2004). Leisure-time physical activity among pregnant women in the US. *Paediatric and Perinatal Epidemiology, 18* (6), 400–407. http://onlinelibrary.wiley.com/doi/10.1111/j.1365-3016.2004.00595.x/full.

129. Symons Downs, D., & Hausenblas, H. A. (2004). Women's exercise beliefs and behaviors during their pregnancy and postpartum. *Journal of Midwifery & Women's Health, 49* (2), 138–144. http://www.sciencedirect.com/science/article/pii/S1526952303004951.

130. Evenson, K. R., & Pompeii, L. A. (2010). Obstetrician practice patterns and recommendations for physical activity during pregnancy. *Journal of Women's Health, 19* (9), 1733–1740. http://online.liebertpub.com/doi/abs/10.1089/jwh.2009.1833.

131. Artal, R., et al., Guidelines of the American College of Obstetricians and Gynecologists for exercise during pregnancy and the postpartum period.

132. Evenson, K. R., Savitz, A., & Huston, S. L., Leisure-time physical activity among pregnant women in the US.

133. For completeness in cataloging off-limits activities, heavy weightlifting and diving also get the red light.

Artal, R., et al., Guidelines of the American College of Obstetricians and Gynecologists for exercise during pregnancy and the postpartum period; Camporesi, E. M. 1996. Diving and pregnancy. *Seminars in Perinatology 20*, 292–302. www.sciencedirect.com/science/article/pii/S014600059680022X.

134. Davies, G. A., Wolfe, L. A., Mottola, M. F., & MacKinnon, C. (2003). Joint SOGC/CSEP clinical practice guideline: exercise in pregnancy and the postpartum period. *Canadian Journal of Applied Physiology, 28* (3), 329–341. http://www.nrcresearchpress.com/doi/abs/10.1139/h03-024#.WcxbSnaGPIU.

135. Madsen, M., Jørgensen, T., Jensen, M. L., Juhl, M., Olsen, J., Andersen, P. K., & Nybo Andersen, A. M. (2007). Leisure time physical exercise during pregnancy and the risk of miscarriage: a study within the Danish National Birth Cohort. *BJOG: An International Journal of Obstetrics & Gynaecology, 114* (11), 1419–1426. http://onlinelibrary.wiley.com/doi/10.1111/j.1471-0528.2007.01496.x/full.

92,671 pregnant women were interviewed about their exercise habits throughout their pregnancies. The researchers found no relationship at all between exercise and miscarriage after 18 weeks. In terms of earlier pregnancy, amongst the group of 2,500 women who had very early miscarriages and were only interviewed afterward, there appeared to be a relationship between miscarriage and ~1–4 hours of high-impact exercise [jogging, ball games, and racquet sports] per week. But this could have been partly driven by recall bias, because when they analyzed the full group of women, including those interviewed prior to miscarrying, "hardly any statistically significant results emerged."

136. Wolfe, L. A., & Davies, G. (2003). Canadian guidelines for exercise in pregnancy. *Clinical Obstetrics and Gynecology, 46* (2), 488–495. www.researchgate.net/publication/10707481_Canadian_guidelines_for_exercise_in_pregnancy.

137. Nascimento, S. L., Surita, F. G., & Cecatti, J. G. (2012). Physical exercise during pregnancy: a systematic review. *Current Opinion in Obstetrics and Gynecology, 24* (6), 387–394. https://www.researchgate.net/profile/Fernanda_Surita/publication/231213702_Physical_exercise_during_pregnancy_A_systematic_review/links/0912f506b54f2b9a41000000.pdf.

138. Drinkwater, B. L. (Ed.). (2008). *Women in sport, volume 8 of the encyclopaedia of sports medicine: an IOC Medical Commission Publication.* Oxford: Wiley-Blackwell. http://books.google.co.uk/books?id=rPXr-0PUk5gC.

139. Calguneri, M., Bird, H. A., & Wright, V. (1982). Changes in joint laxity occurring during pregnancy. *Annals of the Rheumatic Diseases, 41* (2), 126–128. http://ard.bmj.com/content/41/2/126.full.pdf.

This might be a specific adaptation that helps with labor, or it could simply be a side effect of the changes in hormones.

140. Drinkwater, B. L., *Women in sport*; Davies, G. A., et al., Joint SOGC/CSEP clinical practice guideline: exercise in pregnancy and the postpartum period.

141. Artal, R., et al., Guidelines of the American College of Obstetricians and Gynecologists for exercise during pregnancy and the postpartum period.

142. Yeo, S., Davidge, S., Ronis, D. L., Antonakos, C. L., Hayashi, R., & O'Leary, S. (2008). A comparison of walking *versus* stretching exercises to reduce the incidence of preeclampsia: a randomized clinical trial. *Hypertension in Pregnancy, 27* (2), 113–130. http://informa-healthcare.com/doi/abs/10.1080/10641950701826778.

143. Yeo, S. (2010). Prenatal stretching exercise and autonomic responses: preliminary data and a model for reducing preeclampsia. *Journal of Nursing Scholarship, 42* (2), 113–121. www.ncbi.nlm.nih.gov/pmc/articles/PMC2904621/.

144. Gilleard, W. L., & Brown, J. M. M. (1996). Structure and function of the abdominal muscles in Primigravid subjects during pregnancy and the immediate postbirth period. *Physical Therapy, 76* (7), 750–762. https://academic.oup.com/ptj/article/76/7/750/2633092/Structure-and-Function-of-the-Abdominal-Muscles-in.

144. Boissonnault, J. S., & Blaschak, M. J. (1988). Incidence of diastasis recti abdominis during the childbearing year. *Physical Therapy, 68* (7), 1082–1086. https://academic.oup.com/ptj/article-abstract/68/7/1082/2728381.

145. Banerjee, A., Mahalakshmi, V., & Baranitharan, R. (2013). Effect of antenatal exercise program with and without abdominal strengthening exercises on diastasis rectus abdominis—a post partum follow up. *Indian Journal of Physiotherapy and Occupational Therapy—An International Journal, 7* (4), 123–126. www.indianjournals.com/ijor.aspx?target=ijor:ijpot&volume=7&issue=4&article=02.

146. Drinkwater, B. L., *Women in sport*.

147. Creager, C. C. 2003. The core of postpartum training. *Inspire women to fitness.* San Diego, CA: IDEA Health and Fitness Association, 63. https://books.google.co.uk/books?id=cfb4cBIHhKoC&dq.

148. Davies, G. A., et al., Joint SOGC/CSEP clinical practice guideline: exercise in pregnancy and the postpartum period.

149. McDonald, D. 1987. Postpartum sit-ups. *Physical Therapy, 67* (11), 1765.

150. Gilleard, W. L., et al., Structure and function of the abdominal muscles in Primigravid subjects during pregnancy and the immediate postbirth period.

151. Nascimento, S. L., et al., Physical exercise during pregnancy: a systematic review.

152. Zavorsky, G. S., & Longo, L. D. (2011). Adding strength training, exercise intensity, and caloric expenditure to exercise guidelines in pregnancy. *Obstetrics & Gynecology, 117* (6), 1399–1402. http://journals.lww.com/co-obgyn/Abstract/2012/12000/ Physical_exercise_during_pregnancy___a_systematic.6.aspx.

153. Babbar, S., Parks-Savage, A. C., & Chauhan, S. P. (2012). Yoga during pregnancy: a review. *American Journal of Perinatology, 29* (6), 459. https://www.thieme-connect.com/products/ ejournals/html/10.1055/s-0032-1304828.

154. Moretti, M. E., Bar-Oz, B., Fried, S., & Koren, G. (2005). Maternal hyperthermia and the risk for neural tube defects in offspring: systematic review and meta-analysis. *Epidemiology, 16* (2), 216–219. http://journals.lww.com/epidem/Abstract/2005/03000/Maternal_ Hyperthermia_and_the_Risk_for_Neural_Tube.10.aspx.

155. Harvey, M. A. S., McRorie, M. M., & Smith, D. W. (1981). Suggested limits to the use of the hot tub and sauna by pregnant women. *Canadian Medical Association Journal, 125* (1), 50. www.ncbi.nlm.nih.gov/pmc/articles/PMC1862577/pdf/canmedaj01346-0052.pdf.

156. Pleet, H., Graham, J. M., & Smith, D. W. (1981). Central nervous system and facial defects associated with maternal hyperthermia at four to 14 weeks' gestation. *Pediatrics, 67* (6), 785–789. http://pediatrics.aappublications.org/content/67/6/785.short, as cited in Harvey, M. A. S., et al., Suggested limits to the use of the hot tub and sauna by pregnant women.

157. Milunsky, A., Ulcickas, M., Rothman, K. J., Willett, W., Jick, S. S., & Jick, H. (1992). Maternal heat exposure and neural tube defects. *JAMA, 268* (7), 882–885. www.ncbi.nlm. nih.gov/pubmed/1640616.

158. Li, D. K., Janevic, T., Odouli, R., & Liu, L. (2003). Hot tub use during pregnancy and the risk of miscarriage. *American Journal of Epidemiology, 158* (10), 931–937. http://aje.oxford-journals.org/content/158/10/931.short.

160. Chambers, C. D. (2006). Risks of hyperthermia associated with hot tub or spa use by pregnant women. *Birth Defects Research Part A: Clinical and Molecular Teratology, 76* (8), 569–573. http://onlinelibrary.wiley.com/doi/10.1002/bdra.20303/full.

161. Hertz-Picciotto, I., & Howards, P. P. (2003). Invited commentary: hot tubs and miscarriage—methodological and substantive reasons why the case is weak. *American Journal of Epidemiology, 158* (10), 938–940. http://aje.oxfordjournals.org/content/158/10/938.full.

162. Chambers, C. D., Risks of hyperthermia associated with hot tub or spa use by pregnant women.

163. The AAP Committee on Fetus and Newborn and the ACOG Committee on Obstetric Practice. (2007). Chapter 4: antepartum care. *Guidelines for perinatal care*, (6th ed.). The American Academy of Pediatrics and the American College of Obstetricians and Gynecologists. www.acog.cl/descargar.php?4f5268d7f2c2d57cd085e3054d6905df.

164. Andrews, E. (2000, September 24). Sauna-of-the-month club. NYTimes.com. www. nytimes.com/2000/09/24/travel/sauna-of-the-month-club.html?pagewanted=all&src=pm.

165. Hillila, B. (2003). *The sauna is.* Iowa City, IA: Penfield Books. As cited in Sylver, N., *The holistic handbook of sauna therapy.* South Lake Tahoe, CA: BioMed Publishing Group. www.lymebook.com/history-of-sauna-therapy.

166. Andrews, E., Sauna-of-the-month club.

   Finnish women ordinarily stay in the sauna 6–12 minutes (Harvey, M. A. S., et al., Suggested limits to the use of the hot tub and sauna by pregnant women), with the temperature 140–212 degrees Farenheit (Culture of Finland. [n.d.]. Wikipedia. http:// en.wikipedia.org/wiki/Culture_of_Finland).

167. Rapola, J., Saxen, L., & Granroth, G. (1978). Anencephaly and the sauna. *The Lancet, 311* (8074), 1162.

168. Granroth, G., Hakama, M., & Saxen, L. (1977). Defects of the central nervous system in Finland: I. variations in time and space, sex distribution, and parental age. *British Journal of Preventive & Social Medicine, 31* (3), 164–170. www.ncbi.nlm.nih.gov/pmc/articles/PMC479017/pdf/brjprevsmed00027-0028.pdf.

169. Harvey, M. A. S., et al., Suggested limits to the use of the hot tub and sauna by pregnant women.

170. Uhari, M., Mustonen, A., & Kouvalainen, K. (1979). Sauna habits of Finnish women during pregnancy. *British Medical Journal, 1* (6172), 1216. www.ncbi.nlm.nih.gov/pmc/articles/PMC1599303/pdf/brmedj00071-0062a.pdf.

171. Saxén, L., Holmberg, P. C., Nurminen, M., & Kuosma, E. (1982). Sauna and congenital defects. *Teratology, 25* (3), 309–313. http://onlinelibrary.wiley.com/doi/10.1002/tera.1420250307/full.

172. Hannuksela, M. L., & Ellahham, S. (2001). Benefits and risks of sauna bathing. *The American Journal of Medicine, 110* (2), 118–126. http://butler.cc.tut.fi/~trantala/popular/MinnaH-SaunaReview.pdf.

173. The AAP Committee on Fetus and Newborn and the ACOG Committee on Obstetric Practice, Chapter 4: antepartum care.

174. Finnish sauna, Wikipedia.

175. Ando, Y., & Hattori, H. (1970). Effects of intense noise during fetal life upon postnatal adaptability (statistical study of the reactions of babies to aircraft noise). *The Journal of the Acoustical Society of America, 47* (4B), 1128–1130. http://asa.scitation.org/doi/abs/10.1121/1.1912014.

176. Jones, F. N., & Tauscher, J. (1978). Residence under an airport landing pattern as a factor in teratism. *Archives of Environmental Health: An International Journal, 33* (1), 10–12. www.tandfonline.com/doi/abs/10.1080/00039896.1978.10667300.

177. Knipschild, P., Meijer, H., & Sallé, H. (1981). Aircraft noise and birth weight. *International Archives of Occupational and Environmental Health, 48* (2), 131–136. http://link.springer.com/article/10.1007/BF00378433#.

178. Ando, Y., & Hattori, H. (1973). Statistical studies on the effects of intense noise during human fetal life. *Journal of Sound and Vibration, 27* (1), 101–110. www.sciencedirect.com/science/article/pii/0022460X73900382.

179. Schell, L. M. (1981). Environmental noise and human prenatal growth. *American Journal of Physiology and Anthropolology, 1981* (56), 63–70. http://onlinelibrary.wiley.com/doi/10.1002/ajpa.1330560107/full.

180. Nurminen, T., & Kurppa, K. (1989). Occupational noise exposure and course of pregnancy. *Scandinavian Journal of Work, Environment & Health,* 117–124. www.sjweh.fi/download.php?abstract_id=1873&file_nro=1.

181. Rocha, E. B., Azevedo, M. F. D., & Ximenes Filho, J. A. (2007). Study of the hearing in children born from pregnant women exposed to occupational noise: assessment by distortion product otoacoustic emissions. *Revista Brasileira de Otorrinolaringologia, 73* (3), 359–369. www.scielo.br/scielo.php?script=sci_arttext&pid=S0034-72992007000300011&lng=en&nrm=iso&tlng=en.

182. Lalande, N.M., Hetu, R., Lambert, J. (1986). Is occupational noise exposure during pregnancy a risk factor of damage to the auditory system of the fetus? *American Journal of Industrial Medicine, 10* (4), 427–435. http://onlinelibrary.wiley.com/doi/10.1002/ajim.4700100410/abstract.

183. Hartikainen, A. L., Sorri, M., Anttonen, H., Tuimala, R., & Läärä, E. Effect of occupational noise on the course and outcome of pregnancy. *Scandinavian Journal of Work,*

184 | Lifestyle

Environment & Health, 444–450. www.sjweh.fi/download.php?abstract_id=1376&file_nro=1. DS: did you need to delete this?

184. Niemtzow, R. C. (1993). Loud noise and pregnancy. *Military Medicine, 158* (1), 10–12. http://journals.lww.com/obgynsurvey/abstract/1993/09000/loud_noise_and_pregnancy.5.aspx.

185. Hepper, P. G., & Shahidullah, S. (1994). Noise and the foetus: a critical review of the literature. Sudbury, Suffolk, London: HSE Books. www.hse.gov.uk/research/crr_pdf/1994/crr94063.pdf.

186. Hetu, R., & Fortin, M. (1995). Potential risk of hearing damage associated with exposure to highly amplified music. *Journal of the American Academy of Audiology, 6* (5), 378–386. www.ncbi.nlm.nih.gov/pubmed/8547701.

187. National Institute on Deafness and Other Communication Disorders. (2014, April 9). Noise-induced hearing loss. National Institutes of Health. www.nidcd.nih.gov/health/hearing/pages/noise.aspx.

188. Von Sydow, K. 1999. Sexuality during pregnancy and after childbirth: a metacontent analysis of 59 studies. *Journal of Psychosomatic Research, 47* (1), 27–49. http://www.sciencedirect.com/science/article/pii/S0022399998001068.

189. Reasons to abstain included bleeding, abdominal pains, ruptured membranes, premature dilation of the cervix, or a heightened risk of premature labor. Women with vaginal colonization with certain bacteria (*Trichomonas vaginalis, Mycoplasma hominis,* or bacterial vaginosis) also have a slightly higher risk of pregnancy complications, but frequent intercourse was not significantly associated with preterm delivery in women with these infections (Read, J. S., & Klebanoff, M. A. [1993]. Sexual intercourse during pregnancy and preterm delivery: effects of vaginal microorganisms. *American Journal of Obstetrics and Gynecology, 168* [2], 514–519. www.sciencedirect.com/science/article/pii/000293789390484Z). You may have heard that sex can be helpful inducing labor if the baby is overdue. But according to a review, this remains unproven: "there is not enough evidence to show whether sexual intercourse is effective or to show how it compares with other methods. More research is needed" (Kavanagh, J., Kelly, A. J., & Thomas, J. [2001]. Sexual intercourse for cervical ripening and induction of labour. *Cochrane Database of Systematic Reviews, 2001* (2): CD003093. http://onlinelibrary.wiley.com/doi/10.1002/14651858.CD003093/full; Von Sydow, K., Sexuality during pregnancy and after childbirth).

190. Hotmilk maternity and nursing UK. (n.d.). www.hotmilklingerie.com.

191. It's worth mentioning STDs here, as infections can sometimes be asymptomatic but nevertheless cause problems during pregnancy. If you think you're at high risk (e.g., a large number of prior sexual partners), it would be worth proactively requesting a test for gonorrhea specifically.

According to a review (McDonald, H. M., Brocklehurst, P., & Gordon, A. [2007]. Antibiotics for treating bacterial vaginosis in pregnancy. *Cochrane Database of Systematic Reviews, 2007* (1): CD000262. https://www.ncbi.nlm.nih.gov/pmc/articles/PMC4164464/), there are five STDs for which there is good evidence of an increased risk of preterm birth:

1. **Asymptomatic bacteriuria (urinary tract infection without any symptoms):** This is a relatively common phenomenon, affecting between 2 percent and 10 percent of all pregnancies (Smaill, F., & Vazquez, J. C. [2007]. Antibiotics for asymptomatic bacteriuria in pregnancy. *Cochrane Database of Systematic Reviews, 2015* (8): CD000490. http://onlinelibrary.wiley.com/doi/10.1002/14651858.CD000490.pub3/full). Fortunately, standard prenatal care in the US includes a urine test to check for the presence of bacteria (The American College of Obstetricians and Gynecologists. [2014, January]. Routine

tests in pregnancy. Frequently Asked Questions, FAQ133: Pregnancy. www.acog.org/
publications/faq/faq133.pdf).

2. *Neisseria gonorrhoeae:* The rate of gonorrhea infection among women of childbearing age is between 0.33% and 0.9% (Datta, S. D., Sternberg, M., Johnson, R. E., Berman,
S., Papp, J. R., McQuillan, G., & Weinstock, H. [2007]. Gonorrhea and chlamydia in
the United States among persons 14 to 39 years of age, 1999 to 2002. *Annals of Internal
Medicine, 147* [2], 89–96. http://annals.org/article.aspx?articleid=735575; Van Der Pol, B.
[2007]. *Trichomonas vaginalis* infection: the most prevalent nonviral sexually transmitted
infection receives the least public health attention. *Clinical Infectious Diseases, 44* [1],
23–25. http://cid.oxfordjournals.org/content/44/1/23.full), and ~50% of infected women
are asymptomatic (Platt, R., Rice, P. A., & McCormack, W. M. [1983]. Risk of acquiring
gonorrhea and prevalence of abnormal adnexal findings among women recently exposed
to gonorrhea. *JAMA, 250* [23], 3205–3209. http://jama.jamanetwork.com/article.aspx?ar-
ticleid=389055; Wallin, J. [1975]. Gonorrhoea in 1972: a 1-year study of patients attending the VD Unit in Uppsala. *The British Journal of Venereal Diseases, 51* [1], 41–47. www.
ncbi.nlm.nih.gov/pmc/articles/PMC1045109/pdf/brjvendis00055-0047.pdf). Routine
prenatal care only includes a test for gonorrhea for high-risk women, e.g., those who are
25 or younger or live in an area where gonorrhea is common (The American College of
Obstetricians and Gynecologists, Routine tests in pregnancy). Therefore, if you think you
have a high risk of infection for other reasons, it would be worth proactively requesting a
test. Treating gonorrhea with antibiotics reduces the likelihood of health complications
(Gonorrhea—CDC fact sheet. [Last updated 2014, January 29]. US Centers for Disease
Control and Prevention. www.cdc.gov/std/gonorrhea/STDFact-Gonorrhea.htm).

3. *Chlamydia trachomatis:* This infection is routinely screened for as part of standard
prenatal testing (The American College of Obstetricians and Gynecologists, Routine tests
in pregnancy.)

4. *Trichomonas vaginalis:* This infection is not routinely screened for as stan-
dard prenatal testing (Ibid.), but "treatment of pregnant women with asymptomatic
Trichomoniasis does not prevent preterm delivery," so "routine screening and treat-
ment of asymptomatic pregnant women for this condition cannot be recommended"
(Klebanoff, M. A., Carey, J. C., Hauth, J. C., Hillier, S. L., Nugent, R. P., Thom, E.
A., & Leveno, K. J. [2001]. Failure of metronidazole to prevent preterm delivery
among pregnant women with asymptomatic *Trichomonas vaginalis* infection. *New
England Journal of Medicine, 345* [7], 487–493. http://www.nejm.org/doi/full/10.1056/
NEJMoa003329#t=article).

5. **Bacterial vaginosis (BV):** BV is an imbalance of the normal vaginal bacteria
(including overgrowth of *Gardnerella vaginalis, Mycoplasma hominis,* and *Mobiluncus*),
and 25 percent of women of childbearing age have this condition without realizing—29.2
percent of women ages 14–49 tested had BV, with 84 percent reporting no symptoms
(Koumans, E. H., Sternberg, M., Bruce, C., McQuillan, G., Kendrick, J., Sutton, M.,
& Markowitz, L. E. [2007]. The prevalence of bacterial vaginosis in the United States,
2001–2004: associations with symptoms, sexual behaviors, and reproductive health.
Sexually Transmitted Diseases, 34 [11], 864–869. http://journals.lww.com/stdjournal/
Abstract/2007/11000/The_Prevalence_of_Bacterial_Vaginosis_in_the.6.aspx). BV
during pregnancy has been linked to pregnancy complications, including premature
birth (STDs during pregnancy—CDC fact sheet. [Last updated 2016, November 10].
US Centers for Disease Control and Prevention. www.cdc.gov/std/pregnancy/STDFact-
Pregnancy.htm). But according to a review, "antibiotics given to pregnant women
reduced this overgrowth of bacteria, but did not reduce the numbers of babies who were
born too early" (McDonald, H. M., Brocklehurst, P., & Gordon, A. [2007]. Antibiotics for
treating bacterial vaginosis in pregnancy. *Cochrane Database of Systematic Reviews, 2007*
(1): CD000262. https://www.ncbi.nlm.nih.gov/pmc/articles/PMC4164464/), perhaps

because individual susceptibility to preterm birth or intrauterine infection, or both, may be increased by specific genes.

In addition to these five, there are three other infections also worth mentioning:

1. **Genital herpes (herpes simplex virus 2 or HSV-2)** can lead to miscarriage, premature birth, fatal infection in newborns (CDC fact sheet: incidence, prevalence, and cost of sexually transmitted infections in the United States. [2013, February]. US Centers for Disease Control and Prevention. www.cdc.gov/std/stats/sti-estimates-fact-sheet-feb-2013.pdf), and longer-term symptoms such as brain damage or eye problems (The American College of Obstetricians and Gynecologists. [2011, May]. Genital herpes. Frequently Asked Questions, FAQ054: Gynecologic Problems. www.acog.org/~/media/For%20Patients/faq054.ashx). And you may have it without realizing: a full 70 percent of mothers of infants with neonatal HSV infections are asymptomatic at delivery, with no history of genital lesions (Kulhanjian, J. A., Soroush, V., Au, D. S., Bronzan, R. N., Yasukawa, L. L., Weylman, L. E., Arvin, A., & Prober, C. G. [1992]. Identification of women at unsuspected risk of primary infection with herpes simplex virus type 2 during pregnancy. *New England Journal of Medicine, 326* [14], 916–920. www.nejm.org/doi/pdf/10.1056/NEJM199204023261403). Luckily, "the greatest risk of transmission to the fetus and the newborn occurs in case of an initial maternal infection contracted in the second half of pregnancy," so as long as you're not sleeping around while pregnant, you're at lower risk of adverse effects (Straface, G., Selmin, A., Zanardo, V., De Santis, M., Ercoli, A., & Scambia, G. [2012]. Herpes simplex virus infection in pregnancy. *Infectious Diseases in Obstetrics and Gynecology, 2012* (2012), 385697. www.ncbi.nlm.nih.gov/pmc/articles/PMC3332182/). And according to the US Preventive Services Task Force, there currently isn't value in screening for HSV-2, since there's only limited evidence that interventions can reduce the risk of transmitting the infection to the fetus (Genital herpes: screening, recommendation summary. [2005, March]. US Preventative Services Task Force. www.uspreventiveservicestaskforce.org/uspstf05/herpes/herpesrs.htm).

2. **Group B Strep (GBS)** can be transferred to the baby during birth, but testing for GBS is part of routine medical care (Reingold, A., Gershman, K., & Petit, S. [2007]. Perinatal group B streptococcal disease after universal screening recommendations—United States, 2003–2005. *Morbidity and Mortality Weekly Report, 56* [28], 701–705. www.ncbi.nlm.nih.gov/pubmed/17637595). "Among term deliveries, lack of screening contributed to only a small portion of the early-onset disease burden; only a small percentage of term infants with group B streptococcal disease were born to mothers from key subgroups of unscreened women, such as women with inadequate prenatal care or women with a history of drug use" (Van Dyke, M. K., Phares, C. R., Lynfield, R., Thomas, A. R., Arnold, K. E., Craig, A. S., Mohle-Boetani, J., Gershman, K., Schaffner, W., Petit, S., Zansky, S. M., Morin, C. A., Spina, N. L., Wymore, K., Harrison, L. H., Shutt, K. A., Bareta, J., Bulens, S. N., Zell, E. R., Schuchat, A., & Schrag, S. J. [2009]. Evaluation of universal antenatal screening for group B streptococcus. *New England Journal of Medicine, 360* [25], 2626–2636. www.nejm.org/doi/full/10.1056/NEJMoa0806820).

3. **Syphilis** is another STD which can cause problems in pregnancy, but fortunately, it is increasingly rare: "Syphilis during pregnancy in the Western world is rare today. In this era, the prevalence of seropositivity in pregnancy is between 0.02–4.5% in northern Europe and the United States after accounting for biological false reactive tests. Thanks to effective intervention strategies and the availability of penicillin, few of these pregnancies result in congenital syphilis—for example, an average of 30 cases per 100,000 live births in the United States in 1996. The demographic profile of women who deliver syphilitic babies represents that of women with other sexually transmitted diseases (STDs) as well as those who fail to get adequate prenatal care" (Genç, M., & Ledger, W. J. [2000]. Syphilis in pregnancy. *Sexually Transmitted Infections, 76* [2], 73–79. http://sti.bmj.com/content/76/2/73.full).

5

LEGEND OF THE SUPER BABY

Good Influences

hy produce an ordinary baby when you could produce a super baby? That's right—by simply enriching your baby's prenatal environment with a graded course of heart-rhythm sounds, you could boost your child's intelligence level by 25–50 percent. Does this sound too good to be true? It's not, according to the author of parenting advice book *Super Baby*.[1] The key is a product called BabyPlus, available at a retailer near you. According to the company's website: "BabyPlus is an audio device that introduces patterns of sound to prenatal children in the only language they understand, the maternal heartbeat. As a baby discriminates the simple rhythmic sounds of BabyPlus from those of the mother, learning begins. . . . BabyPlus children have an intellectual, developmental, creative, and emotional advantage from the time they are born."[2]

This all sounds promising, but why stop at heartbeat sounds? Why not implement an entire course of prenatal instruction? Here's a description of the program one family implemented under the guidance of a pair of prenatal experts:

> Every ten-minute session, morning and evening, would begin with the 'Hi Baby!' megaphone greeting. . . . The lesson introduced different kinds of contact—patting, rubbing, squeezing, shaking, stroking, tapping—and the accompanying verbs, delivered via paper megaphone. Jeannine [the mother] would stand up, sit down, sway, or rock and say the appropriate verbs. She would drink hot and cold liquids and label the sensation for Lisel [the fetus]. Tony [the father] would turn on a radio speaker ("Music!") or a vacuum cleaner ("Noise!"), or shine a flashlight on and off ("Light!" "Dark!" "Light!" "Dark!")[3]

It's hard not to laugh at the antics of such hyperactive parents. But perhaps some small corner of your mind is secretly wondering whether maybe, just maybe, you've already fallen behind in the competitive sport of parenting. Have you missed your chance to give your baby an edge? Let me put your mind at ease: there's no evidence whatsoever to back up claims of even a small increase in intelligence from prenatal stimulation, let alone an improvement of 25–50 percent. Here's what we do know, as outlined by a recent review:[4] according to one relatively well-designed study, babies whose mothers read them a passage twice a day for six weeks before birth seemed to suck differently when they heard that same passage after birth.[5] And two other studies have suggested that babies prefer their mother's voice over another female voice,[6,7] although neither controlled for the fact that the babies in question could have learned their mother's voice in the few days since being born.

Only one researcher, Dr. Donald Shetler, claims to have attempted any long-term follow-up of supposed prenatal learning.[8] He suggests that fetal learning persists for months, perhaps even years. But he doesn't provide any detail on his research methods, which is hardly confidence-inspiring. Keep in mind that any parents who are motivated enough to implement a fetal-stimulation program will also likely provide their children with lots of stimulation once they're born. That makes it hard to measure the impact without a properly controlled, randomized trial.

So when it comes to prenatal instruction, I suggest you relax and let your bump be. But flashlights aside, there must be other ways to help your baby while he or she is still in the womb. What about music? Health food? Those prenatal vitamins your doctor prescribed? Maybe there's some truth to the legend of the super baby. Let's take a tour through the world of potential positive influences for Junior to find out.

Benefit level for prenatal instruction: Very low

The Mozart Effect: Music

January 1998: Georgia governor Zell Miller makes a controversial proposal. He would like to use state funding to purchase 100,000 Bach and Mozart CDs each year to send home with every newborn child. Why? Because "listening to soothing music helps those trillions of brain connections to develop." The governor said he had a stack of research on the subject but also that his experiences growing up in the mountains of north Georgia had proved convincing: "Musicians were folks that not only could play a fiddle, but they also were good mechanics. They could fix your car."[9] So if you want your child to grow up to be an intelligent, fiddle-playing car mechanic, no problem. A couple of eighteenth-century musicians to the rescue.

Governor Zell isn't alone in his excitement over the transformational potential of music. Florida has also passed a law mandating that classical music be played to toddlers in all state-run classrooms.[10] And parents across the country have been eagerly embracing the "Mozart effect": sales of classical music have skyrocketed.

But if the effect of music is so powerful, why even wait until birth? Why not serenade your fetus? Fortunately, mothers-to-be no longer need to stretch headphones awkwardly around their bellies. There's the Nuvo Ritmo, an "advanced and complete system for delivering quality and safe sound to prenatal listeners."[11] There's the Lullabelly, "an ultra-soft, adjustable, lightweight, machine-washable prenatal music belt you can wear over your clothes or directly against your belly."[12] Or how about Bellybuds, "two modular bellyphones that gently adhere to the varying curvature of a growing belly with skin-safe, form-fitting hydrogel adhesive rings"?[13]

The problem is, Zell's claim to have "stacks of research" is a bit hard to verify. Let's go back to the original study that launched the storm of media hype. In 1993, three researchers split a group of thirty-six college students at the University of California at Irvine into three groups. One group listened to a Mozart sonata, one group to a relaxation tape, and the last group to nothing at all. They then gave the students a spatial IQ test, which involved imagining unfolding a piece of paper that had been folded several times and cut up. Those who had listened to Mozart scored 9 points better on the test than those in the two nonmusical groups.[14]

But here's the catch, or rather, here are the many catches. First, mentally unfolding a piece of paper is a very narrowly defined task, not a full IQ test. Second, these were college students, not young children, and certainly not fetuses. Third, the effect lasted only ten to fifteen minutes, after which the influence of the music disappeared. And finally, when the same researchers repeated the experiment a few years later with more subjects over several days, the effect showed up only on the first day and disappeared thereafter. The initial study was an intriguing result that launched a media circus, but the scientific community quickly concluded that the results didn't generalize to broader intelligence (or performance as a mechanic, for that matter).

Ultimately the primary author of the study, Frances Rauscher, had to weigh in, publishing a response in the journal *Nature*: "Our results have generated much interest but several misconceptions . . . the most common of these: that listening to Mozart enhances intelligence. We made no such claim. The effect is limited to spatial-temporal tasks involving mental imagery and temporal ordering."[15] Rauscher also attempted to set the record straight with the public. In response to Miller's budget proposal, she told *The New York Times*: "I don't think it can hurt. I'm all for exposing children to wonderful cultural experiences. But I do think the money could be better spent on music education programs."[16]

Rauscher isn't the only scientist to have had her results on the topic of brain stimulation mangled by the media. Dr. William Greenough spent his career investigating the effects of exposing rats to enriched environments and concluded that rats are capable of solving mazes more rapidly after various forms of mental stimulation. Since publication, his work has been broadly cited as evidence for the importance of enrichment programs for children. He ultimately protested, "I spent most of thirty years demonstrating that that's not true" and pointed out that "the 'rich' environment for a rat is actually the normal environment for a child."[17]

Has anyone actually investigated the impact of serenading babies in the womb specifically? There's little doubt Junior is listening and even capable of remembering what he's heard. For example, newborns exposed to the theme song of a popular TV program during pregnancy "exhibited changes in heart-rate, number of movements, and behavioral state 2–4 days after birth" upon hearing the same tune.[18] Floundering around in this strange new world outside the womb, perhaps the babies were calmed by hearing a familiar sound. (If Mozart is more your cup of tea, you may be questioning the benefits of your fetus memorizing a television jingle, but still). The study wasn't randomized, however, and didn't control for the possibility that the babies could have been exposed to the tune in the 2–4 days since birth. Regardless, the babies didn't appear to retain the memory for long: evidence of learning had disappeared within 20 days.

Another, better-designed study from 2002 has also concluded that newborns can recognize music they heard in the womb. But the authors specifically caveat that "there is no information that such effects are either long lasting or beneficial. Most of the evidence that we have on pre-birth experiences affecting later childhood or adulthood is anecdotal, unscientific, and based on subjective interpretation."[19]

In conclusion, it would be quite a stretch to believe there's a magical window of musical exposure in the womb. By all means, listen to Mozart if it happens to please you, but save the money you'd have spent on the absurd fetal iPod. Your child will be pestering you for his or her own iPod soon enough.

Benefit level for music: Very low

Eat Your Peas, Please: Taste Preferences

NPR 2011: "Want your child to love veggies? Start early. Very early. Research shows that what a woman eats during pregnancy not only nourishes her baby in the womb, but may shape food preferences later in life."[20] Sounds promising, doesn't it? What pregnant woman wouldn't consider eating more vegetables if this could help avoid future battles with a stubborn toddler over spinach and peas?

We all know that kids aren't supposed to enjoy eating their vegetables. From popular culture (Calvin of *Calvin & Hobbes* battling heroically with the unidentified green goo on his plate) to real-life individuals (George Bush Sr. with his well-publicized hatred of broccoli),[21, 22] examples of picky eaters are everywhere. And childhood aversion to healthy foods is no theoretical concern. By the age of two, a full 50 percent of children are labeled picky eaters by their parents.[23]

Fortunately, in this case, there does seem to be evidence that we can start influencing our children's taste preferences as early as pregnancy. There's little doubt that certain tastes make their way into the womb. For example, if you eat garlic or spicy foods, your amniotic fluid will start to reek soon after.[24, 25] A handful of studies also suggest that babies have a preference for tastes they acquired in utero. For example, newborns are more likely to prefer the odor of anise if their mothers consumed that flavor while pregnant, and mothers who were randomly assigned to drink lots of carrot juice during pregnancy had an easier time feeding their six-month-old babies carrot-flavored cereal.[26, 27]

But there's no unique window of opportunity during pregnancy. You can also pass along taste preferences to your baby by consuming foods while breastfeeding or by simply introducing the foods early in weaning, before your child's food aversions start kicking in.[28, 29] So if the thought of eating even a single brussels sprout makes you queasy, never fear—the vicious cycle of vegetable hatred can yet be broken.

**Benefit level for shaping prenatal taste preferences:
Very low**

Horse Pills for Breakfast: Vitamins

Rapunzel's mother may have gotten into trouble by craving a nutritious leafy green vegetable,[30] but most of us aren't quite so virtuous. Our primary cravings during pregnancy are for dairy and sweets.[31, 32] So if there's one pregnancy topic everyone agrees on, it's the daily vitamin supplement, the one-stop-shop for nutrients. (I use the term "vitamin" to cover vitamins, minerals, and trace elements.) Pregnant women everywhere are dutifully popping a pill every morning with their breakfast, and I challenge you to find a single pregnancy website that doesn't tout the benefits of vitamins as the ultimate prenatal insurance plan. Having trouble swallowing your daily dosage? No problem. Liquid and gummy vitamins to the rescue. Foul-smelling ingredients making you nauseous? Try the Bellybar Complete Prenatal Chocolate Vitamin, a "delicious fortified chocolate ball with a soft nougat center." The benefits don't even stop with your fetus: Gwyneth Paltrow and Mindy Kaling have both revealed that prenatal multivitamins are supposedly the secret to their luxurious tresses.[33]

Movie-star hair may be a nice (although questionable) side benefit, but we're really hoping to protect our babies. And we know exactly what we're getting in those horse pills: our daily dose of folic acid, along with some other good stuff we presumably must need. What is folic acid, exactly? I'll admit that during my pregnancies, I never really knew the answer to that question. I figured I would get plenty of it if I ate muesli for breakfast and kale for lunch—but I didn't eat that way. So instead I downed my folic acid and other essential nutrients in one quick, convenient swallow. And I was following seemingly sound advice—it's not just the baby websites that tout the benefits of supplements. The CDC, the American Academy of Pediatrics, the National Healthy Mothers/Healthy Babies Coalition, and the Institute of Medicine all agree that any woman who is even thinking of becoming pregnant should start taking folic acid daily to prevent birth defects (specifically, neural tube defects like spina bifida, which can cause difficulties walking, bladder and bowel problems, abnormal curvature of the spine, and learning disabilities, among other symptoms).[34, 35, 36, 37]

While technically correct, it turns out upon further inspection that all of this well-meaning advice is more than a decade out of date. No matter what the websites tell you, you are very unlikely to be suffering from a folic acid deficiency. In a wise bid to improve public health, the FDA ruled that as of January 1, 1998, breads, cereals, flours, cornmeals, pastas, rice, and other grain products had to be fortified with folic acid. The strategy has by now produced dramatic results: "Before fortification, folate deficiency was about 10–12 percent in women of childbearing age, but after fortification, folate deficiency dropped to less than 1 percent."[38] The vast majority of us are getting plenty of folic acid every day, even if we don't realize it. That's important, because neural tube defects form in the first four weeks—often before a woman even realizes she's pregnant.[39, 40] But after the first 4–6 weeks of pregnancy, folic acid becomes irrelevant.

Does that mean we're off the hook? Can we throw away our smelly multivitamins? Not so fast. Do you smoke or have a secret predilection for alcohol or drugs? Are you a vegan? Pregnant with twins? Do you suffer from iron-deficiency anemia, or eat a poor-quality diet? (No, you don't automatically fall into this category just because you hate green vegetables. This is more about socioeconomic status and overall access to a balanced diet. In low-income, urban women with insufficient access to nutrient-rich food, prenatal supplements may reduce infant mortality.)[42] If the answer to any of these questions is yes, the American Dietetic Association recommends taking multivitamin/mineral supplements. But this same association seems curiously blasé about everyone else: "The consumption of more food and the increased absorption and efficiency of nutrient utilization in pregnancy are generally adequate to meet the needs for most nutrients."[43]

So why is your GP advising you to take a supplement? Why can't the experts get their story straight? As with so many pregnancy topics on which there is seemingly universal agreement, the answer when you dig deeper is that the effect of supplements on pregnancy outcomes . . . hasn't been sufficiently studied yet. According to a recent review, "Health care providers generally recommend that pregnant women consume a standard prenatal supplement as insurance against inadequate micronutrient intake. Interestingly, however, evidence to support a benefit from this practice for most women in developed countries such as the United States is weak."[44]

What is the evidence? A few preliminary studies suggest that taking a multivitamin while pregnant may slightly decrease the risk of certain birth defects,[45, 46] preeclampsia (a disorder involving high blood pressure, which if untreated can occasionally lead to life-threatening complications),[47] and preterm birth.[48] But the authors of the review point out various limitations of these studies and conclude that more research is needed to confirm the findings.[49] Other studies have found no effects. One study of ~1,000 women in the UK concluded there was "no evidence that the use of supplements would improve infant and placental growth,"[50] and another study of 5,500 women found no observable effects of supplements on pregnancy outcome.[51]

In other words, we still have no idea how important vitamin supplements are. The problem is, more than three-quarters of pregnant women are already taking a regular multivitamin, so it's hard to justify a randomized trial asking women *not* to take their supplement.[52] But in the face of such inconclusive findings, it's tough to understand all the hoopla over prenatal vitamins. I began to develop a sneaking suspicion that pregnant women, myself included, were behaving like lemmings. I decided to look deeper.

When you focus on individual vitamins, minerals, and trace elements, the story becomes clearer. Looking at national data on nutrient levels, some of us are indeed deficient in certain nutrients, at least before we realize we're pregnant and start bingeing on supplements. Here's a chart showing nutrient status for American women of childbearing age (all women, not specifically pregnant ones).[53] I've looked at proportions rather than absolute amounts, so we can compare all the nutrients on the same scale. The black line is the minimum recommended level, and the bars show how much the bottom fifth or tenth percentile of the population is actually getting.

According to the data, there are six different nutrients that at least 5 percent and sometimes at least 10 percent of women aren't getting enough of, and that's before even taking into account any extra nutritional requirements of pregnancy. But surprisingly, only two of these—iron and iodine—are universally recommended as supplements during pregnancy.[54] So let's see how much each of these six nutrients actually matters.

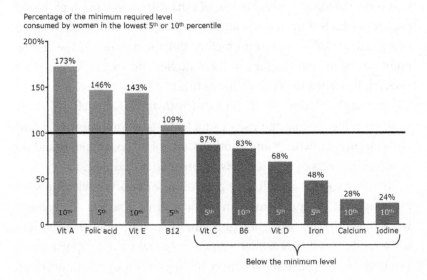

Percentage of the minimum required level consumed by women in the lowest 5th or 10th percentile

Salty Seaweed: Iodine

Here's a tricky and morbid trivia question: What's the number one cause of preventable intellectual disability worldwide? I'll give you a hint—it's not malnourishment or contaminated water. It has nothing to do with exposure to lead, mercury, or any other kind of pollution. It's not related to child abuse or domestic violence. The answer? Iodine deficiency.[55] Yes, iodine, that yellow stuff your mom might have painted on your scraped knees as a child.

I'm sure you're immediately picturing deprived children in remote parts of the world, and you're partially right: this is primarily a problem in faraway places like Siberia and Iraq. But before you make a complacent assumption that living here in the first world protects you, I have another factoid for you. According to the National Health and Nutrition Examination Survey (NHANES), more than half of pregnant American women aren't getting as much iodine as they supposedly need,[56] and 5 percent of American women have levels that actually fall below the guidelines set by the World Health Organization.[57]

If iodine, of all random things, is such a problem, why haven't we heard about it before? If you happened to search for "iodine" on one of the typical parenting websites (I know, why would you?), it would tell you, "You probably won't need to take a supplement because it's easy to meet your requirement through food."[58] But the good people at the American Thyroid Association, who spend a lot of their time thinking about this issue, would beg to differ. They currently recommend that all pregnant and breastfeeding women in the United States start taking 150 micrograms (μg) of supplementary iodine per day.[59]

So has all that time spent thinking about thyroids made them slightly paranoid, or should we be rushing out to the pharmacy ASAP for little yellow supplements? There is no doubt that extreme iodine deficiency can have a severe effect on your baby (a condition actually called "cretinism"!), and supplementation clearly helps prevent such cases.[60, 61] But to this day, no one truly knows whether the millions of American women with mild deficiency are doing any harm to their babies, since this issue hasn't been properly studied. Scientists speculate that deficiency could lead to lower IQs,[62] and one study in Spain showed some potential benefit from giving iodine supplements to a randomly chosen group of pregnant women.[63] But most of the studies so far are "limited due to lack of randomization and small sample sizes,"[64] and the American Thyroid Association itself freely admits the need for a better study.[65]

Perhaps, despite the lack of definitive evidence, you'd like to ensure you're getting the minimum level. The solution seems easy: only about half of us use iodized salt.[66] So if you use fancy-schmancy sea salt, just switch to the ordinary iodized kind. Unfortunately, if you're an average American adult, you'd have to triple the amount of table salt you use to get the amount of iodine recommended during pregnancy. This definitely wouldn't be advisable, as most of us are eating far too much salt already.[67]

Maybe you're thinking that your pregnancy multivitamin has it covered. Nope. The American Thyroid Association recommends that all prenatal vitamins contain 150 μg of iodine.[68] But a recent survey of prenatal multivitamins showed that half did not bother to include any iodine at all and those that did often contained far less than was claimed on the label.[69] (It's not that they're trying to cheat anyone—it's just that the usual source of iodine in vitamins is seaweed, which contains variable amounts.) So if you want to protect against deficiency, you'll have to add yet another pill to your morning regimen. Or start eating kelp for breakfast—I hear it's quite tasty sprinkled with a bit of iodized table salt.

Benefit level for iodine supplements: Very low[70]

Iron Woman: Iron

To earn the prestigious title of Ironman, participants must complete a 2.4-mile swim, a 112-mile bicycle ride, and a 26.2-mile run within a fixed time frame.[71] As a result of the intense training required to accomplish such a feat, the typical elite endurance athlete develops a blood volume 35–40 percent higher than that of normal adults.[72] But Ironmen of the world, take note: training for an Ironman is nothing compared to growing a baby. When a woman is pregnant, the volume of blood in her body gets pumped up by a full 50 percent.[73]

Increasing the blood supply by that kind of magnitude is a massive physiological change. And iron, as you may remember from biology class, is a critical ingredient in making blood (part of hemoglobin, the molecule in red blood cells that carries the oxygen around). So it's unsurprising that there's almost universal agreement that all women should take supplemental iron during pregnancy. The World Health Organization recommends 60 mg per day.[74, 75] The CDC recommends 30 mg per day.[76] The American Academy of Pediatrics, the

American College of Obstetricians and Gynecologists,[77] the Institute of Medicine,[78] and the Department of Agriculture[79] all agree: take an iron supplement! All these many august institutions, so the proof must be watertight, right?

As usual, the answer is: not really. The premise behind supplementation is perfectly logical: if you measure a woman's iron level throughout her pregnancy, you'll see it dropping steadily. Iron supplementation reverses that trend. It helps bring iron levels back up[80, 81, 82, 83, 84] and even appears to reduce the risk of iron-deficiency anemia,[85] which can be problematic during pregnancy.[86] And giving iron supplements to low-income, higher-risk women has been shown to help improve pregnancy outcomes.[87, 88, 89]

The problem is, these studies have primarily involved women who had higher-risk pregnancies to begin with.[90] Perhaps it's perfectly normal and acceptable for iron levels to drop in healthy women. In fact, a significant number of clinical trials have all found no improvements in pregnancy outcomes from giving women routine iron supplements.[91, 92, 93, 94, 95, 96, 97, 98, 99] Studies following children longer term have also shown no beneficial effects—e.g., on IQ at age four[100] or on later behavior in school.[101] Various reviews of the field similarly conclude there are no proven benefits[102] and acknowledge that there are "many gaps in our knowledge about the adverse effects of maternal anemia and iron deficiency on pregnancy outcome."[103] Even the US Preventative Services Task Force concluded, "most clinical trials of iron supplementation have not demonstrated significant improvements in maternal or neonatal outcomes," although "sample sizes in these trials are small, and thus are inadequate to prove that iron supplementation is ineffective."[104]

We may never know for sure how important iron supplements are, because we've made it impossible to study the topic any further here at home. A full ~80 percent of us take supplements with iron while pregnant, which makes randomized trials difficult to justify.[105, 106, 107] Furthermore, blood tests for anemia are a routine part of prenatal care,[108] so anyone who gets regular checkups has little chance of slipping through the cracks.

In conclusion, those of us who already eat well-balanced diets and get prenatal care are dutifully taking our iron supplements. But the women at highest risk of iron deficiency (e.g., low-income and minority women not receiving prenatal care) remain the least likely to take them.[109] Distressingly ironic—if you'll excuse the bad pun.

Benefit level for iron supplements: Very low[110]

Sheep Grease and Sunshine: Vitamin D

Did you know that you're regularly consuming sheep grease with your food? Milk, cereals, juice, and margarine are all frequently fortified with vitamin D, which is produced by shining ultraviolet radiation on either yeast or lanolin, the oily coating from sheep's wool.

We've had to come up with these cunning methods of fortifying our food because so many of us live in areas where the sun simply doesn't shine strongly enough to give us vitamin D all year round. Technically, none of us should require vitamin D from food, because we've evolved a photosynthetic mechanism in our skin to produce the vitamin from sunlight. But while UVA (the "tanning ray") shines down all day, the amount of UVB (the burning and vitamin D ray) you're getting depends on the angle of the sun's rays. So if you live in a city like Chicago, Boston, or Seattle, you may enjoy some bright and sunny days during the winter, but your body isn't producing any vitamin D between late October and early March. Even if you live as far south as Atlanta, you're missing out on vitamin D from November to February.[111] So that pasty complexion you develop in the winter isn't just a cosmetic problem you can fix with bronzer. To make matters worse, many of us no longer live where our ancestors lived, and darker skin that evolved to provide protection from harsh sun in the tropics may not let in enough UVB in colder climes. Fortification helps, but you'd need to drink at least five glasses of milk a day just to hit the daily recommended intake for vitamin D, which is why at least five percent of pregnant women are still deficient.[112]

Does this matter? In countries that are farther north like Canada and the UK, probably, but in the United States, probably not.[113] The Institute of Medicine and the National Academy of Sciences both concluded in the '90s that there was no need for routine supplementation with vitamin D during pregnancy, except for vegans and other women who drank very little fortified milk.[114, 115] More than twenty years later, not much has changed. Cases of children with rickets (deformed bones as a result of insufficient vitamin D, which helps the body absorb calcium) remain very rare in the United States. There's some preliminary research about a possible link between vitamin D and asthma,[116] and a suggestion that low vitamin D may be a risk factor in preeclampsia,[117] but no definitive conclusions. According to the American Congress of Obstetricians and Gynecologists in 2011, "Recommendations concerning routine vitamin D supplementation during pregnancy beyond that contained in a prenatal vitamin [400 international units] should await the completion of ongoing randomized clinical trials."[118] In other words, we still haven't finished the research that would put the question to rest, but there's no strong case for supplementation at the moment.

It's hard to get rid of the nagging suspicion that it can't be good for five percent of us to be vitamin D–deficient during pregnancy. In a study in the (northern, not very sunny) UK, pregnant women who took vitamin D supplements during the winter had children with slightly higher bone mass on average at age nine. So particularly if you're dark-skinned or living in Seattle or Anchorage, it could theoretically be worthwhile to try to boost your levels.

How to do so? The body accumulates stores of vitamin D over the summer to tide us over through the winter (vitamin D is stored in body fat), so it might be tempting (financial considerations aside) to grab the sarong and flip-flops and splurge on a flight to Miami. But although a single beach vacation will indeed boost your levels, it won't let you stock up on all the vitamin D you'd need for nine months in one efficient swoop. First, there's a maximum amount you can absorb from the sun each day,[119] and any further vitamin D simply gets degraded[120, 121] (we've evolved an efficient system to prevent ourselves from overdosing).[122] Second, vitamin D isn't stored in the body indefinitely. The half-life appears to be approximately two months, based on studies of men who spent prolonged periods in submarines.[123] So when it comes to sun exposure, "little and often is best."[124]

If flying to the Bahamas every couple of months isn't exactly feasible, you might consider the local tanning salon. Although tanning beds provide a lower percentage of vitamin D rays (UVB) rays than ordinary sunshine, they do increase vitamin D levels.[125] Such behavior, of course, would have the melanoma experts in a fury of righteous indignation at your recklessness. The CDC makes the point: why increase your risk of skin cancer when there's a much safer way without the side effects?[126] If you're worried about being deficient (despite the lack of definitive evidence), simply take a supplement. Or plan a trip to the countryside to lick some sheep.

Benefit level for vitamin D supplements: Very low[127]

The Unmemorable Vitamin: Vitamin B$_6$

Vitamin B$_6$ is a nutrient that's quite obscure. We all know vitamin C comes from citrus fruit and prevents scurvy and calcium comes from milk and builds up bones. But here's a list of some foods that are good sources of B$_6$: wheat bran, raw garlic, pistachios, chili powder, liver, and molasses. A pretty random list if I ever saw one, although it might make a good witches' brew. And here are some symptoms of B$_6$ deficiency: "a seborrhoeic dermatitis-like eruption, atrophic glossitis with ulceration, angular cheilitis, conjunctivitis, intertrigo, and neurologic symptoms of somnolence, confusion, and neuropathy." Right.

Does this unmemorable vitamin require supplementation in pregnancy? Probably not. According to a review from 2015, "there's not enough evidence to detect clinical benefits of vitamin B$_6$ supplementation in pregnancy other than one trial suggesting protection against dental decay."[128] And according to a book published by the Institute of Medicine on nutrition in pregnancy, "most clinical trials of routine [vitamin B$_6$] supplementation of pregnant women have failed to demonstrate any differences in pregnancy outcome."[129] Furthermore, there's unlikely to be more news on this topic anytime soon, since most pregnant women in the United States are already consuming multivitamins containing vitamin B$_6$, making the topic difficult to study.[130]

I should mention the one quality of this elusive vitamin that may be memorable to you after all: B_6 can help alleviate nausea in early pregnancy.[131, 132, 133, 134] So at least you won't be sick on B_6.[135]

Benefit level for vitamin B_6 supplements: Very low

Lemons, Limes, and Clementines: Vitamin C

A cure for a scurvy sailor stranded at sea? Most certainly. A cure for the common cold? Probably not. Vitamin C did get an early PR boost from Nobel Prize winner Linus Pauling, who was convinced of its effectiveness in warding off the sniffles. But his theory has been mostly discredited.[136] Nevertheless, many of us still don't think twice about popping vitamin C in large quantities whenever we feel a cold coming on. It comes from citrus fruits—it must be healthy!

The question is, do we need to worry about vitamin C during pregnancy? The same answer applies: probably not. Despite a number of studies, there's no compelling evidence that it's helpful. In 1999, a study of vitamin supplementation in ~700 women of high socioeconomic status in the UK noted, "Vitamin C was the only micronutrient independently associated with birth weight," but this was only a small effect, and the authors concluded that "concern over the impact of maternal nutrition on the health of the infant [in industrialized nations] has been premature."[137] And a recent review concluded that "taking vitamin C supplements during pregnancy does not help to prevent problems in pregnancy including stillbirth, the death of the baby, preterm birth, preeclampsia or low birthweight babies."[138] No exciting news there.

So while there's no need to urgently flush your supplements down the toilet, there's also no need to keep taking them. Go ahead and eat your morning grapefruit with gusto, but skip the C supplements. Your baby may be afloat in the sea of your womb, but he or she is unlikely to end this particular voyage suffering from scurvy.

Benefit level for vitamin C supplements: Very low

Vampire Baby: Calcium

Drink your milk! Eat your cheese! Guzzle yogurt! Otherwise, your vampire baby will suck the calcium right out of your very bones, leaving you with a rickety skeleton. Here's the conventional wisdom from a typical parenting website: "If you don't get enough calcium in your diet when you're pregnant, your baby will draw it from your bones, which may impair your own health later on. . . . Most American women don't get nearly enough of this important mineral."[139] Insufficient calcium may not harm your baby, but no sensible mother would give herself osteoporosis unnecessarily. Besides, I've already mentioned this phenomenon in the section about lead, so what exactly might there be to quibble with? Turns out: plenty.

On the second point, the conventional wisdom is technically correct. As we've seen from the vitamin chart at the beginning of this section, many women aren't getting the recommended levels of calcium.[140] On the first point, they're also technically correct. According to a review of the topic from 2002, "There seems to be good evidence that calcium is mobilized from the maternal skeleton to that of the developing fetus during pregnancy."[141] So our babies are calcium vampires after all.

On the question of whether you'll impair your own health later on, however, the prevailing view is treading on much thinner ice. Of the studies that have evaluated the effect of having a baby on bone density, none have found a link between more pregnancies and lower bone density.[142, 143] A review of the field concludes, "No long-term adverse clinical effects have been noted in healthy women who had at least one ongoing pregnancy."[144] And the Institute of Medicine agrees.[145, 146] Your bones appear to simply return to normal once you're finished with pregnancy and breastfeeding.[147] Perversely, it's childlessness, rather than having children, that appears to be the true risk factor for developing osteoporosis later in life.[148]

What if you're lactose-intolerant and can't bring yourself to eat tofu? Even then, there seems to be little cause for worry about your bones. According to a study of vitamin-deficient women in South

Africa, "Multiple pregnancies and long lactations in both Bantu and Caucasian mothers were not accompanied by evidence of significant bone loss, in spite of a relatively low calcium intake."[149] Your skeleton will be just fine.

But we haven't closed the file on calcium yet. There's a reason to take calcium supplements, and it has nothing to do with skeletons. A review from 2011 concluded that taking at least 1,000 mg of supplemental calcium per day can reduce your risk of preterm birth because of calcium's ability to help control high blood pressure.[150] The authors support the use of calcium supplementation during pregnancy, particularly for those with low dietary intake.[151] And those with low dietary intake are not a small minority: at least half of American women of childbearing age have a dietary intake of less than 900 mg per day, the default threshold used in the review.[152]

You won't solve the problem with a standard prenatal vitamin, because the common brands don't contain anywhere near 1000 mg,[153] so it's yet another little white pill to add to the daily routine. Or, actually, two—calcium should ideally be taken in two daily doses, since your body absorbs calcium best in amounts ≤500 mg.[154] Or you could always start eating yogurt for breakfast, brunch, lunch, dinner, and bedtime snack. Fortunately, it comes in lots of flavors.

Benefit level for calcium supplements: Medium[155]

Conclusions: A Head Start

If you have the misfortune to live in a city where the elite nursery schools require application essays and parents are hiring admissions coaches for two-year-olds, it may sometimes feel as if competition starts in the womb.[156] Companies selling baby headphones would certainly like you to believe so. But as common sense would dictate, there's no magic pill or prenatal instructional gadget that will give your baby a head start before birth. Every mother-to-be should be consuming fish oil daily, as discussed in Chapter 2, and calcium supplements may also be worth adding to the daily routine. But when it comes to providing your child with mental stimulation, you have a good eighteen-plus years of parenting ahead in which to do so. That should be more than enough time, even for the most motivated of hyper-parents. For now, you're better off getting started on those nursery school applications.

Notes

1. Brewer, S. (1998). *Super baby: boost your baby's potential from conception to year one.* Thorsons.

2. BabyPlus. (n.d.). BabyPlus Pre-natal Education System. http://babyplus.com/wp-content/uploads/2016/11/HealthDigest10-08.pdf.

3. Van de Carr, R., & Lehrer, M. (1997). *While you are expecting: creating your own prenatal classroom.* Atlanta: Humanics; Diamond, M., & Hopson, J. L. (1999). *Magic trees of the mind: how to nurture your child's intelligence, creativity, and healthy emotions from birth through adolescence.* New York: Plume. Both books cited in Story, L. (2003). A head start in life? Prenatal parenting and the discourse of fetal stimulation. *Critical Studies in Gender, Culture & Social Justice, 27* (2), 41–48. http://forms.msvu.ca/atlantis/vol/272all/272story.PDF.

4. James, D. K., Spencer, C. J., & Stepsis, B. W. (2002). Fetal learning: a prospective randomized controlled study. *Ultrasound in Obstetrics & Gynecology, 20* (5), 431–438. http://onlinelibrary.wiley.com/doi/10.1046/j.1469-0705.2002.00845.x/pdf.

5. DeCasper, A. J., & Spence, M. J. (1986). Prenatal maternal speech influences newborns' perception of speech sounds. *Infant Behavior and Development, 9* (2), 133–150. http://earlyexperience.unsw.wikispaces.net/file/view/DeCasper1986.pdf/351993426/DeCasper1986.pdf.

6. DeCasper, A. J., & Fifer, W. P. (1980). Of human bonding: newborns prefer their mothers' voices. *Science, 208* (4448), 1174–1176. http://bernard.pitzer.edu/~dmoore/psych199s03articles/Of_Human_Bonding.pdf.

7. Fifer, W. P., & Moon, C. (1989, October). Psychobiology of newborn auditory preferences. *Seminars in Perinatology, 13* (5), 430–433. https://www.researchgate.net/publication/20340774_Psychobiology_of_newborn_auditory_Preferences.

8. Shetler, D. J. (1989). The inquiry into prenatal musical experience: a report of the Eastman project 1980–1987. *Journal of Prenatal & Perinatal Psychology & Health.* http://psycnet.apa.org/psycinfo/1989-32440-001.

9. Sack, K. (1998, January 15). Georgia's governor seeks musical start for babies. NYTimes.com. www.nytimes.com/1998/01/15/us/georgia-s-governor-seeks-musical-start-for-babies.html.

10. Goode, E. (1999, August 3). Mozart for baby? Some say, maybe not. NYTimes.com. www.nytimes.com/1999/08/03/science/mozart-for-baby-some-say-maybe-not.html.

11. Nuvo Ritmo pregnancy sound system. (n.d.). Amazon.com. www.amazon.com/Nuvo-Ritmo-Pregnancy-Sound-System/dp/B002XFE894.

12. Lullabelly Prenatal music belt. (n.d.). www.lullabelly.com/.

13. Bellybuds Baby-Bump sound system. (n.d.). Amazon.com. www.amazon.com/Bellybuds-V2-BBDLX-Bellybuds%C2%AE-Baby-Bump-System/dp/B0097F3YES/ref=sr_1_1?ie=UTF8&qid=1415745657&sr=8-1&keywords=bellybuds.

14. Rauscher, F. H., Shaw, G. L., & Ky, K. N. (1993). Music and spatial task performance: a causal relationship. *Nature, 365* (6447), 611. https://files.eric.ed.gov/fulltext/ED390733.pdf.

15. Rauscher, F. H. (1999). Reply: prelude or requiem for the 'Mozart effect'?. *Nature, 400* (6747), 827–828. http://libres.uncg.edu/ir/asu/f/Steele_KM_1999_Prelude_or_Requiem. pdf.

16. Goode, E., et al., Mozart for baby?

17. Ibid.; Spinks, S. (n.d.). The "first years" fallacy: Mozart, mobiles and the myth of critical windows. PBS Frontline. www.pbs.org/wgbh/pages/frontline/shows/teenbrain/science/ firstyears.html.

18. Hepper, P. G. (1991). An examination of fetal learning before and after birth. *The Irish Journal of Psychology, 12* (2), 95–107. http://psycnet.apa.org/psycinfo/1992-19350-001.

19. James, D. K., et al., Fetal learning: a prospective randomized controlled study.

20. Cuda-Kroen, G. (2011, August 8). Baby's palate and food memories shaped before birth. NPR.org. www.npr.org/2011/08/08/139033757/ babys-palate-and-food-memories-shaped-before-birth.

21. Watterson, B. (2009, October 12). *Calvin and Hobbes.* GoComics.com. www.gocomics. com/calvinandhobbes/2008/10/12/.

22. Dowd, M. (1990, March 23). "I'm president," so no more broccoli. NYTimes.com. www. nytimes.com/1990/03/23/us/i-m-president-so-no-more-broccoli.html.

23. Carruth, B. R., Ziegler, P. J., Gordon, A., & Barr, S. I. (2004). Prevalence of picky eaters among infants and toddlers and their caregivers' decisions about offering a new food. *Journal of the American Dietetic Association, 104* (Supplement 1), S57–S64. www.science direct.com/science/article/pii/S0002822303014925.

24. Mennella, J. A., Johnson, A., & Beauchamp, G. K. (1995). Garlic ingestion by pregnant women alters the odor of amniotic fluid. *Chemical Senses, 20* (2), 207–209. http://chemse. oxfordjournals.org/content/20/2/207.short.

25. Hauser, G. J., Chitayat, D., Berns, L., Braver, D., & Muhlbauer, B. (1985). Peculiar odours in newborns and maternal prenatal ingestion of spicy food. *European Journal of Pediatrics, 144* (4), 403. http://link.springer.com/article/10.1007/BF00441788.

26. Schaal, B., Marlier, L., & Soussignan, R. (2000). Human foetuses learn odours from their pregnant mother's diet. *Chemical Senses, 25* (6), 729–737. http://chemse.oxfordjournals. org/content/25/6/729.long.

27. Mennella, J. A., Jagnow, C. P., & Beauchamp, G. K. (2001). Prenatal and postnatal flavor learning by human infants. *Pediatrics, 107* (6), e88. http://pediatrics.aappublications.org/ content/107/6/e88.short.

28. Mennella et al., Prenatal and postnatal flavor learning by human infants.

29. Carruth, B. R., et al., Prevalence of picky eaters among infants and toddlers and their caregivers' decisions about offering a new food.

30. Turnip, Rampion Rapunzel, Heirloom Seeds 2016. (2014, November 11). CherryGal.com. www.cherrygal.com/turniprampionrapunzelheirloomseeds2014-p-7164.html.

31. King, J. C. (2000). Physiology of pregnancy and nutrient metabolism. *The American Journal of Clinical Nutrition, 71* (5), 1218s–1225s. http://ajcn.nutrition.org/content/71/5/1218s.full.

32. Hook, E. B. (1978). Dietary cravings and aversions during pregnancy. *The American Journal of Clinical Nutrition, 31* (8), 1355–1362. http://ajcn.nutrition.org/content/31/8/1355.short.

33. Dumas, D. (2011, October 31). Should we all be taking prenatal vitamins? Mindy Kaling reveals unlikely hair care tip. DailyMail.co.uk. www.dailymail.co.uk/femail/article-2055706/ Should-taking-prenatal-vitamins-Mindy-Kaling-reveals-unlikely-hair-care-tip.html

34. Folic acid recommendations. (2012, January 13). Centers for Disease Control and Prevention. www.cdc.gov/ncbddd/folicacid/recommendations.html.

35. Desposito, F., Cunniff, C., Frias, J. L., Panny, S. R., Trotter, T. L., & Wappner, R. S. (1999). Folic acid for the prevention of neural tube defects. *Pediatrics, 104* (2). http://pediatrics. aappublications.org/content/104/2/325.full.

36. Preconceptional consumption of folic acid. (2007, June). Association of Women's Health, Obstetric and Neonatal Nurses.

37. Institute of Medicine, Hellwig, J. P., Otten, J. J., & Meyers, L. D. (Eds.). (2006). *Dietary reference intakes: the essential guide to nutrient requirements.* Washington, DC: National Academies Press, 245. https://www.nap.edu/read/11537/chapter/26#245.

38. National Center for Environmental Health, Division of Laboratory Sciences, (2012). Second national report on biochemical indicators of diet and nutrition in the U.S. population. Centers for Disease Control and Prevention. https://www.cdc.gov/nutritionreport/pdf/ Nutrition_Book_complete508_final.pdf.

39. Holmes, L. B. (1988). Does taking vitamins at the time of conception prevent neural tube defects? *JAMA, 260* (21), 3181. http://jama.jamanetwork.com/article.aspx?articleid=375392.

40. Botto, L. D., Moore, C. A., Khoury, M. J., & Erickson, J. D. (1999). Neural-tube defects. *New England Journal of Medicine, 341* (20), 1509–1519. http://www.nejm.org/doi/full/10.1056/ NEJM199911113412006.

41. Milunsky, A., Jick, H., Jick, S. S., Bruell, C. L., MacLaughlin, D. S., Rothman, K. J., & Willett, W. (1989). Multivitamin/folic acid supplementation in early pregnancy reduces the prevalence of neural tube defects. *JAMA, 262* (20), 2847–2852. www.sjsu.edu/faculty/gerstman/ eks/Milunsky1989.pdf.

42. Scholl, T. O., Hediger, M. L., Bendich, A., Schall, J. I., Smith, W. K., & Krueger, P. M. (1997). Use of multivitamin/mineral prenatal supplements: influence on the outcome of pregnancy. *American Journal of Epidemiology, 146* (2), 134–141. http://aje.oxfordjournals. org/content/146/2/134.full.pdf.

43. Kaiser, L. L., & Allen, L. (2002). Position of the American Dietetic Association: nutrition and lifestyle for a healthy pregnancy outcome. *Journal of the American Dietetic Association, 102* (10), 1479–1490. www.ncbi.nlm.nih.gov/pubmed/12396171.

44. Picciano, M. F., & McGuire, M. K. (2009). Use of dietary supplements by pregnant and lactating women in North America. *The American Journal of Clinical Nutrition, 89* (2), 663S–667S. http://ajcn.nutrition.org/content/89/2/663S.full.pdf+html.

45. Czeizel, A. E. (1996). Reduction of urinary tract and cardiovascular defects by periconceptional multivitamin supplementation. *American Journal of Medical Genetics, 62* (2), 179–183. https://www.researchgate.net/profile/Andrew_Czeizel/publication/14325305_ Reduction_of_urinary_tract_and_cardiovascular_defects_by_periconceptional_vitamin_ supplementation/links/55f0144d08ae199d47c0489a.pdf.

46. Lammer, E. J., Shaw, G. M., Iovannisci, D. M., & Finnell, R. H. (2004). Periconceptional multivitamin intake during early pregnancy, genetic variation of acetyl-*N*-transferase 1 (NAT1), and risk for orofacial clefts. *Birth Defects Research Part A: Clinical and Molecular Teratology, 70* (11), 846–852. http://onlinelibrary.wiley.com/doi/10.1002/ bdra.20081/abstract;jsessionid=596102FAAB61113AF0F461204081FAFC. do4to3?deniedAccessCustomisedMessage=&userIsAuthenticated=false.

47. Bodnar, L. M., Tang, G., Ness, R. B., Harger, G., & Roberts, J. M. (2006). Periconceptional multivitamin use reduces the risk of preeclampsia. *American Journal of Epidemiology, 164* (5), 470–477. http://aje.oxfordjournals.org/content/164/5/470.full.

48. Vahratian, A., Siega-Riz, A. M., Savitz, D. A., & Thorp, J. M. (2004). Multivitamin use and the risk of preterm birth. *American Journal of Epidemiology, 160* (9), 886–892. http://aje. oxfordjournals.org/content/160/9/886.full.

49. Picciano, M. F., et al., Use of dietary supplements by pregnant and lactating women in North America.

50. Mathews, F., Youngman, L., & Neil, A. (2004). Maternal circulating nutrient concentrations in pregnancy: implications for birth and placental weights of term infants. *The American Journal of Clinical Nutrition, 79* (1), 103–110. http://ajcn.nutrition.org/content/79/1/103. full.

51. **Beyond the effects of folic acid, as the study was done in 1994, in the era pre-fortification.**

    Czeizel, A. E., Dudas, I., & Metneki, J. (1994). Pregnancy outcomes in a randomised controlled trial of periconceptional multivitamin supplementation. *Archives of Gynecology and Obstetrics, 255* (3), 131–139. www.springerlink.com/content/jg5654w694477630/.

52. Sullivan, K. M., Ford, E. S., Azrak, M. F., & Mokdad, A. H. (2009). Multivitamin use in pregnant and nonpregnant women: results from the Behavioral Risk Factor Surveillance System. *Public Health Reports, 124* (3), 384. www.ncbi.nlm.nih.gov/pmc/articles/ PMC2663874/.

53. **Data for US women aged 20–39. Data points for all nutrients except calcium are based on women age 20–39 and taken from a 2012 report from the CDC; data point for calcium is based on women age 25–50 from a 1997 report drawing on data from the Continuing Survey of Food Intakes by Individuals, conducted by the United States Department of Agriculture. The CDC report used biochemical indicators in urine and blood, but calcium intake cannot be measured this way. (National Center for Environmental Health, Second national report on biochemical indicators of diet and nutrition in the U.S. population; Park, Y. K., Yetley, E. A., & Calvo, M. S. [1997]. Calcium intake levels in the United States: issues and considerations. *Food Nutrition and Agriculture*, 34–43. www.fao. org/docrep/W7336T/w7336to6.htm).**

54. Picciano, M. F., et al., Use of dietary supplements by pregnant and lactating women in North America.

55. Stagnaro-Green, A., Sullivan, S., & Pearce, E. N. (2012). Iodine supplementation during pregnancy and lactation. *JAMA, 308* (23), 2463–2464. http://jama.jamanetwork.com/article. aspx?articleid=1486839.

56. Obican, S. G., Jahnke, G. D., Soldin, O. P., & Scialli, A. R. (2012). Teratology public affairs committee position paper: iodine deficiency in pregnancy. *Birth Defects Research Part A: Clinical and Molecular Teratology, 94* (9), 677–682. http://onlinelibrary.wiley.com/ doi/10.1002/bdra.23051/full. Citing: Caldwell, K. L., Makhmudov, A., Ely, E., Jones, R. L., & Wang, R. Y. (2011). Iodine status of the US population, National Health and Nutrition Examination Survey, 2005–2006 and 2007–2008. *Thyroid, 21* (4), 419–427. http://online. liebertpub.com/doi/abs/10.1089/thy.2010.0077.

57. Becker, D. V., Braverman, L. E., Delange, F., Dunn, J. T., Franklyn, J. A., Hollowell, J. G., Lamm, S. H., Mitchell, M. L., Pearce, E., Robbins, J., & Rovet, J. F. (2006). Iodine supplementation for pregnancy and lactation—United States and Canada: recommendations of the American Thyroid Association. *Thyroid, 16* (10), 949–951. www.thyroid.org/wp-content/uploads/statements/ATAIodineRec.pdf.

58. Iodine in your pregnancy diet. (n.d.). babycenter.com. www.babycenter.com/o_iodine-in-your-pregnancy-diet_667.bc.

59. Becker, D. V., et al., Iodine supplementation for pregnancy and lactation—United States and Canada: recommendations of the American Thyroid Association.

60. Berbel, P., Obregon, M. J., Bernal, J., Rey, F. E. D., & Escobar, G. M. D. (2007). Iodine supplementation during pregnancy: a public health challenge. *Trends in Endocrinology & Metabolism, 18* (9), 338–343. www.sciencedirect.com/science/article/pii/ S1043276007001555.

61. Berbel, P., Mestre, J. L., Santamaría, A., Palazón, I., Franco, A., Graells, M., González-Torga, A., & De Escobar, G. M. (2009). Delayed neurobehavioral development in children born to pregnant women with mild hypothyroxinemia during the first month of gestation: the importance of early iodine supplementation. *Thyroid, 19* (5), 511–519. http://online.liebert-pub.com/doi/abs/10.1089/thy.2008.0341.

62. George Washington University. (2012, December 18). Critical need for iodine supplements during pregnancy and while nursing. ScienceDaily.com. www.sciencedaily.com/releases/2012/12/121218161836.htm.

63. Velasco, I., Carreira, M., Santiago, P., Muela, J. A., García-Fuentes, E., Sanchez-Munoz, B., Garriga, M. J., González-Fernández, M. C., Rodríguez, A., Caballero, F. F., Machado, A., González-Romero, S., Anarte, M. T., & Soriguer, F. (2009). Effect of iodine prophylaxis during pregnancy on neurocognitive development of children during the first two years of life. *The Journal of Clinical Endocrinology & Metabolism, 94* (9), 3234–3241. http://jcem.endojournals.org/content/94/9/3234.full.

64. Stagnaro-Green, A., et al., Iodine supplementation during pregnancy and lactation.

65. Stagnaro-Green, A., Abalovich, M., Alexander, E., Azizi, F., Mestman, J., Negro, R., Nixon, A., Pearce, E. N., Soldin, O. P., Sullivan, S., & Wiersinga, W. (2011). Guidelines of the American Thyroid Association for the diagnosis and management of thyroid disease during pregnancy and postpartum. *Thyroid, 21* (10), 1081–1125. https://www.ncbi.nlm.nih.gov/pmc/articles/PMC3472679/.

66. Trumbo, P., Yates, A. A., Schlicker, S., & Poos, M. (2001). Dietary reference intakes: vitamin A, vitamin K, arsenic, boron, chromium, copper, iodine, iron, manganese, molybdenum, nickel, silicon, vanadium, and zinc. *Journal of the American Dietetic Association, 101* (3), 294–301. http://jandonline.org/article/S0002-8223(01)00078-5/fulltext.

67. American adults consistently consume on average about 3,700 milligrams of sodium a day (Bernstein, A. M., & Willett, W. C. [2010]. Trends in 24-h urinary sodium excretion in the United States, 1957–2003: a systematic review. *The American Journal of Clinical Nutrition, 2010* [92], 1172–1180. http://ajcn.nutrition.org/content/92/5/1172.full.pdf), equivalent to about 1.6 teaspoons of salt, well over the dietary guidelines of a teaspoon of salt per day (For consumers: lowering salt in your diet. [2010, May 18]. US Food and Drug Administration. www.fda.gov/ForConsumers/ConsumerUpdates/ucm181577.htm). According to the FDA, "About 75 percent of our total salt intake comes from salt added to processed foods by manufacturers and salt that cooks add to foods at restaurants and other food service establishments. The salt we add at the table or while cooking adds another 5 to 10 percent." (Ibid.). The sodium used in processed and restaurant foods typically contains little to no iodine (Dasgupta, P. K., Liu, Y., & Dyke, J. V. [2008]. Iodine nutrition: iodine content of iodized salt in the United States. *Environmental Science & Technology, 42* [4], 1315–1323. http://pubs.acs.org/doi/abs/10.1021/es0719071). So if we generously assume 10 percent of our intake is coming from table salt, that's 16 percent of a teaspoon of table salt per day. According to the American Thyroid Association, "One teaspoon of iodized salt contains approximately 400 µg iodine" (Iodine deficiency: what is iodine deficiency? [2012, June 4]. American Thyroid Assocation. www.thyroid.org/iodine-deficiency/). So switching from non-iodized to iodized table salt would give you an extra 64 µg of iodine per day, just over a third of the recommended level of 150 µg per day.

68. Stagnaro-Green, A., et al., Guidelines of the American Thyroid Association for the diagnosis and management of thyroid disease during pregnancy and postpartum.

69. Leung, A. M., Pearce, E. N., & Braverman, L. E. (2009). Iodine content of prenatal multivitamins in the United States. *New England Journal of Medicine, 360* (9), 939–940. www.nejm.org/doi/full/10.1056/NEJMc0807851.

70. Benefit score: 5% (probability, since 5% of American women have levels below the guidelines set by the WHO, as discussed in the main text) x 100 (impact: statistically detectable impairment—lowered IQ) x 1/1000 (certainty: unproven) = .005.

71. Ironman Triathlon. (n.d.). Wikipedia.org. http://en.wikipedia.org/wiki/Ironman_Triathlon.

72. Heinicke, K., Wolfarth, B., Winchenbach, P., Biermann, B., Schmid, A., Huber, G., Friedmann, B., & Schmidt, W. (2001). Blood volume and hemoglobin mass in elite athletes of different disciplines. *International Journal of Sports Medicine, 22* (7), 504–512. www.ncbi.nlm.nih.gov/pubmed/11590477.

73. Hytten, F. (1986). Blood volume changes in normal pregnancy. *Obstetrical & Gynecological Survey, 41* (7), 426–428. www.ncbi.nlm.nih.gov/pubmed/4075604.

74. Standards for maternal and neonatal care: Iron and folate supplementation. (2007). World Health Organization. www.who.int/entity/reproductivehealth/publications/maternal_perinatal_health/iron_folate_supplementation.pdf.

75. Stoltzfus, R. J., & Dreyfuss, M. L. (1998). Guidelines for the use of iron supplements to prevent and treat iron deficiency anemia. Washington, DC: Ilsi Press, 18–21. wwwlive.who.int/entity/nutrition/publications/micronutrients/guidelines_for_Iron_supplementation.pdf.

76. Yip, R., Parvanta, I., Cogswell, M. E., McDonnell, S. M., Bowman, B. A., Grummer-Strawn, L. M., & Trowbridge, F. L. (1998). Recommendations to prevent and control iron deficiency in the United States. *Morbidity and Mortality Weekly Report: Recommendations and Reports, 47* (RR-3), 1–36. www.cdc.gov/mmwr/preview/mmwrhtml/00051880.htm.

77. Hauth, J. C., & Merenstein, B. B., (eds.). (1997). *Guidelines for perinatal care* (4th ed.). Elk Grove Village, IL: American Academy of Pediatrics and American College of Obstetricians and Gynecologists.

78. Panel on Micronutrients, Subcommittees on Upper Reference Levels of Nutrients and of Interpretation and Uses of Dietary Reference Intakes, and the Standing Committee on the Scientific Evaluation of Dietary Reference Intakes; Food & Nutrition Board; & the Institute of Medicine (US). (2001). Dietary reference intakes for vitamin A, vitamin K, arsenic, boron, chromium, copper, iodine, iron, manganese, molybdenum, nickel, silicon, vanadium, and zinc. Washington, DC: National Academies Press. https://www.nap.edu/read/10026/chapter/1.

79. 2010 Dietary Guidelines Advisory Committee. (2010). Report of the Dietary Guidelines Advisory Committee on the dietary guidelines for Americans. USDA Agricultural Research Service. https://www.nutriwatch.org/05Guidelines/dga_advisory_2010.pdf.

80. Makrides, M., Crowther, C. A., Gibson, R. A., Gibson, R. S., & Skeaff, C. M. (2003). Efficacy and tolerability of low-dose iron supplements during pregnancy: a randomized controlled trial. *The American Journal of Clinical Nutrition, 78* (1), 145–153. http://ajcn.nutrition.org/content/78/1/145.long.

81. Taylor, D. J., Mallen, C., McDougall, N., & Lind, T. (1982). Effect of iron supplementation on serum ferritin levels during and after pregnancy. *BJOG: An International Journal of Obstetrics & Gynaecology, 89* (12), 1011–1017. http://onlinelibrary.wiley.com/doi/10.1111/j.1471-0528.1982.tb04656.x/abstract.

82. Thomsen, J. K., Prien-Larsen, J. C., Devantier, A., & Fogh-Andersen, N. (1993). Low dose iron supplementation does not cover the need for iron during pregnancy. *Acta Obstetricia et Gynecologica Scandinavica, 72* (2), 93–98. http://informahealthcare.com/doi/abs/10.3109/00016349309023419.

83. Svanberg, B., Arvidsson, B., Norrby, A., Rybo, G., Solvell, L. (1975). Absorption of supplemental iron during pregnancy: a longitudinal study with repeated bone-marrow studies and absorption measurements. *Acta Obstetrica et Gynecologica Scandinavica, 54* (Suppl. 48), 87–108. http://informahealthcare.com/doi/abs/10.3109/00016347509156332.

84. Puolakka, J., Jäne, O., Pakarinen, A., Järvinen, P. A., & Vihko, R. (1980). Serum ferritin as a measure of iron stores during and after normal pregnancy with and without iron supplements. *Acta Obstetricia et Gynecologica Scandinavica, 59* (S95), 43–51. http://onlinelibrary. wiley.com/doi/10.3109/00016348009156379/abstract.

85. Screening for iron deficiency anemia—including iron prophylaxis. (1996). US Preventive Services Task Force. https://www.uspreventiveservicestaskforce.org/Home/GetFile/1/800/ ironscr/pdf.

86. Just to clarify, iron deficiency and anemia aren't actually one and the same. One is measured by the level of iron circulating in the blood ("serum ferritin level"), while the other is measured by the concentration of red blood cells ("hematocrit level"). Most cases of anemia aren't actually caused by iron deficiency—only ~12 percent of pregnant women suffering from anemia have low iron stores; the rest have insufficient red blood cells for other reasons. Ultimately, though, it's the specific cases of anemia caused by iron deficiency that are most worrisome during pregnancy: "the odds of low birth weight were tripled and of preterm delivery more than doubled with iron deficiency, but were not increased with anemia from other causes." Klebanoff, M. A., Shiono, P. H., Selby, J. V., Trachtenberg, A. I., & Graubard, B. I. (1991). Anemia and spontaneous preterm birth. *American Journal of Obstetrics and Gynecology, 164* (1), 59–63. http://europepmc. org/abstract/MED/1986627; Scholl, T. O., Hediger, M. L., Fischer, R. L., & Shearer, J. W. (1992). Anemia vs iron deficiency: increased risk of preterm delivery in a prospective study. *The American Journal of Clinical Nutrition, 55* (5), 985–988. http://ajcn.nutrition. org/content/55/5/985.full.pdf.

87. Cogswell, M. E., Parvanta, I., Ickes, L., Yip, R., & Brittenham, G. M. (2003). Iron supplementation during pregnancy, anemia, and birth weight: a randomized controlled trial. *The American Journal of Clinical Nutrition, 78* (4), 773–781. http://ajcn.nutrition.org/content/ 78/4/773.long.

88. Siega-Riz, A. M., Hartzema, A. G., Turnbull, C., Thorp, J., McDonald, T., & Cogswell, M. E. (2006). The effects of prophylactic iron given in prenatal supplements on iron status and birth outcomes: a randomized controlled trial. *American Journal of Obstetrics and Gynecology, 194* (2), 512–519. www.ajog.org/article/S0002-9378(05)01251-2/abstract.

89. Scholl, T. O., Hediger, M. L., Bendich, A., Schall, J. I., Smith, W. K., & Krueger, P. M. (1997). Use of multivitamin/mineral prenatal supplements: influence on the outcome of pregnancy. *American Journal of Epidemiology, 146* (2), 134–141. http://aje.oxfordjournals. org/content/146/2/134.full.pdf.

90. US Preventive Services Task Force. (1993). Routine iron supplementation during pregnancy. *JAMA: The Journal of the American Medical Association, 270* (23), 2846–2848. http://jama.jamanetwork.com/article.aspx?articleid=409796.

91. Hemminki, E., & Rimpelä, U. (1991). A randomized comparison of routine versus selective iron supplementation during pregnancy. *Journal of the American College of Nutrition, 10* (1), 3–10. http://www.tandfonline.com/doi/abs/10.1080/07315724.1991.10718119.

92. Paintin, D. B., Thomson, A. M., & Hytten, F. E. (1966). Iron and the haemoglobin level in pregnancy. *BJOG: An International Journal of Obstetrics & Gynaecology, 73* (2), 181–190. http://onlinelibrary.wiley.com/doi/10.1111/j.1471-0528.1966.tb05144.x/abstract.

93. Willoughby, M. L. N. (1967). An investigation of folic acid requirements in pregnancy. II. *British Journal of Haematology, 13* (s1), 503–509. www.ncbi.nlm.nih.gov/pmc/articles/ PMC1944952/pdf/brmedj02373-0036.pdf.

94. Primbs K. (1973). Eisenbehandlung wahrend der Schwangerschaft eine Vergleichsstudie [English abstract: Iron treatment during pregnancy, a comparative study]. *Geburtshilfe und Frauenheilkunde, 33,* 552–559.

95. Fleming, A. F., Martin, J. D., Hahnel, R., Westlake, A. J. (1974). Effects of iron and folic acid antenatal supplements on maternal haematology and fetal well-being. *Medical Journal of Australia, 2*, 429–436; Taylor and Lind 1976 Abstract. https://www.cabdirect.org/cabdirect/abstract/19752700375.

96. Makrides, M., Crowther, C. A., Gibson, R. A., Gibson, R. S., & Skeaff, C. M. (2003). Efficacy and tolerability of low-dose iron supplements during pregnancy: a randomized controlled trial. *The American Journal of Clinical Nutrition, 78* (1), 145–153. http://ajcn.nutrition.org/content/78/1/145.long.

97. Hemminki, E., et al., A randomized comparison of routine versus selective iron supplementation during pregnancy.

98. Hemminki, E., & Meriläinen, J. (1995). Long-term follow-up of mothers and their infants in a randomized trial on iron prophylaxis during pregnancy. *American Journal of Obstetrics and Gynecology, 173* (1), 205–209. www.sciencedirect.com/science/article/pii/0002937895901914.

99. Screening for iron deficiency anemia—including iron prophylaxis, US Preventive Services Task Force.

100. Zhou, S. J., Gibson, R. A., Crowther, C. A., Baghurst, P., & Makrides, M. (2006). Effect of iron supplementation during pregnancy on the intelligence quotient and behavior of children at 4 y of age: long-term follow-up of a randomized controlled trial. *The American Journal of Clinical Nutrition, 83* (5), 1112–1117. http://ajcn.nutrition.org/content/83/5/1112.long.

101. Parsons, A. G., Zhou, S. J., Spurrier, N. J., & Makrides, M. (2008). Effect of iron supplementation during pregnancy on the behaviour of children at early school age: long-term follow-up of a randomised controlled trial. *British Journal of Nutrition, 99* (05), 1133–1139. www.ncbi.nlm.nih.gov/pubmed/17967217.

102. Rasmussen, K. M. (2001). Is there a causal relationship between iron deficiency or iron-deficiency anemia and weight at birth, length of gestation and perinatal mortality? *The Journal of Nutrition, 131* (2), 590S–603S. http://jn.nutrition.org/content/131/2/590S.full.pdf.

103. Allen, L. H. (2000). Anemia and iron deficiency: effects on pregnancy outcome. *The American Journal of Clinical Nutrition, 71* (5), 1280s–1284s. http://ajcn.nutrition.org/content/71/5/1280s.full.

104. US Preventive Services Task Force, Routine iron supplementation during pregnancy.

105. Cogswell, M. E., Kettel-Khan, L., & Ramakrishnan, U. (2003). Iron supplement use among women in the United States: science, policy and practice. *The Journal of Nutrition, 133* (6), 1974S–1977S. http://jn.nutrition.org/content/133/6/1974S.full.

106. Mei, Z., Cogswell, M. E., Looker, A. C., Pfeiffer, C. M., Cusick, S. E., Lacher, D. A., & Grummer-Strawn, L. M. (2011). Assessment of iron status in US pregnant women from the National Health and Nutrition Examination Survey (NHANES), 1999–2006. *The American Journal of Clinical Nutrition, 93* (6), 1312–1320. http://ajcn.nutrition.org/content/93/6/1312.full.

107. Black, R. E. (2001). Micronutrients in pregnancy. *British Journal of Nutrition, 85* (S2), S193–S197. http://journals.cambridge.org/production/action/cjoGetFulltext?fulltextid=891312.

108. The American College of Obstetricians and Gynecologists. (2014, January). Routine tests in pregnancy. Frequently Asked Questions, FAQ133: Pregnancy. www.acog.org/~/media/For%20Patients/faq133.pdf?dmc=1&ts=20131204T0617036726.

109. Cogswell, M. E., et al., Iron supplement use among women in the United States: science, policy and practice.

110. Benefit score for women who are not in the high-risk category (low-income and minority women skipping prenatal care): 5% (probability that a pregnant woman is iron deficient, as shown in the Horse Pills for Breakfast chart; this is an upper bound, as women not in the high-risk category are less likely to fall into this bucket) x 100 (impact: statistically detectable impairment) x 1/1,000 (certainty: unproven) = .005.

111. Holick, M. F. (2007). Vitamin D deficiency. New England Journal of Medicine, 357 (3), 266–281. http://www.nejm.org/doi/full/10.1056/NEJMra070553.

112. One 8-ounce glass of milk has ~120 IU, so you'd need 5 glasses a day to get the DRI of 600 IU.

113. In the UK, which is farther north than any point in the US and where foods such as milk are not routinely supplemented with vitamin D, the Department of Health recommends a daily supplement of 10 micrograms of vitamin D (NHS Choices. [2012, November 26]. Vitamins and minerals—vitamin D. UK National Health Service.www.nhs.uk/Conditions/vitamins-minerals/Pages/Vitamin-D.aspx), while the National Institute for Health and Clinical Excellence (NICE) takes a more wishy-washy approach, leaving it as a decision for each woman to make for herself: "All women should be informed about the importance for their own and their baby's health of maintaining adequate vitamin D stores during pregnancy and whilst breastfeeding. In order to achieve this, women may choose to take 10 micrograms of vitamin D per day" (National Institute for Health and Clinical Excellence. [2008]. Antenatal care: routine care for the healthy pregnant woman (2nd ed.). London: RCOG Press. www.nice.org.uk/nicemedia/pdf/CG062NICEguideline. pdf). In Canada, according to the Canadian Paediatric Society in 2007, reaffirmed in 2013, "consideration should be given to administering 2000 IU of vitamin D daily to pregnant and lactating women, especially during the winter months, to maintain vitamin D sufficiency. The effectiveness of this regimen and possible side effects should be checked with periodic assays for vitamin D and calcium" (First Nations, I. A. M. H. C. [2007]. Vitamin D supplementation: recommendations for Canadian mothers and infants. Paediatrics and Child Health, 12 [7], 583. www.cps.ca/documents/position/vitamin-d).

114. Institute of Medicine, Subcommittee on Dietary Intake & Nutrient Supplements during Pregnancy. (1990). Nutrition during pregnancy: part I, weight gain: part II, nutrient supplements. Chapter 16. Washington, DC: National Academy Press. www.nap.edu/openbook.php?record_id=1451&page=328.

115. Specker, B. L. (1994). Do North American women need supplemental vitamin D during pregnancy or lactation? The American Journal of Clinical Nutrition, 59 (2), 484S–490S. http://ajcn.nutrition.org/content/59/2/484S.short.

116. A group of researchers has been investigating whether vitamin D deficiency in pregnancy might be linked to the rise in childhood asthma in the UK and US. One of their studies in Massachusetts (Camargo, C. A., Rifas-Shiman, S. L., Litonjua, A. A., Rich-Edwards, J. W., Weiss, S. T., Gold, D. R., Kleinman, K., & Gillman, M. W. [2007]. Maternal intake of vitamin D during pregnancy and risk of recurrent wheeze in children at 3 y of age. The American Journal of Clinical Nutrition, 85 [3], 788–795. http://ajcn. nutrition.org/content/85/3/788.short) does provide some preliminary evidence that even women living in the US could benefit from further supplements. But others have hypothesized that vitamin D could actually make asthma worse, so the researchers caveat that the jury is still out, and "determining the role of vitamin D in asthma will require comprehensive multidisciplinary studies." (Litonjua, A. A., & Weiss, S. T. [2007]. Is vitamin D deficiency to blame for the asthma epidemic? Journal of Allergy and Clinical Immunology, 120 [5], 1031–1035. www.jacionline.org/article/S0091-6749(07)01600-4/fulltext).

117. Bodnar, L. M., Catov, J. M., Simhan, H. N., Holick, M. F., Powers, R. W., & Roberts, J. M. (2007). Maternal vitamin D deficiency increases the risk of preeclampsia. *The Journal of Clinical Endocrinology & Metabolism, 92* (9), 3517–3522. http://jcem.endojournals.org/content/92/9/3517.long.

118. ACOG Committee on Obstetric Practice. (2011). ACOG committee opinion no. 495— Vitamin D: Screening and supplementation during pregnancy. *Obstetrics and Gynecology, 118* (1), 197. https://www.acog.org/Resources-And-Publications/Committee-Opinions/Committee-on-Obstetric-Practice/Vitamin-D-Screening-and-Supplementation-During-Pregnancy.

119. ~10,000–20,000 IU, after which the concentrations of vitamin D precursors produced in the skin reach an equilibrium. (Holick, M. F. [1997]. Chapter 2: Photobiology of vitamin D. In: Feldman, D., Pike, W. J., & Adams, J. S. *Vitamin D* (3rd ed.). London: Elsevier, 33–39. https://books.google.co.uk/books?id=w7hMAFmsM84C; Vieth, R. [1999]. Vitamin D supplementation, 25-hydroxyvitamin D concentrations, and safety. *The American Journal of Clinical Nutrition, 69* [5], 842–856. http://ajcn.nutrition.org/content/69/5/842.short).

120. NIH Office of Dietary Supplements. (2014, November 10). Vitamin D: fact sheet for professionals. National Institutes of Health. https://ods.od.nih.gov/factsheets/VitaminD-HealthProfessional/.

121. Holick, M. F. (1995). Environmental factors that influence the cutaneous production of vitamin D. *The American Journal of Clinical Nutrition, 61* (3), 638S–645S. http://ajcn.nutrition.org/content/61/3/638S.short.

122. To produce that maximum amount, the sunlight you need is pretty minimal, equivalent to "a light pinkness of the skin." (Holick, M. F., Photobiology of vitamin D.). How long does this take? According to one estimate, "at noon in June in Boston, Mass, a fair-skinned individual will maximize his or her vitamin D photosynthesis in well less than 5 minutes, and additional sun exposure will produce only photodamage." (Holick, M. F., & Jenkins, M. [2005]. The UV advantage. As quoted in: Wolpowitz, D., & Gilchrest, B. A. [2006]. The vitamin D questions: how much do you need and how should you get it? *Journal of the American Academy of Dermatology, 54* [2], 301–317. http://www.sciencedirect.com/science/article/pii/S0190962205045962). According to another, "light skinned people need 10–20 minutes of exposure while dark skinned people need 90–120 minutes." (Matsuoka, L. Y., Wortsman, J., Haddad, J. G., Kolm, P., & Hollis, B. W. [1991]. Racial pigmentation and the cutaneous synthesis of vitamin D. *Archives of Dermatology, 127* [4], 536–538. http://archderm.ama-assn.org/cgi/reprint/127/4/536.pdf). Concerned that people will go overboard, several large UK health organizations have recently published a joint statement about balancing sun benefits (vitamin D) vs. risks (skin cancer): "The time required to make sufficient vitamin D is typically short and less than the amount of time needed for skin to redden and burn. Regularly going outside for a matter of minutes around the middle of the day without sunscreen should be enough." (Consensus vitamin D position statement. [2010, December 9]. The British Association of Dermatologists, Cancer Research UK, Diabetes UK, the Multiple Sclerosis Society, the National Heart Forum, the National Osteoporosis Society, and the Primary Care Dermatology Society. www.cancerresearchuk.org/prod_consump/groups/cr_common/@nre/@sun/documents/generalcontent/cr_052628.pdf). The key is how much of your body surface is exposed—more is better. Simply walking around in normal clothes may provide enough sunlight if you're out every day. But your face and hands have a small surface area and are the most prone to skin cancer, given how much of the time they're exposed. So a better plan would actually be to spend 5–10 minutes lying around in a bathing suit sometime between 10:00 and 2:00 each day and then cover up or wear sunscreen.

123. Jones, G. (2008). Pharmacokinetics of vitamin D toxicity. *The American Journal of Clinical Nutrition, 88* (2), 582S–586S. www.ncbi.nlm.nih.gov/pubmed/18689406; Feldman, D., Glorieux, F., Pike, J.W. (Eds.). (2005). Vitamin D (2nd ed.). Elsevier, San Diego, CA, Chapter 61. www.direct-ms.org/pdf/VitDVieth/Vieth%20CHAPTER%2061.pdf. And in a study of women from Scotland, the effects of going on a sunny holiday were still noticeable after three months but not after six months (Mavroeidi, A., Aucott, L., Black, A. J., Fraser, W. D., Reid, D. M., & Macdonald, H. M. [2013]. Seasonal variation in 25 [OH] D at Aberdeen [57° N] and bone health indicators—could holidays in the sun and cod liver oil supplements alleviate deficiency? *PloS One, 8* [1], e53381. www.plosone.org/article/info%3Adoi%2F10.1371%2Fjournal.pone.0053381).

124. The British Association of Dermatologists, Consensus vitamin D position statement.

125. Tangpricha, V., Turner, A., Spina, C., Decastro, S., Chen, T. C., & Holick, M. F. (2004). Tanning is associated with optimal vitamin D status (serum 25-hydroxyvitamin D concentration) and higher bone mineral density. *The American Journal of Clinical Nutrition, 80* (6), 1645–1649. http://ajcn.nutrition.org/content/80/6/1645.long.

126. Indoor tanning is not safe. (2014, July 15). Centers for Disease Control and Prevention. www.cdc.gov/cancer/skin/basic_info/indoor_tanning.htm.

127. If you're going to supplement, there is some controversy about how much to take. In the United States, the official recommended intake for vitamin D during pregnancy was tripled in 2010 from 200 to 600 IU per day (Del Valle, H. B., Yaktine, A. L., Taylor, C. L., & Ross, A. C. [Eds.]. [2011]. *Dietary reference intakes for calcium and vitamin D.* Washington, DC: National Academies Press. https://books.google.com/books?hl=en&lr=&id=ZsMPp6I59VwC&oi=fnd&pg=PR1&dq. But if you're vitamin D–deficient, even 600 IU per day may not be enough. According to one study, "mothers who were vitamin D–deficient at the beginning of their pregnancy were still deficient at the end of their pregnancy after being supplemented with 800–1600 IU vitamin D per day throughout their pregnancy" (Datta, S., Alfaham, M., Davies, D. P., Dunstan, F., Woodhead, S., Evans, J., & Richards, B. [2002]. Vitamin D deficiency in pregnant women from a non-European ethnic minority population—an interventional study. *BJOG: An International Journal of Obstetrics & Gynaecology, 109* [8], 905–908. http://onlinelibrary.wiley.com/doi/10.1111/j.1471-0528.2002.01171.x/full, as discussed in: Hollis, B. W., & Wagner, C. L. [2004]. Assessment of dietary vitamin D requirements during pregnancy and lactation. *The American Journal of Clinical Nutrition, 79* [5], 717–726. http://ajcn.nutrition.org/content/79/5/717.long). In the words of one researcher who clearly feels strongly about the topic, "It appears that the current Dietary Reference Intake (DRI) for adults are woefully inadequate, misleading, and potentially harmful . . . 600 IU/[day] is extraordinarily low compared with production during sun exposure. Reexamination of the requirements for vitamin D is clearly merited and may likely reveal the need for vitamin D intakes exceeding 2000 IU per day for adults" (Hollis, B. W. [2005]. Circulating 25-hydroxyvitamin D levels indicative of vitamin D sufficiency: implications for establishing a new effective dietary intake recommendation for vitamin D. *The Journal of Nutrition, 135* [2], 317–322. http://jn.nutrition.org/content/135/2/317.long). The issue is that vitamin D is stored in the body, so it's technically possible to overdose. But many researchers believe even the maximum value, currently set at 4,000 IU per day, is unnecessarily conservative (Del Valle, H. B., et al., Dietary reference intakes for calcium and vitamin D). For example, one review supports increasing the maximum allowed to 10,000 IU per day (Hathcock, J. N., Shao, A., Vieth, R., & Heaney, R. [2007]. Risk assessment for vitamin D. *The American Journal of Clinical Nutrition, 85* [1], 6–18. http://ajcn.nutrition.org/content/85/1/6.long). Another study has suggested that "the easiest method of correcting vitamin D deficiency is to give the patient one pill that contains 50,000 IU vitamin D once a week for 8 weeks" (Heaney, R. P., Dowell, M. S., Hale, C. A., & Bendich, A. [2003]. Calcium

absorption varies within the reference range for serum 25-hydroxyvitamin D. *Journal of the American College of Nutrition, 22* [2], 142–146. http://www.tandfonline.com/doi/abs /10.1080/07315724.2003.10719287). And another points out that the lowest intake of vitamin D that has ever been linked to toxicity involved ingesting 40,000 IU per day for three months (Vieth, R., Vitamin D supplementation, 25-hydroxyvitamin D concentrations, and safety).

128. Salam, R. A., Zuberi, N. F., & Bhutta, Z. A. (2015). Pyridoxine (vitamin B_6) supplementation during pregnancy or labour for maternal and neonatal outcomes. *Cochrane Database of Systematic Reviews, 2015*, (6): CD000179. http://onlinelibrary.wiley.com/ doi/10.1002/14651858.CD000179.pub3/full.

129. Institute of Medicine (US), Nutrition during pregnancy: part I, weight gain: part II, nutrient supplements.

130. Ibid.

131. Sahakian, V., Rouse, D., Sipes, S., Rose, N., & Niebyl, J. (1991). Vitamin B_6 is effective therapy for nausea and vomiting of pregnancy: a randomized, double-blind placebo-controlled study. *Obstetrics & Gynecology, 78* (1), 33–36. http://journals.lww.com/greenjournal/ abstract/1991/07000/vitamin_b6_is_effective_therapy_for_nausea_and.7.aspx.

132. Vutyavanich, T., Wongtra-ngan, S. & Ruangsri, R. (1995). Pyridoxine for nausea and vomiting of pregnancy, a randomized, double-blind, placebo-controlled trial. *American Journal of Obstetrics and Gynecology, 173*, 881–884. www.sciencedirect.com/science/article/ pii/0002937895903593.

133. Chittumma, P., Kaewkiattikun, K., & Wiriyasiriwach, B. (2007). Comparison of the effectiveness of ginger and vitamin B_6 for treatment of nausea and vomiting in early pregnancy: a randomized double-blind controlled trial. *Journal of the Medical Association of Thailand, 90* (1), 15. http://www.imuneksfarma.com/wp-content/uploads/2014/07/EME-5.pdf.

134. Sripramote, M., & Lekhyananda, N. (2003). A randomized comparison of ginger and vitamin B_6 in the treatment of nausea and vomiting of pregnancy. *Journal of the Medical Association of Thailand (Chotmaihet thangphaet), 86* (9), 846–853. http://europepmc.org/ abstract/med/14649969http://cat.inist.fr/?amodele=affichen&cpsidt=15504666.

135. According to a review of interventions for nausea and vomiting in early pregnancy, "Pyridoxine (vitamin B_6) 10 to 25 mg three times a day is the least likely to cause side-effects [vs. other available drugs]. According to standard therapeutic practice, it would seem wise to start treatment with the lower dose. Recent evidence that fresh ginger root is beneficial is encouraging. . . . The evidence on P6 acupuncture or acupressure is mixed. It has not been shown to be clearly more effective than sham or dummy acupressure, or than standard dietary and lifestyle advice. Rest and small amounts of carbohydrate, such as biscuits, are widely believed to be helpful" (Jewell, D., & Young, G. [2003]. Interventions for nausea and vomiting in early pregnancy. *Cochrane Database of Systematic Reviews, 2003*, (4): CD000145. http://onlinelibrary.wiley.com/ doi/10.1002/14651858.CD000145/full). Since publication of the above in 2003, another double-blind randomized placebo-controlled trial has confirmed the effectiveness of ginger in reducing nausea during pregnancy (Willetts, K. E., Ekangaki, A., & Eden, J. A. [2003]. Effect of a ginger extract on pregnancy-induced nausea: a randomised controlled trial. *Australian and New Zealand Journal of Obstetrics and Gynaecology, 43* [2], 139–144. http://onlinelibrary.wiley.com/doi/10.1046/j.0004-8666.2003.00039.x/full), and a further study has suggested that ginger may be even more effective than B_6 (Chittumma, P., et al., Comparison of the effectiveness of ginger and vitamin B6 for treatment of nausea and vomiting in early pregnancy). It's also possible that a standard multivitamin can be effective in reducing nausea (Czeizel, A. E., Dudas, I., Fritz, G., Técsöi, A., Hanck, A., & Kunovits, G. [1992]. The effect of periconceptional multivitamin-mineral

supplementation on vertigo, nausea and vomiting in the first trimester of pregnancy. *Archives of Gynecology and Obstetrics, 251* [4], 181–185. https://link.springer.com/article/10.1007%2FBF02718384?LI=true).

136. Douglas, R. M., & Hemilä, H. (2005). Vitamin C for preventing and treating the common cold. *PLoS Medicine, 2* (6), e168. www.plosmedicine.org/article/info%3A-doi%2F10.1371%2Fjournal.pmed.0020168.

137. Mathews, F., Yudkin, P., & Neil, A. (1999). Influence of maternal nutrition on outcome of pregnancy: prospective cohort study. *BMJ, 319* (7206), 339–343. www.ncbi.nlm.nih.gov/pmc/articles/pmc28185/.

138. Rumbold, A., Ota, E., Nagata, C., Shahrook, S., & Crowther, C. A. (2015). Vitamin C supplementation in pregnancy. *Cochrane Database of Systematic Reviews, 2015*, (9): CD004072. http://onlinelibrary.wiley.com/doi/10.1002/14651858.CD004072.pub3/full.

139. Babycenter Medical Advisory Board. (Last reviewed 2016, June). Calcium in your pregnancy diet. Babycenter.com. www.babycenter.com/0_calcium-in-your-pregnancy-diet_665.bc.

140. Bailey, R. L., Dodd, K. W., Goldman, J. A., Gahche, J. J., Dwyer, J. T., Moshfegh, A. J., Sempos, C. T., & Picciano, M. F. (2010). Estimation of total usual calcium and vitamin D intakes in the United States. *The Journal of Nutrition, 140* (4), 817–822. http://jn.nutrition.org/content/140/4/817.long.

141. Ensom, M. H., Liu, P. Y., & Stephenson, M. D. (2002). Effect of pregnancy on bone mineral density in healthy women. *Obstetrical & Gynecological survey, 57* (2), 99–111. http://journals.lww.com/obgynsurvey/Abstract/2002/02000/Effect_of_Pregnancy_on_Bone_Mineral_Density_in.22.aspx.

142. Karlsson, C., Obrant, K. J., & Karlsson, M. (2001). Pregnancy and lactation confer reversible bone loss in humans. *Osteoporosis International, 12* (10), 828–834. http://link.springer.com/article/10.1007/s001980170033#.

143. Ensom, M. H., et al., Effect of pregnancy on bone mineral density in healthy women.

144. Ibid.

145. Institute of Medicine, Nutrition during pregnancy: part I, weight gain: part II, nutrient supplements.

146. Del Valle, H. B., et al., Dietary reference intakes for calcium and vitamin D.

147. More, C., Bettembuk, P., Bhattoa, H. P., & Balogh, A. (2001). The effects of pregnancy and lactation on bone mineral density. *Osteoporosis International, 12* (9), 732–737. https://link.springer.com/article/10.1007%2Fs001980170048?LI=true.

148. The likely reason for the link is that hormone levels influence bone density, and women who have children are exposed to different levels of hormones over the course of their lives than women who remain childless. (Stevenson, J. C., Lees, B., Devenport, M., Cust, M. P., & Ganger, K. F. [1989]. Determinants of bone density in normal women: risk factors for future osteoporosis? *BMJ: British Medical Journal, 298* [6678], 924. http://www.bmj.com/content/298/6678/924.short; Hillier, T. A., Rizzo, J. H., Pedula, K. L., Stone, K. L., Cauley, J. A., Bauer, D. C., & Cummings, S. R. [2003]. Nulliparity and fracture risk in older women: the study of osteoporotic fractures. *Journal of Bone and Mineral Research, 18* [5], 893–899. http://onlinelibrary.wiley.com/doi/10.1359/jbmr.2003.18.5.893/full).

149. Walker, A. R. P., Richardson, B., & Walker, F. (1972). The influence of numerous pregnancies and lactations on bone dimensions in South African Bantu and Caucasian mothers. *Clinical Science, 42* (2), 189–196. http://www.clinsci.org/content/42/2/189.

150. Hofmeyr, G. J., Atallah, A. N., & Duley, L. (2006). Calcium supplementation during pregnancy for preventing hypertensive disorders and related problems. *Cochrane*

Database Systematic Reviews, 2006 (3): CD001059. http://onlinelibrary.wiley.com/doi/10.1002/14651858.CD001059.pub2/full.

151. Or high risk of preeclampsia, a condition involving high blood pressure which can lead to life-threatening seizures (eclampsia) if left untreated. Supplementation halved the risk of preeclampsia; fortunately, this condition only affects about 3 percent of pregnancies in the United States (Wallis, A. B., Saftlas, A. F., Hsia, J., & Atrash, H. K. [2008]. Secular trends in the rates of preeclampsia, eclampsia, and gestational hypertension, United States, 1987–2004. *American Journal of Hypertension, 21* [5], 521–526. www.preeclampsia.org/pdf/saftlas_wallis%5B2%5D.pdf). The medical website UptoDate does not recommend routine calcium supplementation to prevent preeclampsia, but it does acknowledge that supplementation may be beneficial for women who eat a low calcium diet (August, P. [2012]. Preeclampsia: prevention. In: Lockwood, C. J. [Ed.]. UpToDate. Waltham, MA: Wolters Kluwer. www.uptodate.com/contents/preeclampsia-prevention).

152. Bailey, R. L., et al., Estimation of total usual calcium and vitamin D intakes in the United States.

153. CVS prenatal vitamins contain 300 mg of calcium, Nature Made prenatal vitamins contain 250 mg, One-a-Day prenatal vitamins contain 300 mg, and Nature's Bounty prenatal vitamins contain 200 mg (CVS.com. [n.d.]. www.cvs.com).

154. Del Valle, H. B., et al., Dietary reference intakes for calcium and vitamin D.

155. Benefit score is 50% x 24% x 8.15%. Probability: as discussed in the main text, half of American women of childbearing age have a dietary intake of less than 900 mg per day, supplements reduce the risk of preterm birth by 24%, according to the review from 2011 (Hofmeyr, G. J., et al., Calcium supplementation during pregnancy for preventing hypertensive disorders and related problems), and the baseline incidence of low birth weight in the population as of 2010 was 8.15%, according to the CDC (www.cdc.gov/nchs/data/nvsr/nvsr61/nvsr61_01.pdf) x 100 impact: statistically detectable impairment x 1 certainty: well proven = 1.0.

156. Moody, E. (2013, June 18). Secrets of a preschool admissions coach. Forbes.com. www.forbes.com/sites/learnvest/2013/06/18/secrets-of-a-preschool-admissions-coach/.

6

OUT OF CONTROL

Unavoidable Risks

J mentioned upfront that I'd focus on factors you could control. If you're reading this book, you're presumably pregnant, so you can hardly change your age or pre-pregnancy weight, for example. On the other hand, I'd be remiss not to address a few critical factors that will enable us to put the importance of the controllable risks in perspective. If you prefer not to feel momentarily helpless, feel free to skip this chapter.

Fluorescent Milk: Dioxins

It was a classic example of human ingenuity gone wrong. Manufacturers needed to keep electrical equipment cool, and a class of compounds called polychlorinated biphenyls, or PCBs, did the trick perfectly. These chemicals were soon filling fluorescent light fittings and cooling transformers and capacitors (ubiquitous electrical components that power up our daily life).

Unfortunately, PCBs had one problematic property: they didn't break down easily. And as we began relegating our old fluorescent lights and transformers and capacitors to the junk heap, the PCBs began to leach out. The United States Congress caught on to the problem and banned their production in 1979, but PCBs had already spread throughout the environment and begun accumulating in the air and water supply. By now, PCBs can be found all over the world, including Antarctica.[1] And just like mercury, they've started accumulating in the food chain. According to the FDA, more than 95 percent of your exposure comes from eating animal fat.[2]

Who sits at the very top of the food chain, receiving the biggest dose? Our babies, of course: "The baby, before birth and when breast-fed, is the highest animal in the food chain, consuming the most concentrated amount of PCBs in his/her daily fat intake."[3] So while it may be an exaggeration to say your milk is fluorescent, breast milk does in fact contain chemicals that originally leached out of fluorescent lights, among other sources.

It turns out PCBs are just one example of a broader class of similar, related chemicals that also includes dioxins and furans (released into the environment from burning trash and fossil fuels) and certain flame retardants.[4] All these chemicals, often collectively called *dioxins*, have now been internationally banned through a global treaty called the Stockholm Convention on Persistent Organic Pollutants, which has also banned a number of other harmful chemicals that persist in the environment.[5] But this treaty came too late to prevent widespread pollution.

There's little doubt that dioxins are harmful to human health. Remember the disturbing pictures of Ukrainian President Victor Yushchenko's pockmarked face after he was poisoned in 2004? The poison in question was a potent dose of a dioxin called TCDD. No surprise, then, that dioxins in sufficient doses would also be harmful to a developing fetus. For example, in a study of pregnant women who had eaten fish from Lake Michigan contaminated with PCBs, investigators found that "PCB exposure predicted lower birth weight and smaller head circumference."[6] Even more worryingly, when the same children were tested again at age eleven, "the IQ scores of the most highly exposed group averaged 6.2 points lower than those of the other four groups."[7] Similarly, a 2010 study found that children with the highest concentrations of a type of dioxin in their umbilical cord blood at birth scored 5.5 to 8 points lower on IQ tests at age four.[8] And the CDC references a recent study suggesting that PCBs may cause certain birth defects.[9, 10]

So dioxins are nasty chemicals that we want to avoid in high doses, and if you happen to have a predilection for Lake Michigan sport fish, it's probably best to steer clear from now on. But even exposure to the background levels of dioxins drifting pervasively around the planet may be problematic. A pair of scientists studied a group of 930 ordinary pregnant women in North Carolina with no known exposure to any particular chemicals and found negative effects in the 3 to 5 percent of children who happened to have the highest exposure levels in utero.[11] And according to the Environmental Protection Agency, a series of Dutch studies have found that "pre- and early postnatal exposures may impact developmental milestones at levels at or near current average human background exposures."[12] So we all may be at risk.

The good news is that the damage done by these chemicals may not be permanent. Some studies suggest the effects disappear over time,[13] and the UK Committee on the Toxicity of Chemicals (COT) concluded it isn't possible yet to determine whether the cognitive changes in children persist longer term.[14] The jury is still out.

But if these chemicals have even a chance of doing permanent damage, shouldn't you at least try to avoid ingesting any more dioxins now that you're pregnant? I hate to be defeatist, but there's no point. These compounds have been accumulating in your body over a lifetime, and "there are no safe and effective treatments to rid dioxins now in humans. Dioxins metabolize slowly over years."[15] Little did you know that that bit of extra flab on your thighs not only makes you self-conscious but is full of poisonous electrical coolant, too.[16]

If you're considering having more children and want to make a concerted attempt to reduce your dioxin exposure, it's technically possible to do so. If you eat like a typical American, though, it'll require some drastic changes in your diet. Fish are frequently portrayed as the villains, but only freshwater (e.g., lake) and farm-raised fish contain lots of these chemicals; simply trimming off the fat and skin may reduce the total amount of dioxins by ~80 percent.[17] In truth, according to a recent estimate of dioxin levels in foods, dioxin levels are also high in meat and dairy products (see chart).[18]

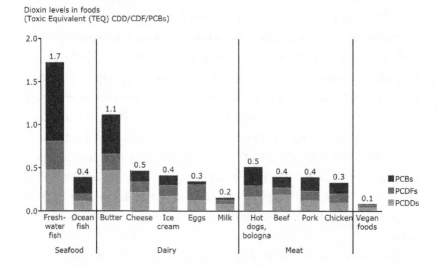

Dioxin levels in foods
(Toxic Equivalent (TEQ) CDD/CDF/PCBs)

If you want to avoid dioxins, your best bet is to become a vegan, or at least a wild-fish-itarian. Just don't bother moving to Antarctica.

Threat level for dioxins: Medium[19]

The American Epidemic: Obesity

Of all the diverse diets in the world, the Western diet is the only one that does not appear to be conducive to human health. Approximately one-third of women of childbearing age in the United States are obese, defined as a Body Mass Index (BMI) ≥ 30.[20] We've already discussed weight gain during pregnancy and concluded it's nothing to worry obsessively about. But the weight at which you start your pregnancy *is* something to worry about. According to the American College of Obstetricians and Gynecologists, "during pregnancy, obese women are at increased risk for several adverse perinatal outcomes," including higher rates of miscarriage and stillbirth.[21]

There's no reason to belabor the point. We all know it's better for our own health to maintain a sensible weight, so it shouldn't be surprising that it's better for our future offspring as well. And who knows—perhaps this knowledge will provide the motivational tipping point you require to get to the gym in advance of baby number two.

Threat level for BMI ≥ 30: Very high[22]

Fountain of Youth: Age

The legendary Fountain of Youth, long sought by the fearless explorers of yore, has finally been discovered. Its location? Somewhere hidden deep in the hills of Hollywood.

We all know celebrities have their tricks for preserving the appearance of perpetual youth, from airbrushing to sadistic personal trainers to high-end plastic surgery. But they're also curiously untethered from the supposedly ruthless biological clock. Here are the ages at which various cultural icons have recently given birth: Jennifer Connelly at forty; Tina Fey, Nicole Kidman, Salma Hayek, Uma Thurman, and Julianne Moore all at forty-one; Mariah Carey, Meryl Streep, and Celine Dion all at forty-two; Marcia Cross at forty-four; Jane Seymour at forty-five; Kelly Preston and Halle Berry both at forty-seven; Geena Davis at forty-six and again at forty-eight, and Laura Linney at age forty-nine.[23, 24]

The highly visible nature of these success stories can give us the impression that giving birth to a healthy child at age forty-plus is imminently doable as long as one has enough money (or some magic water) to throw at the problem. Of course, what we don't see are the backstories of how these stars achieved these feats of biological implausibility (in many cases, probably egg donation)[25] or, equally important, the much longer list of celebrity women who hoped to have children and never succeeded.[26]

Perhaps after this pregnancy you'll have a subsequent child, and there will be a bit of leeway in the decision (or negotiation!) about when to try—right away, or in a year or two or three? Getting pregnant again probably won't be an issue. Once you've had a first child, it's dramatically easier to conceive a second one. If you're between ages thirty-five and thirty-nine, you have only a 4 percent chance of being infertile, and a 7 percent chance between ages forty and forty-four.[27] (The numbers are 23 percent and 27 percent, respectively, for women trying for their first child at the same age).[28] The real issue is carrying the baby to term. This chart shows the percentage of pregnancies that won't result in a live birth. This is primarily due to miscarriage but also includes ectopic pregnancies and stillbirth. These figures aren't based on data from the US because only four states report miscarriages (losses under 20 weeks) to the CDC.[29] Instead, the best data source is from the little Nordic country of Denmark, where ever since 1977, all diagnoses for all patients admitted to all hospitals in the country have been recorded in a single central database.[30] The chart shows the results of all 1.2 million Danish pregnancies recorded over a fifteen-year period.[31]

Percentage of pregnancies with no live birth

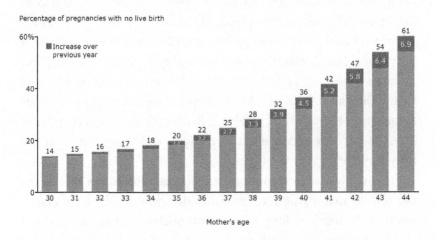

Mother's age

You can see why most official bodies consider age thirty-five to be a fertility tipping point of sorts. If you delay by a year from age thirty-five to thirty-six, you increase the risk of your pregnancy going wrong by about 2 percentage points, while delaying from forty to forty-one raises the risk by approximately 5 percentage points.

What about the miracles of Assisted Reproductive Technology? In vitro fertilization, or IVF, might seem like the obvious solution for defeating the biological clock if you can afford it. Unfortunately, the underlying issue is egg quality, and so the failure rate of IVF for women using their own eggs shows the same unrelenting curve as age increases (data courtesy of the CDC):[32]

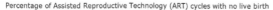

Percentage of Assisted Reproductive Technology (ART) cycles with no live birth

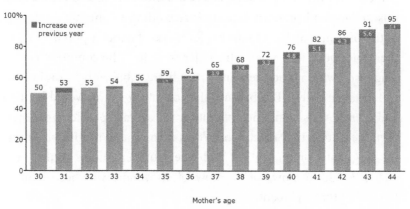

Mother's age

I have no desire to compound the angst you may already be feeling about your biological clock ticking—I'll leave it to your mother to fulfill her role of pestering you about the timing of grandchildren. But I would like to combat simple misinformation. According to a random survey of 500 American women, only 25 percent were aware that fertility begins to decline substantially at age thirty-five, with the majority assuming the decline doesn't begin until forty.[33]

In German, they have a word for the feeling of your biological clock ticking—*Torschlusspanik*, or literally "gate-closing panic." I don't think we need any more *Torschlusspanik* at the moment. But a little more *Torschlusswissen* (knowledge) wouldn't do us any harm.

Threat level for delaying pregnancy by a year: Very high[34]

The Symptomless Disease: Hypothyroidism

In all my reading about thyroids and goiters and cretinism for the iodine section of this book, I stumbled upon a strange fact: approximately two percent of American women appear to suffer from a medical condition that has no outward signs or symptoms.[35] This seems absurd. How can something be considered a medical condition if there are no effects? Because there may be subtle effects during pregnancy. According to one study, having a mildly underactive thyroid, a condition called sub-clinical hypothyroidism, may increase a woman's likelihood of both miscarriage and preterm delivery.[36] According to another study, hypothyroidism may be responsible for a loss of about 4 points of IQ in the babies born to women who suffer from it.[37] The condition can be diagnosed with a blood test and is easily treatable with an oral medication taken daily.[38] But because the cost of screening would be high and thyroid tests would be difficult for the average physician to interpret, the Endocrine Society doesn't yet recommend routine screening for pregnant women, until if and when further studies confirm the effects.[39, 40] So for now, we're simply left to wonder whether we might fall within that 2 percent.

Threat level for hypothyroidism: Low[41]

Mere Mortals: Accidental Death

Pregnancy is a time to celebrate the start of new life, so it feels morbid to dwell on death. I'll therefore keep this section brief. This chart shows the most common causes of accidental death for women ages twenty-five to thirty-four:[42]

Number of accidental deaths by cause
(women age 25–34, 2010)

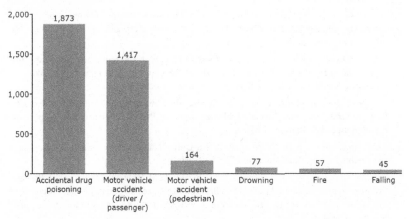

We've already covered driving, and the other categories are small enough to be irrelevant. But accidental poisoning by drugs looks worrisome at the very top of the list. Unfortunately, it's hard to delve into this topic any further, as the majority of deaths in this category are from "exposure to other and unspecified drugs, medicaments, and biological substances"—which isn't very specific. There's also no breakdown based on whether the drugs were being used for legitimate or illegitimate purposes. Are these women drug addicts, absent-minded professors who took the wrong dose by mistake, or victims of doctors' illegible handwriting? It's difficult to know. All that can be said here is that if you're taking medications, be sure to check the doses on your prescriptions carefully.

Threat level from accidental drug poisoning: Medium[43]

Notes

1. Ritter, L., Solomon, K. R., Forget, J., Stemeroff, M., & O'Leary, C. (1995, December). A review of selected persistent organic pollutants: DDT, aldrin, dieldrin, endrin, chlordane, heptachlor, hexachlorobenzene, mirex, toxaphene, polychlorinated biphenyls, dioxins and furans. Prepared for the International Programme on Chemical Safety (IPCS) within the framework of the Inter-Organization Programme for the Sound Management of Chemicals (IOMC). http://www.who.int/ipcs/assessment/en/pcs_95_39_2004_05_13.pdf.

2. Interagency Working Group on Dioxin. (2006). Questions and answers about dioxins. US Food and Drug Administration and the Center for Food Safety and Nutrition.

http://www.nj.gov/dep/passaicdocs/docs/2005DirectiveSupportingDocs/FDAQuestions-AnswersAboutDioxins.pdf.

3. Koppe, J. G. (1995). Nutrition and breast-feeding. *European Journal of Obstetrics & Gynecology and Reproductive Biology, 61* (1), 73–78. www.sciencedirect.com/science/article/pii/002822439502156M.

4. Dioxins: FDA strategy for monitoring, method development, and reducing human exposure. (Last updated 2017, December 12). US Food and Drug Administration. www.fda.gov/food/foodborneillnesscontaminants/chemicalcontaminants/ucm077432.htm.

   The most harmful dioxins are polychlorinated dibenzodioxins, or PCDDs; the most harmful furans are polychlorinated dibenzofurans, or PCDFs. Flame retardants: polybrominated diphenyl ethers, or PBDEs.

5. Stockholm Convention. (n.d.). What are POPs? United Nations Environment Programme. http://chm.pops.int/TheConvention/ThePOPs/tabid/673/Default.aspx.

6. Fein, G. G., Jacobson, J. L., Jacobson, S. W., Schwartz, P. M., & Dowler, J. K. (1984). Prenatal exposure to polychlorinated biphenyls: effects on birth size and gestational age. *The Journal of Pediatrics, 105* (2), 315–320. http://www.sciencedirect.com/science/article/pii/S0022347684801390.

7. Jacobson, J. L., & Jacobson, S. W. (1996). Intellectual impairment in children exposed to polychlorinated biphenyls in utero. *New England Journal of Medicine, 335* (11), 783–789. http://www.nchh.org/Portals/0/Contents/Article0357.pdf.

8. Herbstman, J. B., Sjödin, A., Kurzon, M., Lederman, S. A., Jones, R. S., Rauh, V., Needham, L. L., Tang, D., Niedzwiecki, M., Wang, R. Y., & Perera, F. (2010). Prenatal exposure to PBDEs and neurodevelopment. *Environmental Health Perspectives, 118* (5), 712–719. www.ncbi.nlm.nih.gov/pmc/articles/PMC2866690/.

9. Agency for Toxic Substances and Disease Registry (ATSDR). (2000). Toxicological profile for polychlorinated biphenyls (PCBs). Atlanta, GA: US Department of Health and Human Services, Public Health Service. www.atsdr.cdc.gov/ToxProfiles/tp.asp?id=142&tid=26.

10. Brucker-Davis, F., Wagner-Mahler, K., Delattre, I., Ducot, B., Ferrari, P., Bongain, A., Kurzenne, J. Y., Mas, J. C., & Fénichel, P. (2008). Cryptorchidism at birth in Nice area (France) is associated with higher prenatal exposure to PCBs and DDE, as assessed by colostrum concentrations. *Human Reproduction, 23* (8), 1708–1718. http://humrep.oxford-journals.org/content/23/8/1708.full.

11. Jacobson, J. L., & Jacobson, S. W. (1996). Dose-response in perinatal exposure to polychlorinated biphenyls (PCBs): the Michigan and North Carolina cohort studies. *Toxicology and Industrial Health, 12* (3–4), 435–445. http://tih.sagepub.com/content/12/3-4/435.short.

12. US Environmental Protection Agency (US EPA). (2004). Exposure and human health reassessment of 2,3,7,8-tetrachlorodibenzo-p-dioxin and related compounds. National Academy of Sciences Review Draft. National Center for Environmental Assessment, Office of Research and Development. Washington, DC. https://cfpub.epa.gov/ncea/risk/record isplay.cfm?deid=87843.

13. Koopman-Esseboom, C. (1995). Effects of perinatal exposure to PCBs and dioxins on early human development. Erasmus MC: University Medical Center Rotterdam. http://repub.eur.nl/res/pub/22013/951004_KOOPMAN-ESSEBOOM,%20Corine.pdf.

14. Grigg, J. (2004). Environmental toxins; their impact on children's health. *Archives of Disease in Childhood, 89* (3), 244–250. http://adc.bmj.com/content/89/3/244.full.

15. Questions and Answers about Dioxins (n.d.). US Environmental Protection Agency. https://semspub.epa.gov/work/06/9345339.pdf.

16 . In case you were wondering about breastfeeding, a study in the Netherlands looking at breast milk concluded that short-term dietary changes don't make any difference there either: "short-term dietary measures will not reduce dioxin concentrations in human milk. A lowering of intake of these chemicals must take place years before the mother becomes pregnant." (Koppe, J. G. [1995]. Nutrition and breast-feeding. *European Journal of Obstetrics & Gynecology and Reproductive Biology, 61* [1], 73–78. www.sciencedirect. com/science/article/pii/002822439502156M.)

17. Skea, J. C., Simonin, H. A., Harris, E. J., Jackling, S., Spagnoli, J. J., Symula, J., & Colquhoun, J. R. (1979). Reducing levels of Mirex, Aroclor 1254, and DDE by trimming and cooking Lake Ontario brown trout (*Salmo trutta Linnaeus*) and smallmouth bass (*Micropterus dolomieui Lacepede*). *Journal of Great Lakes Research, 5* (2), 153–159. www.sciencedirect.com/ science/article/pii/S0380133079721411.

18. Schecter, A., Cramer, P., Boggess, K., Stanley, J., Päpke, O., Olson, J., Silver, A., & Schmitz, M. (2001). Intake of dioxins and related compounds from food in the US population. *Journal of Toxicology and Environmental Health Part A, 63* (1), 1–18. www.dioxinnz.com/ pdf-Reports/dioxininfood.pdf.

In 1998, the World Health Organization developed Toxic Equivalency Factors to enable estimates of exposure to dioxins and related compounds to be combined to calculate a total exposure, so the data are presented as "Toxicity Equivalents." (Dioxin analysis results/exposure estimates. [2007, November]. US Food and Drug Administration. www. fda.gov/food/foodborneillnesscontaminants/chemicalcontaminants/ucm077444.htm.)

19. Threat score is 4% (probability, based on the study of women in North Carolina with no known exposure to any particular chemicals which found negative effects in the 3–5% of children who happened to have the highest prenatal exposure levels) x 100 (impact: statistically detectable impairment) x 1 (certainty: well proven) = 4.

20. In 2007–2010, 30.4% of American women 20–34 years old and 37.1% of women 35–44 had a BMI of 30 or more. Since plenty of people don't know their BMI off the top of their heads, here are the weights that represent a BMI of 30 at varying heights, according to the CDC calculator (Adult BMI calculator. [2014, October 21]. Centers for Disease Control and Prevention. www.cdc.gov/healthyweight/assessing/bmi/adult_bmi/english_bmi_calculator/bmi_calculator.html): 4'10" = 144 lbs; 5'0" = 154 lbs; 5'2" = 164 lbs; 5'4" = 175 lbs; 5'6" = 186 lbs; 5'8" = 197 lbs; 5'10" = 209 lbs; 6'0" = 221 lbs.

21. For women with a BMI ≥ 30, the odds ratio for fetal death has been estimated as 1.4 according to a study of 287,000 pregnancies in the UK (Sebire, N. J., Jolly, M., Harris, J. P., Wadsworth, J., Joffe, M., Beard, R. W., Regan, L., & Robinson, S. [2001]. Maternal obesity and pregnancy outcome: a study of 287,213 pregnancies in London. *International Journal of Obesity & Related Metabolic Disorders, 25* [8]. www.ncbi.nlm.nih.gov/ pubmed/11477502), 2.0 according to a study of ~168,000 women in Sweden published in 1998 (Cnattingius, S., Bergström, R., Lipworth, L., & Kramer, M. S. [1998]. Prepregnancy weight and the risk of adverse pregnancy outcomes. *New England Journal of Medicine, 338* (3), 147–152. http://www.nejm.org/doi/full/10.1056/NEJM199801153380302), and 1.79 according to a study of 800,000 women in Sweden published in 2004 (Cedergren, M. I. [2004]. Maternal morbid obesity and the risk of adverse pregnancy outcome. *Obstetrics & Gynecology, 103* (2), 219–224. http://bigbirthas.co.uk/download/studies/ Maternal_Morbid_Obesity_and_the_Risk_of_Adverse.2.pdf), which is an average of 1.73. The probability of stillbirth is ~0.62% (based on 2004 US data as cited in the introduction, there were 6,390,000 pregnancies, 1,222,000 elective abortions, and 1,030,345 miscarriages, which means 4,137,655 later pregnancies, of which 25,655 resulted in fetal deaths). So applying the appropriate conversion formula (Higgins, J. P. T., & Green, S. [eds.]. [2011, March]. Computing absolute risk reduction or NNT from an odds

ratio [OR]. *Cochrane Handbook for Systematic Reviews of Interventions* 12.5.4.3. http://handbook.cochrane.org/chapter_12/12_5_4_3_computing_absolute_risk_reduction_or_nnt_from_an_odds.htm), this equates to an absolute increase in stillbirth of 0.45% attributable to a BMI ≥ 30.

22. Threat score is 0.45% (probability, based on an absolute increase in stillbirth of 0.45% as calculated in the previous footnote) x 100,000 (impact: death) x 1 (certainty: well proven) = 450.

23. Clements, E. (2013, April 10). Older celebrity moms: Halle Berry and other stars who've had children after 40. HuffingtonPost.com. www.huffingtonpost.com/2013/04/10/older-celebrity-moms-halle-berry_n_3055764.html.

24. (2014, January 1). Laura Linney's secret pregnancy revealed. ABCNews.com. http://abcnews.go.com/GMA/video/laura-linney-interview-secret-pregnancy-revealed-21607866.

25. "Fertility experts point to Hollywood's dirty little pregnancy secret: egg donation . . . 'A pregnant actress in her forties gets a page in a magazine,' says Dr. Ric Porter, director of IVF Australia. 'But if those same magazines printed all the stories of all the women who couldn't get pregnant, the magazines would be the size of the yellow pages. These celebrity 'miracle pregnancies' give women ridiculous expectations. I'm yet to see a patient who had viable eggs in her mid-forties. Even with IVF, we've never had a pregnancy after age 45.'" (Freedman, M. [2007, May 31]. Another day, another 47-year-old celebrity pregnant with twins. Mamamia.com. www.mamamia.com.au/entertainment/another-day-another-47-year-old-celebrity-pregnant-with-twins/.)

26. Ingall, M. (2006, December 1). Miraculous moms: open talk on infertility. Forward.com. http://forward.com/articles/9536/miraculous-moms-open-talk-on-infertility/.

27. A couple is classified as "infertile," according to the CDC, if they have not used contraception and not become pregnant for twelve months or more. (Infertility FAQs: what is infertility? [Last updated 2017, March 30]. Centers for Disease Control and Prevention. https://www.cdc.gov/reproductivehealth/infertility/index.htm).

28. Chandra, A., Martinez, G. M., Mosher, W. D., Abma, J. C., & Jones, J. (2005). Fertility, family planning, and reproductive health of US women: data from the 2002 National Survey of Family Growth. *Vital and Health Statistics, Series 23*, (25), 1–160. www.cdc.gov/nchs/data/series/sr_23/sr23_025.pdf.

29. MacDorman, M. F., Kirmeyer, S. E., & Wilson, E. C. (2012). Fetal and perinatal mortality, United States, 2006. *National Vital Statistics Reports, 60* (8), 1–22. www.cdc.gov/nchs/data/nvsr/nvsr60/nvsr60_08.pdf.

30. Andersen, A. M. N., Wohlfahrt, J., Christens, P., Olsen, J., & Melbye, M. (2000). Maternal age and fetal loss: population based register linkage study. *British Medical Journal, 320* (7251), 1708–1712. www.ncbi.nlm.nih.gov/pmc/articles/PMC27416/.

31. This study also provided data on the number of induced abortions but didn't provide the reason for the abortion. If prenatal screening for Down syndrome caused a significant number of women to choose to abort despite wanting a healthy child, this would distort the statistics. Fortunately, that's not the case: there were 285,022 induced abortions in Denmark over the fifteen-year period described, or 19,000 per year. For one example year during that period, thirty-one cases of Down syndrome were diagnosed prenatally (Mikkelsen, M., Fischer, G., Hansen, J., Pilgaard, B., & Nielsen, J. [1983]. The impact of legal termination of pregnancy and of prenatal diagnosis on the birth prevalence of Down syndrome in Denmark. *Annals of Human Genetics, 47* [2], 123–131. http://onlinelibrary.wiley.com/doi/10.1111/j.1469-1809.1983.tb00979.x/abstract), so the proportion is minimal. In the vast majority of studies, including this one, data on the effects of maternal age are reported by five-year age brackets–the 30–34 bracket, the 35–39 bracket, etc.

However, because very few women are making a decision about whether to have a child now or in five years' time, I've plotted a curve to fit the available data points so we can look at the effect of delaying conception by even a single year.

32. National Center for Chronic Disease Prevention and Health Promotion, Division of Reproductive Health. Section 4—ART cycles using donor eggs. (2012, December). *2010 Assisted Reproductive Technologies National Summary and Fertility Clinics Report.* Centers for Disease Control and Prevention, Atlanta, GA. https://www.cdc.gov/art/ART2010/PDFs/ART_2010_National_Summary_Report.pdf.

33. National survey results reveal startling lack of awareness of infertility even as numbers climb to 7.3 million. (2005, October 27). RESOLVE: The National Infertility Association. http://www.businesswire.com/news/home/20051027005541/en/National-Survey-Results-Reveal-Startling-Lack-Awareness.

34. Threat score for waiting from age 25 to 26 is .00495 (probability of miscarriage) x 100,000 (impact: death) x 1 (certainty: well proven) = 495.

   Threat score for waiting from age 30 to 31 is .00775 (probability of miscarriage) x 100,000 (impact: death) x 1 (certainty: well proven) = 775. Threat score for waiting from age 35 to 36 is .02198 (probability of miscarriage) x 100,000 (impact: death) x 1 (certainty: well proven) = 2,198.

35. Hypothyroidism: a booklet for patients and their families. (2013). American Thyroid Association. https://www.thyroid.org/wp-content/uploads/patients/brochures/Hypothyroidism_web_booklet.pdf.

36. Negro, R., Formoso, G., Mangieri, T., Pezzarossa, A., Dazzi, D., & Hassan, H. (2006). Levothyroxine treatment in euthyroid pregnant women with autoimmune thyroid disease: effects on obstetrical complications. *The Journal of Clinical Endocrinology & Metabolism, 91* (7), 2587–2591. http://jcem.endojournals.org/content/91/7/2587.full.

37. Haddow, J. E., Palomaki, G. E., Allan, W. C., Williams, J. R., Knight, G. J., Gagnon, J., O'Heir, C., Mitchell, M. L., Hermos, R. J., Waisbren, S. E., Faix, J. D., & Klein, R. Z. (1999). Maternal thyroid deficiency during pregnancy and subsequent neuropsychological development of the child. *New England Journal of Medicine, 341* (8), 549–555. www.gyncph.dk/procedur/ref/obstet/iq_og_hypothyreose.pdf.

38. American Thyroid Association, Hypothyroidism: a booklet for patients and their families.

39. Chen, I. (2009, March 13). Pregnancy and the thyroid. NYTimes.com. www.nytimes.com/ref/health/healthguide/esn-hypothyroidism-expert.html?pagewanted=all.

40. De Groot, L., Abalovich, M., Alexander, E. K., Amino, N., Barbour, L., Cobin, R. H., Eastman, C. J., Lazarus, J. H., Luton, D., Mandel, S. J., Mestman, J., Rovet, J., & Sullivan, S. (2012). Management of thyroid dysfunction during pregnancy and postpartum: an endocrine society clinical practice guideline. *The Journal of Clinical Endocrinology & Metabolism, 97* (8), 2543–2565. https://academic.oup.com/jcem/article/97/8/2543/2823170/Management-of-Thyroid-Dysfunction-during-Pregnancy.

41. Threat score is 2% (probability of having an underactive thyroid, as referenced in the main text) x 100 (impact: statistically detectable impairment—loss of IQ) x 0.1 (certainty: preliminary) = 0.2.

42. Centers for Disease Control and Prevention. (n.d.). CDC Wonder: About compressed mortality, 1999–2012. http://wonder.cdc.gov/cmf-icd10.html.

43. Threat score: 1,873/20,431,857 (probability, since there were 1,873 deaths out of a total of 20,431,857 pregnancies in the US in 2010) x 100,000 (impact: death) x 1 (certainty) = 9.2.

7

CONCLUSIONS

"Stop! Don't eat that!!" My fork clattered down to my plate. "That's parmesan cheese, isn't it?"

I looked down at the seemingly innocuous white powder on top of my pasta. "Yes?"

"But parmesan is unpasteurized! We found out when my wife was pregnant last year. You really shouldn't eat that." Under the censorious gaze of my colleague, I dumped my spaghetti into the trash, cursing the fact that yet another food was off-limits.

According to the media, our colleagues, and our friends, threats to pregnant women lurk everywhere. But all of this dwelling on the negative may actually be having a perverse effect, since stress itself is harmful in pregnancy, as we saw in Chapter 4. The intent of this book has been to cast aside the scary wives' tales, turning instead to insights based on scientific inquiry and data. I hope most of what you've read has made you feel more relaxed about your pregnancy. Ultimately, my research has convinced me that most pregnancies turn out fine. And when something goes wrong, there's typically very little anyone could have done to prevent it based on the current state of knowledge. But if you are going to worry or change your behavior, you might as well channel your energy in the most productive directions. And no more women should have to experience the unnecessary stress caused by the disapproving waiter or the parmesan police.

The next chart summarizes scores for the various topics we've covered:

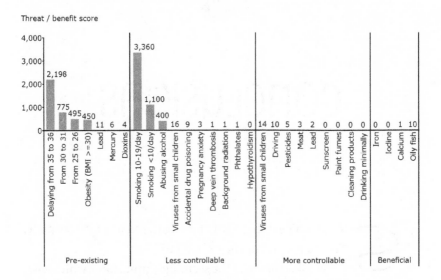

Threat / benefit score

Note: Where factors appear twice, the threat has been split according to how much it is controllable vs. uncontrollable, (e.g., taking calcium supplements can reduce the impact of a high lead burden by 15 percent, so 15 percent of the lead score is controllable, while 85 percent is preexisting.)

Smoking, having children at a later age, and abusing alcohol are the major factors influencing the outcome of pregnancy. These three outweigh all the other factors by a huge order of magnitude. Unfortunately, all three are likely to be out of your direct control. Once you're pregnant, you can't influence your age, and if you're reading a book like this but continuing to drink and smoke while pregnant, you arguably must be having difficulties stopping. So let's zoom in on just the right-hand side, the more controllable factors.

Threat / benefit score

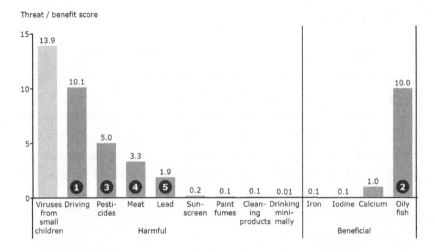

These are the scores I've used to compile the Top Five list in the introduction, and I'll summarize each in turn.

0. Viruses from Small Children

This threat applies only to those who already have children (or who spend time with small children). Although most of us have never heard of cytomegalovirus (CMV) or parvovirus B19, both can cause miscarriage if caught for the first time during pregnancy. If you want to avoid these viruses, ask your GP for blood tests to find out if you're already immune. If you're not, you'll have to watch out for baby drool and wash your hands frequently once your child starts playing with other small children.

1. Driving

While driving is not a risk specific to pregnancy, a major car crash could kill both you and your baby, and even a minor crash could cause injury to a vulnerable fetus. The truth is that driving a car is a fundamentally dangerous activity. So while you probably can't eliminate driving from your life if you live outside a major metropolis, you should theoretically cut down on discretionary trips and drive cautiously if you want to be rationally risk-averse during pregnancy.

2. Oily Fish

Conventional wisdom tells us to limit our fish consumption while pregnant to avoid poisoning our baby with mercury. This advice is completely backward. There's very little we can do about our current accumulation of mercury, and there are significant benefits from eating oily fish daily. Furthermore, the taboo about sushi is completely unfounded: raw fish poses no greater risk to a fetus than most other foods. So while pregnant, eat lots of fish; eat salmon and mackerel in particular.

3. Pesticides

In the United States, we continue to liberally spray our produce with organophosphate pesticides, despite the fact that these chemicals have been proven to reduce IQ in children and have been banned from household use. If you want to avoid exposure during pregnancy, the only sure way is to go organic. Unfortunately, organic produce can be costly. For those on a budget, focus on the worst offenders: green beans and bell peppers.

4. Heat Your Meat

Don't eat a sandwich from the deli (or any other kind of meat, for that matter) without nuking it or thoroughly cooking it first. Every single one of the dangerous pathogens in pregnancy, including, most importantly, *Listeria* and *Toxoplasma gondii*, are found primarily in infected meat.

5. Lead

Lead has long been known to be a potent neurotoxin that lowers the IQ of children exposed in the womb and may even cause miscarriage. Unfortunately, lead is a pervasive environmental contaminant, despite the fact that levels have gradually declined since it was banned from gasoline in 1973. While only 1 in 300 women in the United States today has worryingly high levels, you may not want to take the risk of being one of them. Fortunately, the solution is simple: at your next prenatal checkup, ask your doctor to have your blood tested for lead. If your lead levels are high, calcium supplements could help.

I hope this book, the result of years of dogged research, has helped you have a relaxed and informed pregnancy. For the record, I freely acknowledge that the scores are open to discussion. Let the discussion begin! The result can only be a better-informed population of pregnant women.

In the meantime, please accept my best wishes for a happy, healthy, and successful pregnancy.

EPILOGUE

In Defense of Flip-Flopping

*J*n Woody Allen's comedic film *Sleeper*, the owner of a health food store is cryogenically frozen and awakens 200 years in the future to discover that much has changed during his slumber. Here's a conversation between two of the scientists observing him:

Woman: "This morning for breakfast he requested something called wheat germ, organic honey, and tiger's milk."

Man: "Oh yes, those are the charmed substances that some years ago were thought to contain life-preserving properties."

Woman: "You mean there was no deep fat? No steak or cream pies or hot fudge?"

Man: "Those were thought to be unhealthy . . . precisely the opposite of what we now know to be true."[1]

Although this dialogue was designed to be patently absurd, dramatic reversals of scientific opinion are not without precedent. For example, the theory of plate tectonics was widely rejected before gaining ultimate acceptance.[2] And we've all lived through the confusing reversals of messages about which foods to eat (fat is bad; oh no, actually, certain types of fats are good).

Furthermore, just because a study has been published in a respected academic journal doesn't mean its conclusions are foolproof. A Stanford University epidemiologist recently caused a stir when he published a paper claiming that "most published research findings are probably false," based on a number of factors, including the bias of journals toward publishing claims to have found something new.[3, 4] So while this book summarizes the current state of knowledge about pregnancy, that knowledge will almost certainly continue to evolve.

Unfortunately, as a society, we're not very forgiving of changes in scientific opinion. Politicians like John Kerry may get skewered for changing positions based on seemingly political considerations. But even academics come under fire for changing their minds in light of further evidence. For example, in a debate about childhood sleep, "Sears and Ferber [two experts originally on opposite sides] have moved closer to the middle, to the position that where a child sleeps is not nearly as important as interactions during the transition to and from sleep. However, this has been perceived by the public as experts not being trustworthy because they change their minds and flip positions."[5]

I'd therefore like to proactively reserve the right to "flip-flop" in the future—that is, to publish subsequent editions of this book with different conclusions or recommendations to the ones put forward here. One of the most important qualities in a rational thinker is a willingness to change opinion based on gaining access to further contradictory evidence. But plenty of disturbing studies show that humans have an insidious tendency to value evidence that supports and validates their initial hypotheses and to discount or discard any contradictory evidence (as described, for example, in the excellent book *Thinking, Fast and Slow*[6]). To avoid falling into that trap, I'm committed to never becoming wedded to a conclusion I've previously expressed. I hope that by publishing this book, I'm beginning a dialogue, and I would love to hear from anyone who has a conclusion different from mine and the facts to back it up.

Notes

1. Allen, W. (Director). (2000). Sleeper [motion picture]. United States: MGM Home Entertainment Incorporated.

2. Unfortunately, such reversals of prevailing opinion tend to happen at a glacial pace. The geophysicist who first hypothesized that the world's continents used to be a single land-mass was widely discredited, and it took more than fifty years for the prevailing views of the profession to shift towards acceptance of plate tectonics (Bryson, B., & Roberts, W. [2003]. A short history of nearly everything. New York: Broadway Books).

3. (2013, October 9). Trouble at the lab. Economist.com. www.economist.com/news/briefing/21588057-scientists-think-science-self-correcting-alarming-degree-it-not-trouble.

4. Ioannidis, J. P. (2005). Why most published research findings are false. *PLoS medicine, 2* (8), e124. http://dx.plos.org/10.1371/journal.pmed.0020124.

5. Ramos, K. D., & Youngclarke, D. M. (2006). Parenting advice books about child sleep: cosleeping and crying it out. *Sleep, 29* (12), 1616–23. https://www.ncbi.nlm.nih.gov/pubmed/17252893.

6. Kahneman, D. (2011). Thinking, fast and slow. New York: Farrar, Straus & Giroux.

APPENDIX I

Methodology for Calculating Threats/Benefits

Here's a little hypothetical question. Which of the following would you prefer to endure: getting mauled by a dog, spending nine minutes onboard an aircraft doomed to crash, or giving birth to a stillborn baby? Yes, I know—it's a ghastly question with no obvious answer. But it's not one that I made up. In 2011, a court in New York was grappling with the question of how to value the comparative emotional trauma of stillbirth versus other precedents, for the purposes of awarding damages to a bereaved mother.[1]

Attempting to attach a relative or absolute value to human life or suffering feels intuitively and morally repugnant to most people. If the adage "comparing apples and oranges" ever held, surely it would in the domain of human emotional experience. Yet in practice, every day as a society we are forced to make judgments about the value of life, sometimes implicitly, sometimes explicitly. Courts award damages for suffering; insurance companies decide which medical procedures to cover; government agencies calculate the return on investment of undertaking public health projects; and individual consumers decide how much they're willing to pay for items like extra safety features in their cars. We are confronted with trade-offs whether we like it or not.

The need to make trade-offs is as true during pregnancy as it is at any other stage in our lives. We have a limited amount of time and energy available to devote to changing our behavior for the benefit of our fetus. What we need, then, is a ranked list of the most important things to worry about and the key actions we should take. In other words, we need to compare apples and oranges.

Setting out to write a book about pregnancy, it never occurred to me that I would end up attempting to tackle any thorny moral issues. I was envisioning simply doing some research. The problem is, even I was having trouble drawing conclusions from the data. Take the nuanced answer I mentioned previously, that "eating deli meat gives you a small chance of something really nasty happening, while eating pesticides on your produce gives you a high chance of something relatively minor happening." While true, this just isn't very helpful. We can't avoid asking the natural question: "So which is worse, the meat or the fruit?" To answer such a question, we need to not only estimate a likelihood that some worrying outcome will occur, but also capture the relative severity of that outcome. This will inevitably involve making some hairy subjective comparisons: How much worse is a stillbirth versus a birth defect? Versus a learning difficulty or reduction in IQ?

Fine, I thought. I may be entering the realm of subjectivity, but at least I can base my scale of "badness" on other people's collective judgments, rather than my own. I therefore turned to the US justice system, where many fine legal minds have spent time grappling with the question of how to compare various unfortunate happenings.

When courts consider cases where pregnancies have gone wrong, they may consider the financial costs, the emotional costs, or both. But damages tend to be awarded primarily based on financial costs, as these can be estimated more objectively. For example, the State of

California has attempted to estimate the lifetime costs of caring for children with various types of birth defects.[2]

Calculating the financial burden of an outcome is fine if we want to simply compare different types of birth defects with each other. The problem is that on this dimension, we can't compare stillbirth on one end of the spectrum, which results in no ongoing financial cost of care but is a devastating result, with minor learning difficulties or impaired IQ on the other end, which also have no explicit cost except perhaps lost earning potential for the child (which would be challenging to quantify, depending on whether your child was destined to become a poet or an investment banker).

More importantly, the amount of financial burden doesn't necessarily correspond with our intuition about how bad an outcome might be. If I were to tell you that your child was going to be born with cerebral palsy, I suspect the additional cost burden of caring for that child, while important, would not be the first consideration to spring to mind. It's the emotional cost, first and foremost, that we care about and want to avoid.

On the matter of emotional costs, or "hedonic damages" as they are called in legalese, the courts are unfortunately not particularly consistent, which is unsurprising, given this is a subjective area (although disappointing from the perspective of general fairness and justice in our country). First, there is no national consistency: "U.S. decisions are numerous and divergent because the birth torts [cases] are a state rather than federal matter."[3] For example, in New York State a bereaved mother was recently awarded $1 million in a stillbirth malpractice verdict; in a similar Texas case, the award was $200,000; in Louisiana, $100,000; while in Maine, local law states that hedonic damages cannot even be considered.[4] Moreover, even individual states have changed their approaches over time: "New York courts long prohibited [stillbirth malpractice] suits unless the mother was physically injured. But in its 2004 ruling, the state's Court of Appeals overruled precedent and said it was unfair to leave a devastated woman who lost a baby with no legal recourse, even if she suffered no physical harm."[5] So while there's plenty of legal literature opining on various theoretical approaches to evaluating the emotional cost of traumatic events, there is no consistent data set to turn to in practice.

But to compare my apples and oranges, I really did need a scale of some sort. I therefore decided to create my own scale to use in my calculations for this book, which looks like this:

Impact Scale

Impact	Relative magnitude
Death (miscarriage, stillbirth)	(-) 100,000
Significant impairment (including birth defects)	(-) 10,000
Minor impairment (including very low birth weight)*	(-) 1,000
Statistically-detectable impairment (including low birth weight)**	(-) 100
Statistically-detectable improvement	(+) 100
Minor improvement	(+) 1,000

*I've categorized very low birth weight (<1,500 g or 3.3 lbs) as equivalent to a minor impairment. According to one review, "Very-low-birth-weight participants had a higher incidence of chronic medical conditions . . . lower IQs and academic achievement scores and higher rates of grade repetition."[6] And according to another, "about a quarter of survivors have substantial neurological morbidity . . . Most studies of VLBW infants show continued [outcomes] such as cognitive deficits, academic underachievement, grade failures, and the need for increased remedial assistance during mid-childhood and adolescence . . . Very preterm survivors also have high rates of dysfunction in other cognitive areas, such as attention, visual processing, academic progress, and executive function . . . chronic health disorders remained higher."[7]

**I've categorized low birth weight (<2,500 g or 5.5 lbs) as equivalent to a statistically detectable impairment. According to one review, "Developmental [outcomes] for most low birth weight infants include mild problems in cognition, attention, and neuro-motor functioning . . . adverse consequences of being born low birth weight were still apparent in adolescence."[8]

In other words, according to me, having a baby die is 10 times worse than having a baby with a significant impairment, which is 10 times worse than a minor impairment, and so on. This scale feels intuitively right to me. Perhaps it doesn't feel intuitively right to you; in which case, fair enough, you're welcome to make up your own scale and calculate your own figures on that basis. (The final scores and relative rankings of the risk factors may change, depending on what you decide.)

Even with an impact scale on hand, we're not yet ready to make comparisons. Some potential threats have been observed and studied for decades; there's universal consensus that lead and mercury are harmful to our unborn babies. But other threats (like phthalates) have come to our attention far more recently, and still others (like many of the chemicals in personal care products) have yet to even be studied in humans. So here's my scale for certainty, which you should likewise feel free to adapt:

Certainty Scale

Certainty	Relative magnitude
Well proven	1
Preliminary (supported by existing studies)	1/10
Ambiguous (little studied, or supported by some studies but not others)	1/100
Unproven (biologically plausible but unsupported by studies in humans)	1/1,000

Now that we have our scales on hand, whether yours or mine, we can do the unthinkable—compare apples and oranges. For each potential factor that might influence a pregnancy, we can do research to estimate the probability that it will cause a specific outcome (good or bad), assign an impact and certainty based on the tables above, and then multiply the three together to calculate a "threat score" or "benefit score."[9] This final score doesn't inherently mean anything in and of itself; but it does provide a single, quick "back-of-the envelope" way to compare which threats are most important to worry about.[10] For use within the text, I've grouped my final scores into buckets representing "threat levels": very high >200; high 50–200; medium 1–50; low 0.1–1; and very low <0.2.

As an example, in Appendix IV, I've estimated that there are 9 fetal deaths from *E. coli* each year out of a total of 3,381,000 pregnancies. So the threat score for *E. coli* would be: 9/3,381,000 (probability of death) x 100,000 (impact: death) x 1 (certainty: well proven) = 0.27 [low].

Notes

1. Glaberson, W. (2011, August 23). After stillbirth, courts try to put a price on a mothers' anguish. NYTimes.com. www.nytimes.com/2011/08/24/nyregion/in-stillbirth-malpractice-cases-courts-try-to-put-price-on-mothers-anguish.html?pagewanted=all&_r=0.

2. Waitzman, N. J., Romano, P. S., & Scheffler, R. M. (1994). Estimates of the economic costs of birth defects. Inquiry, 188-205. https://www.researchgate.net/profile/Patrick_Romano/publication/15178269_Estimates_of_the_economic_cost_of_birth_defects/links/54a370760cf257a63604e19d/Estimates-of-the-economic-cost-of-birth-defects.pdf.

3. Stretton, D. (2005). The Birth Torts: Damages for Wrongful Birth and Wrongful Life, The Deakin Law Review, 10, 319. www.austlii.edu.au/au/journals/DeakinLRev/2005/16.html.

4. Glaberson, W. (2011, August 23). After stillbirth, courts try to put a price on a mothers' anguish. NYTimes.com. www.nytimes.com/2011/08/24/nyregion/in-stillbirth-malpractice-cases-courts-try-to-put-price-on-mothers-anguish.html?pagewanted=all&_r=0; www.mainelegislature.org/legis/statutes/24/title24sec2931.html.

5. Ibid.

6. Hack, M., Flannery, D. J., Schluchter, M., Cartar, L., Borawski, E., & Klein, N. (2002). Outcomes in young adulthood for very-low-birth-weight infants. New England Journal of Medicine, 346(3), 149-157. http://www.nejm.org/doi/full/10.1056/NEJMoa010856#t=article.

7. Saigal, S., & Doyle, L. W. 2008. An overview of mortality and sequelae of preterm birth from infancy to adulthood. The Lancet, 371(9608), 261-269.http://www.sciencedirect.com/science/article/pii/S0140673608601361.

8. Hack, M., Klein, N. K., & Taylor, H. G. (1995). Long-term developmental outcomes of low birth weight infants. The future of children, 176-196. www.jstor.org/discover/10.2307/1602514?uid=3738032&uid=2&uid=4&sid=21102905178893.

9. Where there are a variety of potential negative outcomes from a threat, the "threat score" is simply summed together for each potential outcome. For example, if toxoplasmosis can result in death or blindness and mental retardation, the final score would be the probability of death from toxoplasmosis x 10,000 x 1, plus the probability of blindness and mental retardation from toxoplasmosis x 1,000 x 1.

10. I'd like to acknowledge that there are a variety of obvious intellectual critiques of this approach. For example, there's no single point or threshold at which most threats suddenly become dangerous. Exposure to a microscopic amount of lead may have very little consequence, while a big whopping dose is clearly terrible, but it's a gradual scale. So why pick a single point on that spectrum to make a representative calculation of harm? Perhaps picking a point farther up or down the curve would yield a different number; perhaps we should be estimating the point where the maximum occurs and comparing that value, or doing some frequency-weighted calculation to take the entire curve into account. My answer to this critique is pure pragmatism—most studies evaluate a particular exposure level, so we simply don't have a detailed plot of this "curve" in most cases. And even if we did, it would be very complex to compare the shape and slope of these curves with each other in a way that would be consistent across so many different types of risk factors. I have therefore opted for simplicity and transparency over intellectual rigor in calculating "threat scores."

APP€NDiX II

Cataloguing Influences Exhaustively

There are three broad categories of factors that could influence the development of a fetus: genetics, maternal influences, and external influences. We can't change our genes (at least for now), so I haven't bothered to discuss genetics here. Maternal influences include age, physical health, mental health, and behavior (e.g., exercise, driving—specifically, behavior that doesn't result in fetal exposure to an external substance, which is covered elsewhere). With maternal factors, I've ignored preexisting medical conditions, which are the domain of the medical profession and wouldn't have relevance to a general audience. I've also focused primarily on those we can control; but I've included certain topics such as age and causes of accidental death as a basis for putting risks into context.

Third, there are external influences; the dizzying and practically infinite array of different factors that could theoretically influence the outcome of a pregnancy from the outside in (and which could potentially be avoided to some degree if they turned out to be harmful). To develop my long list of external influences to research, I used the following three statements:

Something has the potential to affect the fetus.

Then it reaches the fetus.

Then it causes a health outcome.

I used each of these three lenses to ensure I captured as many relevant factors as possible. Any one lens should theoretically be sufficient; but in practice our current body of research still has plenty of gaps, so I wanted to cast overlapping nets to make sure nothing important would slip through the cracks.

Something has the potential to affect the fetus.

I started by looking for sources that exhaustively listed environmental contaminants with the potential to harm a fetus. Unsurprisingly, the CDC proved to be a good first port of call, and other governmental sources at both the national and state level helped further bulk out the list.[1] International bodies were another important source of input.[2] And finally, there are academic publications that have attempted to summarize environmental threats to fetal development.[3] As a result of this type of substance-focused research, parts of the book are organized by substance (e.g., the section on lead).

Then it reaches the fetus.

Next, I considered potential exposure routes, which I classified as follows:

Exposure routes

	Eaten	Drank	Inhaled	Absorbed
Alive	Bad: • Foodborne infectious diseases Good: • Probiotics	Bad: • Waterborne infectious diseases	Bad: • Airborne infectious diseases	• n/a
Inert	Bad: • Food contaminants (from the environment, food packaging, pesticides, food additives) Voluntary: • Oral recreational drugs Good: • Macronutrients (fat, carbohydrates, protein) • Micronutrients (vitamins, minerals, and trace elements)	Bad: • Water contaminants Voluntary: • Imbibed recreational drugs (alcohol, caffeine) Good: • Fluids	Bad: • Outdoor air contaminants • Indoor air contaminants (from personal care products, household cleaning products) Voluntary: • Cigarette smoke • Other inhaled recreational drugs	Bad: • Soil contaminants • Personal care product ingredients Voluntary: • Injected recreational drugs Bad: • Heat • Radiation • Magnetic fields Voluntary: • Loud noise Good: • Sound (music, human speech)

For each cell of the grid, I brainstormed all the potential influences that might fall within that category. As a result, further chapters in this book are organized around topics such as air, water, or personal care products.

It's worth an aside on why in the "Eaten" section of the grid I've listed macronutrients and micronutrients, instead of listing specific foods. This is not because a list of specific foods would be impractically long, although of course that's true. It's because the vast majority of research in the U.S. on both nutritional intake and the impact of nutrition on health is couched in these terms. For example, using data from NHANES, the government's National Health and Nutrition Examination Survey, it's possible to find an estimate of the number of Americans who are deficient in a particular vitamin, but impossible to find an estimate of the number of Americans who eat a specific food, like sushi. The guide to Nutrition During Pregnancy published by the Institute of Medicine in 1990 focuses its guidelines only on weight gain and vitamin and mineral supplements.[4] And a more recent publication from the IOM in 2006 addressing the full population outlines recommendations for consumption of macronutrients (carbohydrates, fiber, fat, cholesterol, protein and amino acids) as well as vitamins and minerals, but makes little reference to actual foods.[5]

This perverse situation has its roots in a 1970s political battle. As described by Michael Pollan, author of *In Defense of Food*,[6] in 1977 Senator George McGovern convened a set of hearings to look at the American diet, and came out with a set of guidelines.

> McGovern said we're eating too much red meat, and the official advice of the government became eat less red meat. Now, that was a very controversial message. The meat industry, in fact the whole food industry, went crazy, and came down on him like a ton of bricks. That's why McGovern lost in 1980. The beef lobby went after him, and they tossed him out. And so from then on, anyone who would pronounce on the American diet understood you had to speak in this very obscure language of nutrients. You could talk about saturated fat, you could talk about antioxidants, but you couldn't talk about whole foods. So that is the official language in which we discuss nutrition.[7]

Studies from countries such as Norway and Denmark have unsurprisingly found that classically "western" diets are associated with worse pregnancy outcomes,[8] but this could be correlation with a generally less healthy lifestyle overall rather than causation. Unfortunately, no one to my knowledge has yet launched any randomized trials feeding lots of broccoli or kale to one group of women and not another.

Then it causes a health outcome.

Finally, I considered what could ultimately go wrong. Here, I looked for studies that tried to tease out factors that might have increased the odds of various problems occurring, such as miscarriage,[9] fetal death later in the pregnancy,[10] and low birth weight.[11]

By this point, I had a list of all the topics I felt warranted inclusion from a scientific perspective. But I also decided to step back and look at the question through the eyes of the consumer—what topics, rightly or wrongly, might be worrying people, and therefore need to be addressed or debunked? To find out, I consulted common "what to avoid in pregnancy" lists: for example, Babycenter.com and Oprah.com's article "Toxins in Food and Medications to Avoid When You're Pregnant" by Dr. Oz and Dr. Roizen.[12] I looked at a March of Dimes survey on what was worrying pregnant women,[13] and consulted my friends about what had concerned them when they were pregnant. I looked at the publications by advocacy groups such as the Environmental Working group.[14] And I looked for published lists of common environmental contaminants, even those without a pregnancy-specific angle, such as *Time*'s collection of articles on environmental toxins,[15] Listosaur's "Top 10 Most Dangerous Environmental Toxins in the U.S.,"[16] and the "Top 10 most common environmental toxins," by Dr. Mercola.[17]

So is this book exhaustive? Probably not. But it's a start.

Notes

1. Of the ~200 different chemicals or chemical categories listed in the CDC's 2009 "Fourth National Report on Human Exposure to Environmental Chemicals,"[1] the 27 mentioned as having the potential for adverse reproductive or developmental effects went on my list to research (Acrylamide, Disinfection By-Products (Trihalomethanes), Benzophenone, Bisphenol A, 4-tert-Octylphenol, Atrazine, DBP, 2,4,5-Trichlorophenoxyacetic Acid, Carbofuran, DDT, Hexachlorobenzene, Mirex, Chlorpyrifos, Pyrethroid Insecticides, Lead, Mercury, Cadmium, Molybdenum, Perchlorate, Perfluorochemicals, Phthalates, PBDEs, Non-Dioxin-Like Polychlorinated Biphenyls, Dioxin-like chemicals, Toluene, and Xylene).

For example, the US EPA published a report with top 35 pesticides in use in the US,[2] the CDC published a study listing all causes of foodborne illness in the US,[3] and the Office of Health Assessment and Translation publishes opinions on whether various substances are of concern given current knowledge of human exposure levels and health effects;[4] one of their recent presentations listed ten chemicals with "clear evidence of adverse developmental effects"[5] (Acrylamide, Bisphenol A [developmental toxicity at "high" dose], 1-bromopropane, 2-bromopropane [developmental toxicity at "high" dose], Butyl benzyl phthalate, Di-n-butyl phthalate, Di-n-hexyl phthalate, Di-isodecyl phthalate, Genistein, and Methanol).

The California Environmental Protection Agency produces an annual list of chemicals known to cause health effects,[6] which currently includes five substances with a potential health risk of developmental toxicity (DEHA, Diquat, Lead, Nickel, and Perchlorate). And Washington State's guide to Workplace Hazards to Reproduction and Development[7] lists a variety of potential risk factors (Ionizing radiation, advanced maternal age, poor nutrition, inconsistent prenatal care, smoking, alcohol consumption, ethylene oxide, nitrous oxide, formaldehyde, arsenic, organic solvents, toxoplasmosis, dioxins, polychlorinated biphenyls (PCBs), carbon disulfide, solvents, mercury, lead, carbon monoxide, methylene chloride, and heavy physical exertion (e.g., repetitive heavy lifting, stooping, and/or climbing).

1. Centers for Disease Control and Prevention (CDC), & Centers for Disease Control and Prevention (CDC). (2009). Fourth national report on human exposure to environmental chemicals. Atlanta (GA). https://www.cdc.gov/exposurereport/pdf/fourthreport.pdf

2. Grube, A., Donaldson, D., Kiely, T., & Wu, L. (2011). Pesticides industry sales and usage. US EPA, Washington, DC. https://swap.stanford.edu/20140417081610/http://www.epa.gov/opp00001/pestsales/07pestsales/market_estimates2007.pdf

3. Scallan, E., Hoekstra, R. M., Angulo, F. J., Tauxe, R. V., Widdowson, M. A., Roy, S. L., . . . & Griffin, P. M. (2011). Foodborne illness acquired in the United States—major pathogens. Emerg Infect Dis, 17(1). https://www.ncbi.nlm.nih.gov/pmc/articles/PMC3375761/

4. National Institute of Environmental Health Sciences (NIEHS). (2013, June 11). Health assessment and translation: About OHAT. https://www.niehs.nih.gov/research/atniehs/dntp/assoc/ohat/

5. Bucher, J.R., Wolfe, M.S., Thayer, K. (n.d.). National Toxicology Program: Evaluation of Reproductive and Developmental Hazards. https://oehha.ca.gov/media/downloads/proposition-65/presentation/071211ntpcalepadart.pdf

6. Office of Environmental Health Hazard Assessment. (2007). Proposition 65. OEHHA. CA.gov. www.oehha.ca.gov/prop65.html; Office of Environmental Health Hazard Assessment, California Environmental Protection Agency. (2013, February). Health Risk Information for Public Health Goal Exceedance Reports. https://oehha.ca.gov/water/report/phg-exceedance-reports-2013

7. Drozdowsky, S. L., & Whittaker, S. G. (1999). Workplace Hazards to Reproduction and Development: A Resource for Workers, Employers, Health Care Providers, and Health & Safety Personnel. Safety and Health Assessment and Research for Prevention (SHARP), Washington State Department of Labor and Industries. http://www.lni.wa.gov/Safety/Research/files/repro_dev.pdf

2. For example, the Stockholm Convention on Persistent Organic Pollutants, which has agreed on twenty-four internationally banned or controlled substances (Elimination: Aldrin, Chlordane, Chlordecone, Decabromodiphenyl ether (commercial mixture, c-decaBDE, Dieldrin, Endrin, Heptachlor, Hexabromobiphenyl, Hexabromocyclododecane (HBCDD), Hexabromodiphenyl ether and heptabromodiphenyl ether, Hexachlorobenzene, Hexachlorobutadiene, Alpha hexachlorocyclohexane, Beta hexachlorocyclohexane, Lindane, Mirex, Pentachlorobenzene, Pentachlorophenol and its salts and esters, Polychlorinated biphenyls, Polychlorinated naphthalenes) Short-chain chlorinated paraffins (SCCPs), Technical endosulfan and its related isomers, Tetrabromodiphenyl ether and pentabromodiphenyl ether, and Toxaphene. Restriction: DDT, Perfluorooctane sulfonic acid, its salts, and perfluorooctane sulfonyl fluoride. Reduce unintentional release: Hexachlorobenzene (HCB), Hexachlorobutadiene (HCBD), Pentachlorobenzene, Polychlorinated biphenyls (PCB), Polychlorinated dibenzo-p-dioxins, Polychlorinated dibenzofurans, Polychlorinated naphthalenes) Stockholm Convention. (2008). Listing of POPs in the Stockholm Convention. http://chm.pops.int/TheConvention/ThePOPs/ListingofPOPs/tabid/2509/Default.aspx

3. Wigle, D. T., Arbuckle, T. E., Turner, M. C., Berube, A., Yang, Q., Liu, S., & Krewski, D. (2008). Epidemiologic evidence of relationships between reproductive and child health outcomes and environmental chemical contaminants. Journal of Toxicology and Environmental Health, Part B, 11(5-6), 373-517. www.tandfonline.com/doi/pdf/10.1080/10937400801921320; Stillerman, K. P., Mattison, D. R., Giudice, L. C., & Woodruff, T. J. (2008). Environmental exposures and adverse pregnancy outcomes: a

review of the science. Reproductive Sciences, 15(7), 631-650. http://journals.sagepub.
com/doi/abs/10.1177/1933719108322436; Sharpe, R. M., & Irvine, D. S. (2004). How
strong is the evidence of a link between environmental chemicals and adverse effects on
human reproductive health?. Bmj, 328(7437), 447-451. https://www.ncbi.nlm.nih.gov/
pmc/articles/PMC344268/; Grandjean, P., & Landrigan, P. J. (2014). Neurobehavioural
effects of developmental toxicity. The Lancet Neurology, 13(3), 330-338. http://www.
sciencedirect.com/science/article/pii/S1474442213702783 ; Windham, G., & Fenster, L.
(2008). Environmental contaminants and pregnancy outcomes. Fertility and sterility, 89(2),
e111-e116. http://www.sciencedirect.com/science/article/pii/S0015028207043208.

For example, a highly in-depth report from 2008 (Wigle et al., Epidemiologic
evidence of relationships between reproductive and child health outcomes and environmental chemical contaminants) concludes there's sufficient epidemiological evidence for
causal relationships between adverse outcomes and prenatal exposure to several chemicals (Methylmercury, polychlorinated biphenyls and dibenzofurans, and maternal smoking). The National Academy of Sciences published a review of developmental toxicology
in 2000 (National Research Council. (2000). Scientific frontiers in developmental toxicology and risk assessment. www.nap.edu/openbook.php?record_id=9871&page=R9),
and the most recent edition of the "Catalog of Teratogenic Agents" was published in
2004 (Shepard, T. H., & Lemire, R. J. (2004). Catalog of teratogenic agents. JHU Press.
http://books.google.co.uk/books?hl=en&lr=&id=vBIl2OA6BK8C&oi=fnd&pg=PR9&d-
q=Shepard+1998+catalogue+teratogenic&ots=FJD2f96oMu&sig=_9T733DrpvpBB_
ZTEq91WvoaqsY&redir_esc=y#v=onepage&q=Shepard%201998%20catalogue%20
teratogenic&f=false).

4. Institute of Medicine (U.S.). Subcommittee on Dietary Intake, & Nutrient Supplements
during Pregnancy. 1990. Nutrition during pregnancy: part I, weight gain: part II,
nutrient supplements. National Academy Press. http://books.nap.edu/openbook.
php?record_id=1451.

5. Hellwig, J. P., Otten, J. J., & Meyers, L. D. (Eds.). (2006). Dietary Reference Intakes: The
Essential Guide to Nutrient Requirements. National Academies Press. https://www.nap.
edu/read/11537/chapter/1.

6. Pollan, M. 2008. *In defense of food: an eater's manifesto.* Penguin.

7. Goodman, A., & Pollan, M. (2008, February 13). In defense of food: Author, journalist
Michael Pollan on nutrition, food science, and the American diet. DemocracyNow.org.
www.democracynow.org/2008/2/13/in_defense_of_food_author_journalist.

8. Brantsæter, A. L., Haugen, M., Samuelsen, S. O., Torjusen, H., Trogstad, L., Alexander, J., . . .
& Meltzer, H. M. (2009). A dietary pattern characterized by high intake of vegetables, fruits,
and vegetable oils is associated with reduced risk of preeclampsia in nulliparous pregnant
Norwegian women. The Journal of nutrition, 139(6), 1162-1168. http://jn.nutrition.org/
content/139/6/1162.short; Knudsen, V. K., Orozova-Bekkevold, I. M., Mikkelsen, T. B.,
Wolff, S., & Olsen, S. F. (2008). Major dietary patterns in pregnancy and fetal growth.
European journal of clinical nutrition, 62(4), 463-470. www.nature.com/ejcn/journal/v62/
n4/full/1602745a.html.

9. Rai, R., & Regan, L. (2006). Recurrent miscarriage. The Lancet, 368(9535), 601-611.
http://xa.yimg.com/kq/groups/20183361/1414078795/name/Recurrent+miscarriage.
pdf; Stabile, I., Chard, T., & Grudzinskas, G. (2000). Miscarriage. Clinical Obstetrics
and Gynaecology (pp. 15-21). Springer London. http://link.springer.com/chap-
ter/10.1007/978-1-4471-0783-5_4#; García-Enguídanos, A., Calle, M. E., Valero, J., Luna,
S., & Domínguez-Rojas, V. (2002). Risk factors in miscarriage: a review. European Journal
of Obstetrics & Gynecology and Reproductive Biology, 102(2), 111-119. www.science
direct.com/science/article/pii/S0301211501006133; Arck, P. C., Rücke, M., Rose, M.,

Szekeres-Bartho, J., Douglas, A. J., Pritsch, M., . . . & Klapp, B. F. (2008). Early risk factors for miscarriage: a prospective cohort study in pregnant women. Reproductive biomedicine online, 17(1), 101-113. www.sciencedirect.com/science/article/pii/S1472648310603008; Risch, H. A., Weiss, N. S., Clarke, E. A., & Miller, A. B. (1988). Risk factors for spontaneous abortion and its recurrence. American journal of epidemiology, 128(2), 420-430. http://aje. oxfordjournals.org/content/128/2/420.short; Parazzini, F., Bocciolone, L., Fedele, L., Negri, E., La Vecchia, C. A. R. L. O., & Acaia, B. (1991). Risk factors for spontaneous abortion. International journal of epidemiology, 20(1), 157-161. http://ije.oxfordjournals.org/ content/20/1/157.short; Gardella, J. R., & Hill III, J. A. (2000, January). Environmental toxins associated with recurrent pregnancy loss. In Seminars in reproductive medicine (Vol. 18, No. 04, pp. 407-424) https://www.thieme-connect.com/products/ejournals/html/ 10.1055/s-2000-13731 ; Maconochie, N., Doyle, P., Prior, S., & Simmons, R. (2007). Risk factors for first trimester miscarriage—results from a UK-population-based case–control study. BJOG: An International Journal of Obstetrics & Gynaecology, 114(2), 170-186. www. issues4life.org/pdfs/iariskptb027.pdf.

10. Hoyert, D. L. (1996). Medical and life-style risk factors affecting fetal mortality, 1989-90. Vital and health statistics. Series 20, Data from the National Vital Statistics System, (31), 1. http://europepmc.org/abstract/med/9373370; Silver, R. M., Varner, M. W., Reddy, U., Goldenberg, R., Pinar, H., Conway, D., . . . & Stoll, B. 2007. Work-up of stillbirth: a review of the evidence. American journal of obstetrics and gynecology, 196(5), 433-444. www.ncbi. nlm.nih.gov/pmc/articles/pmc2699761/; Fretts, R. C. (2005). Etiology and prevention of stillbirth. American journal of obstetrics and gynecology, 193(6), 1923-1935. http://www. sciencedirect.com/science/article/pii/S0002937805005119.

11. Kramer, M. S. (1987). Determinants of low birth weight: methodological assessment and meta-analysis. Bulletin of the World Health Organization, 65(5), 663. www.ncbi.nlm.nih. gov/pmc/articles/PMC2491072/?page=1; Valero de Bernabé, J., Soriano, T., Albaladejo, R., Juarranz, M., Calle, M. E., Martınez, D., & Domınguez-Rojas, V. (2004). Risk factors for low birth weight: a review. European Journal of Obstetrics & Gynecology and Reproductive Biology, 116(1), 3-15. www.sciencedirect.com/science/article/pii/S0301211504001654; U.S. Environmental Protection Agency. (2015). Report on the environment: Low birth weight. https://cfpub.epa.gov/roe/indicator.cfm?i=78.

12. Oz, Dr. & Roizen, M. (2010, February 6). Toxins in food and medica-tions to avoid when you're pregnant. Oprah.com. www.oprah.com/health/ Foods-and-Toxins-to-Avoid-When-Youre-Pregnant-RealAge#ixzz1d2joNi7H.

13. (2009, December 9). Sushi & breastfeeding join birth defects & preterm birth as leading concerns of moms. March of Dimes. www.marchofdimes.org/news/sushi-and-breastfeeding-join-birth-defects-and-preterm-birth-as-leading-concerns-of-moms.aspx.

14. Houlihan, J., Kropp, T., Wiles, R., Gray, S., & Campbell, C. (2005, July 14). Body Burden—The Pollution in Newborns. Environmental Working Group, Washington, DC. http://www. ewg.org/research/body-burden-pollution-newborns#.WdL65NNSzIU.

15. (n.d.). Environmental toxins: Full list. Time.com. www.time.com/time/specials/packages/ completelist/0,29569,1976909,00.html.

16. Dickenson, D. (2011, September 6). Top 10 Most Dangerous Environmental Toxins in the U.S. Listosaur.com. https://listosaur.com/science-a-technology/ top-10-most-dangerous-environmental-toxins-in-the-us/.

17. Peterson, B. Toxins in our Everyday World. Creative Living Fellowship. http://www.creativelivingfellowship.com/index.php/ministries/ green-faith/85-green-faith-program/139-toxins-in-our-everyday-world.

APPENDIX III

Overall Pregnancy Calculations

In order to calculate certain threat scores, it was necessary to calculate the percentage of the population that's pregnant at any given moment. The following describes my calculations (these figures also form the basis of the chart that appears in the "What Could Go Wrong" section of the introduction):

According to a U.S. National Vital Statistics Report, in 2004 there were 6,390,000 pregnancies minus 1,222,000 intentionally induced abortions, or 5,168,000 pregnancies in the United States.[1] A total of 1,056,000 were then lost, 25,655 of which were after 20 weeks' gestation (fetal death), so an implied 1,030,345 before 20 weeks' gestation (miscarriage), to reach a total of 4,112,055 live births.[2] We can therefore estimate that at any given moment in 2004, the number of women pregnant was approximately 4,112,055 x 40/52 (assuming an average gestation of 40 weeks for live births) + 25,655 x 30/52 (assuming fetal death occurred at an average of 30 weeks) + 1,030,345 x 10/52 (assuming miscarriage occurred at an average of 10 weeks) = 3,380,997, or approximately 3,381,000. According to the U.S. census, the U.S. population was 293,655,404 as of July 1, 2004.[3] Therefore at any given moment, 3,380,997/293,655,404 = 1.15 percent of the population was pregnant.

Notes

1. Ventura, S.J., US Department of Health & Human Services, Centers for Disease Control and Prevention, National Center for Health Statistics. (2008). Estimated pregnancy rates by outcome for the United States, 1990-2004. https://pdfs.semanticscholar.org/5c6f/15e91bcd-98c73ba703e23c1647453436d971.pdf.

2. MacDorman, M. F., Munson, M. L., & Kirmeyer, S. (2007). Fetal and perinatal mortality, United States, 2004. National vital statistics reports, 56(3). https://pdfs.semanticscholar.org/02ec/9107597bf5cf7207e2dcf3aa7db8c238c1e3.pdf.

3. Population Division, U.S. Census Bureau. (2004, January 28). Table 8: Annual Estimates of the Population for the United States, Regions, and Divisions: April 1, 2000 to July 1, 2004. https://www2.census.gov/programs-surveys/popest/tables/2000-2004/state/totals/nst-est2004-08.pdf.

APPENDiX IV

Foodborne Illnesses

*T*he US Centers for Disease Control and Prevention published a study in January 2011 estimating the prevalence of various foodborne illnesses in the US population for the years 2000 to 2008.[1] Below is the breakdown of the 48 million cases of foodborne illness by pathogen:

Breakdown of annual foodborne illness cases by pathogen

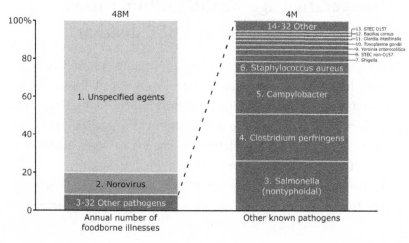

Unfortunately, the proportion of fetuses affected by each pathogen may not be the same as for the general population, for several reasons:

1. Some pathogens may make the mother but not the baby sick, as they do not pass through the placenta and therefore have no negative effect on the fetus, unless the mother becomes gravely ill and dies.

2. Conversely, some foodborne illnesses may make the baby but not the mother sick, as the immature fetus is more vulnerable than the mature mother if both are exposed.

3. Pregnancy itself can actually make a woman more susceptible to contracting certain foodborne illnesses, due to changes in the immune system during pregnancy: "In order to prevent rejection of the fetus by the maternal immune system, cell-mediated immunity must be down-regulated during pregnancy . . . leading to increased susceptibility of the woman and her fetus to infections by intracellular pathogens."[2]

4. The drugs used to treat an infection could be fine for the mother but could present a risk to the fetus.

To estimate the effects of foodborne illness in pregnancy, we therefore need to look at each pathogen in turn and incorporate the above factors to arrive at an estimate of the impact of each foodborne illness.

1. Unspecified agents (38 million cases; 71,878 hospitalizations; 1,686 deaths)

Of the 48 million cases of annual food poisoning, 38 million, or 80 percent, have an unknown cause. These "unspecified" cases involve symptoms of acute gastroenteritis, and most resolve themselves within a few days without any need for medication or hospitalization. Hence in the majority of cases, no definitive diagnosis is ever made as to which pathogen caused the bout of illness.

Fortunately, gastroenteritis rarely has negative impact on pregnancy. In a study of 10,229 mother-infant pairs, "32.5 percent of the mothers suffered from gastroenteritis during pregnancy . . . Gastroenteritis during part of the pregnancy was associated with a shortened pregnancy, but it had no other adverse effects on neonatal outcome. The reduction in the duration of pregnancy is probably of little clinical relevance."[3]

The number of fetuses affected can be estimated simply as the number of pregnant women who die from these unknown pathogens, namely 1,686 deaths estimated in the report x 1.15 percent of the U.S. population pregnant = ~19 pregnant deaths per year in the United States. In actuality, this number will represent an upper bound, as deaths from gastroenteritis are far more likely to occur in elderly or immune-compromised individuals rather than healthy women in their childbearing years.

Threat score: 19/3,381,000 (probability, since there are an estimated 19 maternal deaths out of a total population of 3,381,000 pregnant women) x 100,000 (impact: death) x 1 (certainty: well proven) = 0.57.

Threat level: Low

2. Norovirus (5,462,000 cases; 14,663 hospitalizations; 149 deaths)

Norovirus, also known as Norwalk-like virus, "is an extremely common cause of foodborne illness, though it is rarely diagnosed, because the laboratory test is not widely available. It causes an acute gastrointestinal illness, usually with more vomiting than diarrhea, which resolves within two days."[4] As with unspecified agents, this virus is unlikely to cause problems specific to pregnancy—a review of the literature yields no evidence that noroviruses target pregnant women more frequently or can cross the placenta and affect the fetus, although a conclusive study has not been undertaken. Again, we can simply consider the impact to be only the small number of pregnant individuals who might die from norovirus, namely 149 x 1.15 percent = ~2, where this again represents an upper bound.

Threat score: 2/3,381,000 (probability, since there are an estimated 2 maternal deaths out of a total population of 3,381,000 pregnant women) x 100,000 (impact: death) x 1 (certainty: well proven) = 0.05.

Threat level: Very low

3. *Salmonella* (nontyphoidal; 1,028,000 cases; 19,336 hospitalizations; 378 deaths)

"*Salmonella* is a bacterium that is widespread in the intestines of birds, reptiles and mammals. The illness it causes, salmonellosis, typically includes fever, diarrhea and abdominal cramps. In persons with poor underlying health or weakened immune systems, it can invade the bloodstream and cause life-threatening infections."[5] Fortunately, pregnant women do not fall under this category of increased susceptibility: in "Foodborne Infections during Pregnancy," published in 1999, the author concludes that a pregnant woman has no greater susceptibility to *Salmonella* than the general population.[6]

There is also little risk to the baby of infection crossing the placenta or being transferred during delivery, according to a large-scale study: "Over a 9-year period . . . 30,471 mothers were screened at the time of delivery, and 60 yielded salmonellas, 43 of whom were symptomless excretors. Seven of the 60 babies excreted salmonellas, all of which were the same organism as in the mothers. Five had uncomplicated gastroenteritis in the neonatal period, but no mother or child suffered invasive disease."[7] Furthermore, there have only been 3 cases reported in the literature of intrauterine infection with nontyphoidal species of *Salmonella*.[8] Therefore, we can yet again estimate simply the number of cases in which the mother dies, namely 378 x 1.51 percent = ~4, as the upper bound, given that the majority of deaths occur in immune-compromised individuals. Fortunately, *Salmonella* infections usually resolve in 5–7 days and most do not require treatment other than oral fluids.[9]

Threat score: 4/3,381,000 (probability, since there are an estimated 4 maternal deaths out of a total population of 3,381,000 pregnant women) x 100,000 (impact: death) x 1 (certainty: well proven) = 0.13.

Threat level: Very low

4. *Clostridium perfringens* (966,000 cases; 438 hospitalizations; 26 deaths)

Clostridium perfringens type A is a common and relatively harmless foodborne pathogen that causes a short gastrointestinal illness: "*C. perfringens* food poisoning is characterized by intense abdominal cramps and diarrhoea . . . The illness is usually over within 24 hours."[10] Fortunately, there is no evidence in the literature that this organism targets pregnant women, causes any specific problems in pregnancy, or reaches the fetus. A mild illness with only an estimated 26 deaths per year, this death rate is so low that it is improbable that even one pregnant woman would be affected.

Threat level: Very low

5. *Campylobacter* (845,000 cases; 8,463 hospitalizations; 76 deaths)

"*Campylobacter* is a bacterial pathogen that causes fever, diarrhea, and abdominal cramps. It is the most commonly identified bacterial cause of diarrheal illness in the world.[11] These bacteria live in the intestines of healthy birds, and most raw poultry meat has *Campylobacter* on it. Eating undercooked chicken, or other food that has been contaminated with juices dripping from raw chicken, is the most frequent source of this infection." Almost all persons infected with *Campylobacter* recover without any specific treatment.[12]

Pregnant women fortunately do not face increased susceptibility to contracting *Campylobacter* infection, but the infection can put the fetus at risk.[13] Surprisingly, there has been only a limited amount of research examining outcomes of *Campylobacter* infections during pregnancy. One review of the literature from 1986 cited 20 case histories, stating "18 of 20 pregnancies ended prematurely at 13–32 weeks of gestation. All of the mothers survived, but fetal/neonatal mortality was 80 percent."[14] This approach doesn't necessarily give an accurate reflection of typical outcomes, however, as only the more extreme or noteworthy cases would have been likely to have been written up for publication.

Somewhat more recently, two hospital studies have examined outcomes by screening the records of all women admitted to the hospital within a certain time period for evidence of both pregnancy and *Campylobacter* infection. Cumulatively, these papers present 16 data points:

- In a review of 10 pregnant women admitted to Mount Sinai Hospital in New York City with *Campylobacter* infection, two women were in the second trimester, one of whom lost the baby. Eight women were in the third trimester, and all delivered healthy babies, only one of whom needed antibiotics at birth (three of the mothers were treated with an antibiotic, erythromycin).[15]
- In a review of 6 pregnant women admitted to a Queensland hospital with *Campylobacter* infection, two pregnancies in the second trimester resulted in stillbirths, while of the four pregnancies in the third trimester, two newborns required treatment with antibiotics; the remaining two pregnancies were treated at the time of the infection and had no negative outcomes.[16]

These reviews suggest that infection during the second trimester is dangerous: of the four pregnancies reported in the second trimester, three resulted in stillbirths. But of the twelve pregnancies in the third trimester, all had healthy deliveries, with only three babies needing antibiotics at birth.

Therefore, if 8,463 individuals are hospitalized each year with *Campylobacter* infection, an estimated 1.15 percent x 8,463 = 93 pregnant women would be hospitalized; one-third, or 31, of these would be in the second trimester, so 31 multiplied by a stillbirth rate of 3 out of 4 would imply 24 fetal deaths per year. In addition, there are 76 annual deaths, so an estimated 1.15 percent x 76 = ~1 pregnant death per year.

Campylobacter infection can also be asymptomatic in the mother, but this does not appear to present a risk to the fetus, for two reasons. First, there is a low risk of transmission to the baby: in one study, 12,521 mothers were screened in labor, and 28 tested positive for *Campylobacter* (0.2 percent); however, only 2 of 15 babies tested positive at birth.[17] Second, infection in a baby is rarely serious: "Infection in the newborn usually appears to be manifested only by the passage of blood and mucus per rectum in an otherwise healthy baby"; "Infection in the neonatal period generally seems to cause a much milder gastrointestinal disturbance than that in children and adults. Whether erythromycin treatment is needed in neonatal infections is debatable and a controlled trial is unlikely to be carried out because of the small numbers involved."[18, 19]

Finally, *Campylobacter* infections have the potential to escalate into a rare but serious condition called Guillain-Barré syndrome (GBS), in which the immune system attacks nerve cells, leading to weakness, numbness, and tingling in the feet, hands, and limbs. Fortunately, this condition is not of specific concern in pregnancy: "GBS during pregnancy does not impair fetal or infant development. In addition, treatment of the mother for GBS has no effect on pregnancy or fetal development."[20, 21] Transfer of GBS to the fetus is also extremely rare, with only one such case ever reported in the literature.[22, 23]

Threat score: 25/3,381,000 (probability, since there are an estimated 25 maternal or fetal deaths out of a total population of 3,381,000 pregnant women) x 100,000 (impact: death) x 1 (certainty: well proven) = 0.75.

Threat level: Low

6. *Staphylococcus aureus* (241,000 cases; 1,064 hospitalizations; 6 deaths)

Staphylococcus aureus is a common bacterium found on the skin and in the noses of up to 25 percent of healthy people and animals. . . . As the germ multiplies in food, it produces toxins that can cause illness. Staphylococcal toxins are resistant to heat and cannot be destroyed by cooking. Foods at highest risk of contamination with *Staphylococcus aureus* and subsequent toxin production are those that are made by hand and require no cooking, like sliced meat, puddings, pastries and sandwiches. . . . Symptoms usually develop within one to six hours after eating contaminated food. Patients typically experience nausea, vomiting, stomach cramps, and diarrhea. The illness is usually mild and most patients recover after one to three days.[24]

There is no evidence in the literature that this type of food poisoning causes any specific problems in pregnancy or reaches the fetus.

Threat level: Very low

7. *Shigella* (131,000 cases; 1,456 hospitalizations; 10 deaths)

Shigella is a bacterium that was discovered more than 100 years ago by a Japanese scientist named Shiga. "Most who are infected with *Shigella* develop diarrhea, fever, and stomach cramps starting a day or two after they are exposed to the bacteria. The diarrhea is often bloody. Shigellosis usually resolves in 5 to 7 days. Persons with shigellosis in the United States rarely require hospitalization."[25] Moderate or severe cases can be treated with antibiotics, such as fluoroquinolones, ceftriaxone, and azithromycin.[26, 27] Fluoroquinolones are in pregnancy category C (animal reproduction studies have shown an adverse effect on the fetus and there are no adequate and well-controlled studies in humans, but potential benefits may warrant use of the drug in pregnant women despite potential risks),[28, 29, 30] but the other two are pregnancy category B (animal studies have revealed no evidence of harm to the fetus—however, there are no adequate studies in pregnant women; OR animal studies have shown an adverse effect, but adequate studies in pregnant women have failed to demonstrate a risk to the fetus). Fortunately, pregnant women are not more susceptible to contracting *Shigella*. It doesn't appear to cross the placenta, and has not been identified as a cause of abortion, stillbirth, or premature labor. Finally, infection of the baby during delivery is uncommon.[31]

Threat level: Very low

8. STEC non-O157 (112,752 cases; 271 hospitalizations; 0 deaths)

> Some types of *E. coli* produce a toxin called Shiga toxin which can cause symptoms including stomach cramps, diarrhea (often bloody), and vomiting. These are called 'Shiga toxin-producing' *E. coli*, or STEC for short. . . . The non-O157 STEC are not nearly as well understood, partly because outbreaks due to them are rarely identified. As a whole, the non-O157 serogroup is less likely to cause severe illness than *E. coli* O157, and most people get better within 5–7 days, although on rare occasion the infection can be more severe.[32]

There are no reports on the effects of STEC non-O157 in pregnancy, and the treatment for STEC is primarily hydration.[33]

Threat level: Very low

9. *Yersinia enterocolitica* (97,656 cases; 533 hospitalizations; 29 deaths)

Yersinia enterocolitica is a species of bacteria typically caught from eating undercooked food, particularly pork. According to the CDC:

Infection with *Y. enterocolitica* occurs most often in young children. Common symptoms in children are fever, abdominal pain, and diarrhea, which is often bloody. Symptoms may last 1 to 3 weeks or longer. In older children and adults, right-sided abdominal pain and fever may be the predominant symptoms, and may be confused with appendicitis. In a small proportion of cases, complications such as skin rash, joint pains, or spread of bacteria to the bloodstream can occur. . . . Uncomplicated cases of diarrhea due to *Y. enterocolitica* usually resolve on their own without antibiotic treatment. However, in more severe or complicated infections, antibiotics such as aminoglycosides, doxycycline, trimethoprim-sulfamethoxazole, or fluoroquinolones are useful.[34]

Fluoroquinolones are in pregnancy category C (animal studies show some risk, and evidence in human and animal studies is inadequate, but clinical benefit sometimes exceeds risk),[35] while the remainder are in pregnancy category D (studies in pregnant women have demonstrated a risk to the fetus, but the benefits of therapy in a life-threatening situation or a serious disease may outweigh the potential risk).[36, 37, 38] There do not appear to be any negative effects of contracting yersiniosis during pregnancy. Pregnant women have no increased susceptibility, and there's no evidence of the bacteria being transmitted to the baby either within the womb or at birth.[39]

Threat level: Very low

10. *Toxoplasma gondii* (86,686 cases; 4,428 hospitalizations; 327 deaths)

Toxoplasma gondii is a parasite commonly found in the environment; ~15 percent of women aged 15–44 have antibodies against *T. gondii*, indicating they have been exposed at some point in their lives, according to a large-scale study testing 17,658 individuals in the United States.[40]

When a woman with prior exposure becomes pregnant, her fetus is not at risk of contracting toxoplasmosis even if she is reexposed, as her antibodies provide sufficient protection to stave off further infection. However, a woman exposed to *Toxoplasma gondii* for the first time during pregnancy is at risk of passing the infection along to her fetus, resulting in a serious condition known as congenital toxoplasmosis (or, in rare cases, a stillbirth). Unfortunately, infection is frequently symptomless in the mother: "Infection in the mother is not recognized in approximately 90 percent of cases. Symptoms and signs of acute infection are generally so minor, the woman does not recall the incident. But the infected fetus always shows symptoms—at birth, during infancy, in childhood, in teenage [years], or in adult years."[41]

There have been a variety of studies looking at the long-term effects of congenital toxoplasmosis. Unlike most infections, the symptoms can occasionally remain hidden even throughout childhood, only to emerge in later adolescence:

- In one study of 166 fetuses infected with toxoplasmosis, there were 11 deaths (7 percent), 13 with severe symptoms (8 percent), 22 with mild symptoms (13 percent), and the remaining 120 with no symptoms at birth (72 percent).[42]

- Another study of 542 cases of congenital toxoplasmosis found 7 percent resulted in death, 8 percent in severe symptoms, 12 percent in mild symptoms, and 75 percent in no symptoms at birth. Symptoms categorized as "severe" included chorioretinitis (inflammation in the eye, causing problems with sight), intracranial calcifications (abnormal deposits of calcium in the brain that can cause issues with motor functions, dementia, and other problems), intellectual disability, and neurologic disorders.[43]

- According to a report from the US Department of Agriculture's Economic Research Service working in conjunction with the CDC, an estimated 3 percent of affected children die soon after birth; 11 percent develop serious complications (blindness or intellectual disability); and 86 percent do not show signs of toxoplasmosis at birth but show symptoms by age 17.[44]

The first two studies are in broad agreement, while the figures from the USDA are lower. To be conservative, I have chosen to use the more pessimistic figures from the first two studies in my estimate of the impact.

Toxoplasmosis is "not a nationally reportable disease in the United States, and no reliable data are available at the national level about the number of cases diagnosed each year,"[45] according to the CDC, which provides only a very broad range, stating: "400–4,000 cases of congenital toxoplasmosis occur each year in the U.S."[46] What is a reasonable point estimate within that range? In 1996, economists at the Economic Research Service worked in conjunction with the CDC to estimate that there are 1,581 cases each year of congenital toxoplasmosis.[47] Using the pessimistic assumptions above, this would imply that of the estimated 1,581 annual cases, there would be 106 deaths, 124 serious complications, 201 mild complications, and 1,150 asymptomatic at birth.

This estimate could underrepresent the impact of *Toxoplasma gondii*, as it doesn't take into account miscarriages or abortions. A review of the literature, however, suggests that miscarriage from toxoplasmosis, while possible, is rare: "The earlier the fetus acquires the infection, the more severe the consequences . . . *Toxoplasma gondii* may cause fetal death. However, cases of stillbirth attributed to toxoplasmosis are generally sporadic, and in most developed countries the overall contribution to fetal death is undoubtedly small."[48] This assertion is backed up by a study examining whether *Toxoplasma gondii* is a cause of miscarriage: ~2,000 women with unsuccessful pregnancies were tested for *T. gondii* antibodies during late pregnancy and/or up to 6 weeks after its termination, and there was no association between acute toxoplasmosis and miscarriage.[49]

Threat score: 327 x 1.15 percent (probability of the mother dying, since there are 327 deaths and 1.15 percent of the population is pregnant) x 100,000 (impact: death) x 1 (certainty: well proven) + 106/3,381,000 (probability of the fetus dying) x 100,000 (impact: death) x 1 (certainty: well proven) + 124/3,381,000 (probability) x 10,000 (impact: significant impairment) x 1 (certainty: well proven)

+ 201/3,381,000 (probability) x 1,000 (impact: minor impairment) x 1 (certainty: well proven) = 3.67.

Threat level: Medium

11. *Giardia* (76,840 cases; 255 hospitalizations; 2 deaths)

Giardia is a parasite that's occasionally transmitted through undercooked food, although more typically it is transmitted through contaminated drinking water. *Giardia* causes intestinal symptoms including diarrhea, stomach or abdominal cramps, nausea, and dehydration, which can also lead to weight loss. Symptoms may last 2 to 6 weeks or occasionally longer.[50] Certain drugs can help decrease the amount of time symptoms last, but they aren't recommended during pregnancy because of the potential for adverse effects on the baby.[51]

    Giardia can't pass through the placenta, so the fetus is only affected in rare, severe cases where the mother is so sick she's getting insufficient nutrition, which can affect fetal growth. It's also technically possible for the baby to be infected during birth by fecal contamination, which is unpleasant for a newborn but not life-threatening.[52] Pregnant women may be more likely to experience dehydration from the diarrhea, so the CDC recommends that pregnant women should drink a lot of fluids while ill.[53]

Threat level: Very low

12. *Bacillus cereus* (63,400 cases; 20 hospitalizations; 0 deaths)

Bacillus cereus is a bacterium whose name derives from its shape: *bacillus* means "small rod," and *cereus* means "wax-like."[54] *Bacillus cereus* can be found in a remarkable range of different foods and food ingredients, including rice, dairy products, spices, dried foods, and vegetables.[55] Despite being widespread in foods, it only infrequently causes food poisoning, presumably due to variations among strains.[56] *Bacillus cereus* can produce a variety of different types of toxins, some of which cause diarrhea, others vomiting. In most cases, symptoms are mild and of short duration and don't require any treatment besides hydration.[57] There is no evidence in the literature that *Bacillus cereus* causes any specific harm during pregnancy, with the exception of one case report from 1992 where an infection with *Bacillus* species may have brought on premature labor.[58]

Threat level: Very low

13. STEC O157 (63,153 cases; 2,138 hospitalizations; 20 deaths)

"Some kinds of *E. coli* cause disease by making a toxin called Shiga toxin. The bacteria that make these toxins are called 'Shiga toxin-producing' *E. coli*, or STEC for short. The most commonly identified STEC in North America is *E. coli* O157:H7."[59] Humans are typically infected by consuming food or water that has been contaminated with microscopic amounts of cow feces. The illness usually involves severe and bloody diarrhea and painful abdominal cramps, without much fever, and no specific treatment is recommended beyond hydration.[60]

In a small number of cases, *E. coli* infection can lead to a more serious condition called hemolytic uremic syndrome (HUS), which causes anemia, bleeding, and kidney failure. The majority of cases of HUS occur in children, and there are very few studies that indicate its prevalence in adults; furthermore, HUS in adults shares many similarities with another condition called thrombotic thrombocytopenic purpura, or TTP, and both diseases can be caused by factors other than *E. coli* infection. According to one study of 238 patients hospitalized with *E. coli* infection, however, of the 96 patients aged 15–65, 6 (or 6.25 percent) developed HUS.[61] There have been several relevant studies on the impact of HUS in pregnancy:

- In one retrospective study, the authors reviewed the files of all pregnant women admitted with either TTP or HUS over 25 years (between 1972 and 1997). 13 relevant pregnancies were identified; of these, one woman died in early pregnancy, and two developed severe preeclampsia, but "in general, the response to treatment was prompt."[62]
- In another study, 11 pregnancies resulted in 2 maternal deaths, 1 death of the fetus, 1 stillborn baby, and 7 healthy deliveries (although 5 were premature).[63]
- One case at 18 weeks resulted in a healthy delivery.[64]

In summary, of the 25 pregnancies described, there were three maternal deaths, two fetal deaths, two cases of preeclampsia, and eighteen healthy pregnancies. So to calculate the number of fetuses affected annually, 63,153 cases annually x 1.15 percent of women who are pregnant = 695 pregnant women contract *E. coli* O157, of whom 6.5 percent, or 45, contract HUS; this would imply 5 maternal deaths and 4 fetal deaths per year.

Threat score: 9/3,381,000 (probability) x 100,000 (impact: death) x 1 (certainty: well proven) = 0.27.

Threat level: Low

14. *Cryptosporidium* (57,616 cases; 210 hospitalizations; 4 deaths)

Cryptosporidium is a parasite that can be foodborne, although it's more often transmitted through contaminated drinking water. The most common symptom it causes is watery diarrhea; other symptoms include stomach cramps or pain, dehydration, nausea, vomiting, fever, and weight loss. Symptoms usually last 1 to 2 weeks, although they can come and go for up to 30 days.[65] Most people with healthy immune systems will recover without treatment.

As with *Giardia*, pregnant women are no more susceptible to infection than the rest of the population, and there's no evidence the parasite can be transmitted to the fetus, although it is possible for the baby to be infected during delivery. Pregnant women may be more susceptible to dehydration resulting from diarrhea and are advised to drink plenty of fluids, as fetal distress may occur if the mother's diarrhea is severe.[66, 67]

Threat level: Very low

15. *Vibrio parahaemolyticus* (34,664 cases; 100 hospitalizations; 4 deaths)

As discussed in the section of about oysters, *Vibrio parahaemolyticus* is a bacterium that lives in salt water and is typically caught from eating raw or undercooked shellfish. It causes watery diarrhea and sometimes abdominal cramping, nausea, vomiting, fever, and chills. The illness typically lasts 3 days and is usually self-limited (doesn't require treatment), and severe disease is rare.[68] There's no evidence in the academic literature of any pregnant women or fetuses being specifically affected by *Vibrio* viruses, so it's unlikely that these viruses target pregnant women, pass through the placenta, or cause any specific health outcomes in the fetus.

Threat level: Very low

16. Foodborne ETEC (17,894 cases; 12 hospitalizations; 0 deaths)

"Enterotoxigenic *Escherichia coli*, or ETEC, is the name given to a group of *E. coli* that produce special toxins which stimulate the lining of the intestines, causing them to secrete excessive fluid, thus producing diarrhea."[69] There is little specific risk in pregnancy: "most infected persons will recover within a few days, without requiring any specific treatment" and "virtually all persons recover completely without any long-term consequences."[70]

Threat level: Very low

17. *Vibrio* spp., other (17,564 cases; 83 hospitalizations; 8 deaths)

See the section on oysters for a discussion of *Vibrio* infections.

Threat level: Very low

18. Astroviruses (15,433 cases; 87 hospitalizations; 0 deaths)

Astroviruses derive their name from the five- or six-pointed star shape that can be observed on the particles under an electron microscope. These viruses cause a mild case of self-limiting gastroenteritis that usually lasts for 2 to 9 days. Populations most frequently infected are young children and the elderly, and most American and British children over 10 years of age have antibodies to the virus.[71] There is no evidence in the literature that these viruses target pregnant women or cause any specific problems in pregnancy.

Threat level: Very low

19. Rotaviruses (15,433 cases; 348 hospitalizations; 0 deaths)

These viruses take their name from their similarity in appearance to a wheel (*rota* is Latin for "wheel").[72] Rotaviruses are intestinal viruses that have infected virtually all children by three years of age and are the most common cause of diarrhea in children. Rotavirus illness often also includes fever and vomiting and lasts a week or longer. Most rotavirus infections are mild, but about 1 in 50 cases develop severe dehydration.[73] Fortunately, "The majority of women of childbearing age have preexisting immunity to rotavirus . . . and no evidence exists that rotavirus infection or disease during pregnancy poses any risk to the fetus."[74]

Threat level: Very low

20. Sapoviruses (15,433 cases; 87 hospitalizations; 0 deaths)

These viruses are named after the city of Sapporo, Japan, where the first known outbreak was diagnosed in an orphanage in 1977. They fall within the family of caliciviruses (which also include noroviruses), and they cause self-limited gastroenteritis,[75] which tends to be less severe than with noroviruses.[76] Fortunately, there is no evidence in the literature that sapoviruses target pregnant women or cause any specific problems in pregnancy.

Threat level: Very low

21. Diarrheagenic *E. coli* other than STEC and ETEC (11,982 cases; 8 hospitalizations; 0 deaths)

This category of *E. coli* includes "enteropathogenic *E. coli* (EPEC), enteroinvasive *E. coli* (EIEC), enteroaggregative *E. coli* (EAEC), diffusely adherent *E. coli* (DAEC) and perhaps others that are not yet well characterized."[77] There are no reports on the effects of these types of *E. coli* in pregnancy. With only 8 hospitalizations per year, the likelihood that a material number of pregnant women would be affected is minimal.

Threat level: Very low

22. *Cyclospora cayetanensis* (11,407 cases; 11 hospitalizations; 0 deaths)

Cyclospora cayetanensis is a parasite that spreads through contaminated food or water and causes intestinal infection in humans. Symptoms include watery diarrhea (most common); loss of appetite and weight loss; cramping; bloating; increased gas, nausea, and fatigue; and occasionally vomiting and low-grade fever. Untreated, symptoms can last a month or more. Some symptoms, such as diarrhea, can return, and muscle aches and fatigue may continue after the gastrointestinal symptoms have gone away. The infection usually is not life-threatening.[78]

According to the CDC, the antibiotic trimethoprim-sulfamethoxazole (TMP–SMX) is the treatment of choice, but TMP–SMX should be used during pregnancy only if the potential benefit justifies the potential risk to the fetus and no other highly effective alternatives have been identified.[79] Fortunately, most people who have healthy immune systems will recover without treatment.[80] There's also no evidence that this parasite can cross the placenta or harm the fetus, so it poses little specific risk during pregnancy.

Threat level: Very low

23. *Streptococcus* Group A, foodborne (11,217 cases; 1 hospitalization; 0 deaths)

Group A *Streptococcus* is a bacterium that typically causes the common infection we know as strep throat. In rare cases, Group A *Strep* can also cause a much more serious "invasive" infection, but this occurs only when the bacteria enter through sores or other breaks in the skin, so invasive strep isn't an issue with foodborne infection.[81] Foodborne outbreaks typically arise when an individual infected with strep throat is involved in food preparation.

There are no risks to the fetus from contracting strep throat during pregnancy. Strep throat is treated with one of three standard antibiotics (cephalexin, penicillin, or amoxicillin), all of which are categorized in pregnancy category B (animal reproduction studies have failed to demonstrate a risk to the fetus and there are no adequate and well-controlled studies in pregnant women).[82, 83]

Threat level: Very low

24. *Salmonella enterica* serotype typhi (1,821 cases; 197 hospitalizations; 0 deaths)

Typhoid fever, caused by the bacterium *Salmonella* typhi, causes high fever, delirium, and a variety of other potential complications that can be life threatening if untreated. Most cases in the United States (up to 75 percent) are acquired while traveling internationally, as typhoid fever is still common in the developing world, where it's typically spread via contaminated water used for drinking or washing food. Fortunately, typhoid fever can be treated with antibiotics.[84]

Salmonella typhi can pass through the placenta and infect the fetus during pregnancy or be transmitted to the newborn during delivery.[85] Several studies conducted internationally provide estimates of the likelihood of problems arising with typhoid infection during pregnancy, despite prompt treatment with antibiotics. For example, of 32 women in Chile, there was one case of premature labor and one neonatal death.[86] Of 30 cases in the Mediterranean, 3 cases of abortion and 2 cases of birth defects were reported.[87] On the other hand, in a study of 80 pregnant women in Pakistan, "there were no apparent effects of typhoid fever on pregnancy outcome as measured by gestational age at delivery, pregnancy complications, modes of delivery, neonate gender, birth weight, or birth Apgar scores."[88] So out of a cumulative total of 142 cases across the three studies, there were four deaths, two birth defects, and one case of premature labor reported.

Threat score: 1,821 cases x 25 percent caught in the US x 1.15 percent of the population pregnant x 4/142 fetal death rate/3,381,000 (probability) x 100,000 (impact: death) x 1 (certainty: well proven) = 0.004.

Threat level: Very low

25. *Listeria* (1,591 cases; 1,455 hospitalizations; 255 deaths)

Listeria monocytogenes is a rare but highly dangerous foodborne pathogen. Although it is responsible only for .003 percent of food-borne infections each year, it causes ~8 percent of all foodborne-related deaths. Even worse, it specifically targets pregnant women: according to the CDC, "Pregnant women are about 20 times more likely than other healthy adults to get listeriosis . . . 16.67 percent of listeriosis cases happen during pregnancy."[89]

Listeria infections can have serious consequences if contracted during pregnancy. In a review of the literature from 2002, the authors identified 222 pregnant patients with listeriosis between January 1980 and January 2000:

> Details on the outcome of the pregnancy were available in 178 cases. In 36 of 178 (20.2 percent) of those cases, pregnancy resulted in spontaneous abortion or stillbirth. Among the remaining 142 cases, 97 neonates were infected and 45 were not infected . . . [data were unavailable for 3 of the infected, so using the data for the remaining 94] . . . 59 of 94 infected neonates recovered completely, 23 (13 percent) died, and 12 (7 percent) had neurologic sequelae or other long-term complications.[90]

These figures are in line with a report published in 1990 by the USDA on the cost of foodborne disease, which estimated: "Of the 281 newborn/fetal cases who survive the acute illness, 43 develop chronic complications that leave them with some level of permanent disability."[91] This would imply 15 percent of survivors have complications, while the previous figures above imply a rate of 16 percent if we assume the 3 unknown outcomes were healthy.

The most recent figures from the CDC cited above would imply 265 cases of *Listeria* in pregnancy annually (1,591 total cases x 16.67 percent occurring during pregnancy). However, this figure under-represents the actual impact of listeriosis in pregnancy. Although maternal infection can include symptoms such as fever, muscle aches, and nausea or diarrhea, it can also be asymptomatic but still imperil the fetus. In the previously mentioned 2002 review of the literature on outcomes of listeriosis in pregnancy, the authors found that 55 out of 191 episodes of confirmed listeriosis had no maternal symptoms prior to the diagnosis of the disease in the newborn. Scaling up 265 by this proportion would imply 372 cases affecting fetuses/newborns annually.

These figures are again in line with the USDA report mentioned above, which extrapolated from the most recent large-scale sampling studies at the time and concluded: "The annual number of pregnant women who have listeriosis is estimated at 252. The estimated annual number of newborn/fetal cases ranges between 295 and 360. [The number of newborn/fetal cases is larger than the number of maternal cases, because the mother is often asymptomatic, although she transmits the disease to her infant]." So if we assume 372 cases per year and take the distribution of outcomes described above, this would imply 123 fetal/newborn deaths and 25 babies with long-term complications each year.

Threat score: 255 deaths x 1.15 percent of the population pregnant/3,381,000 (probability of maternal death) x 100,000 (impact: death) x 1 (certainty: well proven) + 123/3,381,000 (probability of fetal death) x 100,000 (impact: death) x 1 (certainty: well proven) + 25/3,381,000 (probability of impairment) x 10,000 (impact: significant disability or impairment) x 1 (certainty: well proven) = 3.72.

Threat level: Medium

26. Hepatitis A virus (1,566 cases; 99 hospitalizations; 7 deaths)

"Hepatitis A is a contagious liver disease that results from infection with the hepatitis A virus. It can range in severity from a mild illness lasting a few weeks to a severe illness lasting several months. Hepatitis A is usually spread when a person ingests fecal matter—even in microscopic amounts—from contact with objects, food, or drinks contaminated by the feces, or stool, of an infected person."[92] Hepatitis A isn't treated with any medications; patients usually require only supportive care.[93]

According to a review, pregnant women have no increased susceptibility to hepatitis A, there have been no reports of transmission across the placenta, and hepatitis A does not increase the risk of spontaneous abortion, stillbirth, or congenital malformation.[94] However, infection may increase the risk of preterm delivery. According to one study of 13 cases of infection during pregnancy, eight of the women gave birth preterm, although "child outcome was favorable in all cases."[95]

Threat score: 1,566 cases x 1.15 percent of the population pregnant x 8/13 /3,381,000 (probability) x 100 (impact: statistically detectable impairment) x 1/10 (certainty: preliminary) = 0.003.

Threat level: Very low

27. *Brucella* (839 cases; 55 hospitalizations; 1 death)

Brucella is a bacterium most commonly contracted by eating or drinking unpasteurized dairy products. Brucellosis can cause of range of signs and symptoms, including fever, sweats, malaise, anorexia, headache, pain in the muscles, joints, and/or back, and fatigue.[96] According to a review, pregnant women have no increased susceptibility to *Brucella*.[97] The bacteria can cause miscarriage if contracted during pregnancy; for example, in one study of 92 pregnant women infected in Saudi Arabia, the incidence of miscarriage was 43 percent.[98] Fortunately, prompt treatment with antibiotics is effective in controlling the infection and protecting the fetus.[99, 100] The two antibiotics commonly used are doxycycline and rifampin.[101] Doxycycline is in pregnancy category D (there is positive evidence of human fetal risk based on adverse reaction data from investigational or marketing experience or studies in humans, but potential benefits may warrant use of the drug in pregnant women despite potential risks), but rifampin is in pregnancy category C (animal reproduction studies have shown an adverse effect on the fetus and there are no adequate and well-controlled studies in humans, but potential benefits may warrant use of the drug in pregnant women despite potential risks).[102, 103]

Threat level: Very low

28. *Trichinella* (156 cases; 6 hospitalizations; 0 deaths)

Trichinella is a species of intestinal worm. Nausea, diarrhea, vomiting, fatigue, fever, and abdominal discomfort are often the first symptoms of trichinellosis. Headaches, fevers, chills, cough, swelling of the face and eyes, aching joints and muscle pains, itchy skin, diarrhea, or constipation may follow the first symptoms. If the infection is heavy, patients may experience difficulty coordinating movements and have heart and breathing problems. Most symptoms subside within a few months. Fatigue, weakness, muscle pain, and diarrhea may last for months.[104] Standard treatment involves using antiparasitic drugs (either mebendazole or albendazole) to kill the worms.[105]

According to two different sources, abortion, stillbirth, and premature labor may occur in the case of maternal *Trichinella* infection, although neither source specifies how frequent these outcomes might be.[106, 107] In one study of four pregnant women infected, "all four gave birth to healthy infants at full term."[108] It's also unclear if *Trichinella* can pass from mother to fetus. In humans, only one possible case of congenital trichinellosis has been reported,[109] and a study done in Laos concluded "our results cannot prove that transmission of trichinellosis occurs from mother to child."[110]

In the case of infection, treatment with drugs can be considered. Data on the use of albendazole and mebendazole in pregnant women are limited, though the available evidence suggests no difference in congenital abnormalities in the children of women who were accidentally treated with either drug during mass prevention campaigns compared with those who were not. The World Health Organization

(WHO) has determined that the benefit of treatment outweighs the risk and allows use of both drugs in the second and third trimesters of pregnancy.[111]

Threat level: Very low

29. *Vibrio vulnificus* (96 cases; 93 hospitalizations; 36 deaths)

See the section on oysters for a discussion of *Vibrio* infections.

Threat level: Very low

30. *Vibrio cholerae*, toxigenic (84 cases; 2 hospitalizations; 0 deaths)

See the section on oysters for a discussion of *Vibrio* infections.

Threat level: Very low

31. *Mycobacterium bovis* (60 cases; 31 hospitalizations; 3 deaths)

Mycobacterium bovis is a bacterium commonly found in cattle, so on rare occasion people can become infected after eating or drinking contaminated, unpasteurized dairy products. This bacterium causes tuberculosis, although a rare form (more than 98 percent of TB cases are caused by a different bacterium, *Mycobacterium tuberculosis*). Symptoms can include fever, night sweats, and weight loss, and gastro-intestinal disease can cause abdominal pain and diarrhea. If untreated, a person can die of the disease.[112]

Mycobacterium bovis poses minimal risk during pregnancy since it can be treated. According to one review, "untreated tuberculosis in pregnancy poses a significant threat to the mother, fetus, and family," but fortunately "all 4 first line drugs [isoniazid, rifampicin (rifampin), ethambutol, and pyrazinamide] have an excellent safety record in pregnancy and are not associated with human fetal malformations."[113] Another review concurs that "none of these drugs in normal dosages are proved teratogens to human fetuses,"[114] and finally, another study suggests "early treatment of the disease during gestation reverts its negative impact on perinatal outcome."[115]

Threat level: Very low

32. *Clostridium botulinum* (55 cases; 42 hospitalizations; 9 deaths)

Clostridium botulinum bacteria produce the most potent food-related toxin known to humans, which causes a serious paralytic illness known as botulism. Foodborne outbreaks of *Clostridium botulinum* are usually caused by foods being improperly canned at home. The classic symptoms of botulism include double vision, blurred vision, drooping eyelids, slurred speech, difficulty swallowing, dry mouth, and muscle weakness. If untreated, these symptoms may progress to cause paralysis and can ultimately be fatal.[116] Botulism is treated with an antitoxin that blocks the action of toxins circulating in the blood.[117] The most recent versions of the antitoxin have not been rated by the FDA for use in pregnancy, but case reports suggest no obvious ill effects.[118] Although there have been only a few documented cases of botulism in pregnancy, the effects on the fetus appear to be surprisingly minimal. According to one review, "Botulism is not known to cause any direct adverse effects on the pregnancy or the fetus" because the toxin molecule is too large to cross the placenta.[119]

Threat level: Very low

Notes

1. Scallan, E., Hoekstra, R. M., Angulo, F. J., Tauxe, R. V., Widdowson, M. A., Roy, S. L., Jones, J. L., & Griffin, P. M. (2011). Foodborne illness acquired in the United States—major pathogens. *Emerging Infectious Diseases, 17* (1). wwwnc.cdc.gov/eid/article/17/1/p1-1101_article.htm.

2. Smith, J. L. (1999). Foodborne infections during pregnancy. *Journal of Food Protection, 62* (7), 818–829. http://jfoodprotection.org/doi/pdf/10.4315/0362-028X-62.7.818?code=fopr-site.

3. Ludvigsson, J. (2001). Effect of gastroenteritis during pregnancy on neonatal outcome. *European Journal of Clinical Microbiology and Infectious Diseases, 20* (12), 843–849. www.ncbi.nlm.nih.gov/pubmed/11837634?dopt=Abstract.

4. Foodborne illness—frequently asked questions. (2005, January 10). US Centers for Disease Control and Prevention. https://stacks.cdc.gov/view/cdc/28126/Share.

5. Ibid.

6. Smith, J. L., Foodborne infections during pregnancy.

7. Roberts, C., & Wilkins, E. G. L. (1987). Salmonella screening of pregnant women. *Journal of Hospital Infection, 10* (1), 67–72.

8. Ault, K. A., Kennedy, M., Seoud, M. A. F., & Reiss, R. (1993). Maternal and neonatal infection with *Salmonella heidelberg*: a case report. *Infectious Diseases in Obstetrics and Gynecology, 1* (1), 46–48. https://www.hindawi.com/journals/idog/1993/623507/abs/.

9. *Salmonella*: diagnosis and treatment. (2015, March 9). Centers for Disease Control and Prevention. www.cdc.gov/salmonella/general/diagnosis.html.

10. US Food and Drug Administration. (2012). Bad bug book—foodborne pathogenic microorganisms and natural toxins. Second Edition. https://wayback.archive-it.org/7993/20170405001300/https://www.fda.gov/downloads/Food/FoodborneIllnessContaminants/UCM297627.pdf.

11. US Centers for Disease Control and Prevention, Foodborne illness—frequently asked questions.

12. National Center for Emerging and Zoonotic Infectious Diseases. (2014, June 3). Campylobacter. US Centers for Disease Control and Prevention. https://www.cdc.gov/campylobacter/index.html.

13. Smith, J. L., Foodborne infections during pregnancy.

14. Simor, A. E., Karmali, M. A., Jadavji, T., & Roscoe, M. (1986). Abortion and perinatal sepsis associated with campylobacter infection. *Review of Infectious Diseases, 8* (3), 397–402. https://academic.oup.com/cid/article-abstract/8/3/397/396030.

15. Simor, A. E., & Ferro, S. (1990). *Campylobacter jejuni* infection occurring during pregnancy. *European Journal of Clinical Microbiology and Infectious Diseases, 9* (2), 142–144.

16. Goh, J., & Flynn, M. (1992). *Campylobacter jejuni* in pregnancy. *Australian and New Zealand Journal of Obstetrics and Gynaecology, 32* (3), 246–248.

17. Youngs, E. R., & Roberts, C. (1985). Campylobacter carriage and pregnancy. *British Journal of Obstetrics and Gynaecology, 92* (5), 541–542.

18. Anders, B. J., Lauer, B. A., & Paisley, J. W. (1981). Campylobacter gastroenteritis in neonates. *American Journal of Diseases of Children, 135* (10), 900–902.

19. Youngs, E. R., Roberts, C., & Davidson, D. C. (1985). Campylobacter enteritis and bloody stools in the neonate. *Archives of Disease in Childhood, 60* (5), 480–481. http://adc.bmj.com/content/60/5/480.full.pdf.

20. Smith, J. L., Foodborne infections during pregnancy.

21. Bolik, A., Wissel, J., & Rolfs, A. (1995). Guillain-Barré syndrome in pregnancy—two case reports and a discussion on management. *Archives of Gynecology and Obstetrics, 256* (4), 199–203.

22. Luijckx, G. J., Vles, J., De Baets, M., Buchwald, B., & Tmost, J. (1997). Guillain-Barré syndrome in mother and newborn child. *The Lancet, 349* (9044), 27.

23. Rolfs, A., & Bolik, A. (1994). Guillain-Barré syndrome in pregnancy: reflections on immunopathogenesis. *Acta Neurologica Scandinavica, 89* (5), 400–402.

24. Staphylococcal food poisoning: frequently asked questions. (Last updated 2016, October 4). US Centers for Disease Control and Prevention. https://www.cdc.gov/foodsafety/diseases/staphylococcal.html.

25. *Shigella*: questions and answers. (Last updated 2017, October 12). US Centers for Disease Control and Prevention. www.cdc.gov/shigella/general-information.html.

26. Christopher, P. R., David, K. V., John, S. M., & Sankarapandian, V. (2010). Antibiotic therapy for Shigella dysentery. *Cochrane Database of Systematic Reviews 2010, 8* (CD006784). http://onlinelibrary.wiley.com/doi/10.1002/14651858.CD006784.pub4/full.

27. US Centers for Disease Control and Prevention, *Shigella*—shigellosis: questions and answers.

28. Schlecht, H. P., & Bruno, C. (2013, October). Fluoroquinolones. *Merck Manuals.* www.merckmanuals.com/professional/infectious_diseases/bacteria_and_antibacterial_drugs/fluoroquinolones.html.

29. Ceftriaxone (injection route). (2014, October 1). US National Library of Medicine, PubMed Health. www.ncbi.nlm.nih.gov/pubmedhealth/PMH0044878/.

30. Azithromycin (oral route). (2014, October 1). US National Library of Medicine, PubMed Health. www.ncbi.nlm.nih.gov/pubmedhealth/PMH0046181/.

31. Smith, J. L., Foodborne infections during pregnancy.

32. *E. coli*: general information. (Last updated 2015, November 6). US Centers for Disease Control and Prevention. www.cdc.gov/ecoli/general/.

33. Ibid.

34. *Yersinia enterocolitica*: questions and answers. (Last updated 2016, May 25). US Centers for Disease Control and Prevention. www.cdc.gov/yersinia/faq.html.

35. Schlecht, H. P., et al., Fluoroquinolones.

36. Schlecht, H. P., & Bruno, C. (2013, October). Aminoglycosides. *Merck Manuals.* www.merckmanuals.com/professional/infectious_diseases/bacteria_and_antibacterial_drugs/aminoglycosides.html.

37. Doxycycline (oral route). (2014, October 1). US National Library of Medicine, PubMed Health. www.ncbi.nlm.nih.gov/pubmedhealth/PMH0044904/.

38. Sulfamethoxazole/trimethoprim (oral route). (2014, October 1). US National Library of Medicine, PubMed Health. www.ncbi.nlm.nih.gov/pubmedhealth/PMH0045169/.

39. Smith, J. L., Foodborne infections during pregnancy.

40. Jones, J. L., Kruszon-Moran, D., Wilson, M., McQuillan, G., Navin, T., & McAuley, J. B. (2001). *Toxoplasma gondii* infection in the United States: seroprevalence and risk factors. *American Journal of Epidemiology, 154* (4), 357–365. http://courses.washington.edu/zepi526/Papers/Toxoplasma.pdf.

41. Smith, J. L., Foodborne infections during pregnancy.

42. Remington, J. S., McLeod, R., & Desmonts, S. G. (1995). Toxoplasmosis. In: Remington, J. S., & Klein, J. O. (1995). *Infectious diseases of the fetus and newborn infant*. Philadelphia: WB Saunders, 140–267.

43. Desmonts, G., & Couvreur, J. (1979). Congenital toxoplasmosis: a prospective study of the offspring of 542 women who acquired toxoplasmosis during pregnancy. In: Thalhammer, O., Pollak, A., & Baumgarten, K. (Eds.). Pathophysiology of congenital disease. *Perinatal Medicine*, Sixth European Congress, Stuttgart, Georg Thieme (51–60).

44. Buzby, J. C., & Roberts, T. (1996). ERS updates US foodborne disease costs for seven pathogens. *FoodReview, 19* (3), 20–25. https://www.researchgate.net/publication/246089508_ERS_Updates_US_Foodborne_Disease_Costs_for_Seven_Pathogens.

45. Hughes, J. M., Colley, D. G., Lopez, A., Dietz, V. J., Wilson, M., Navin, T. R., & Jones, J. L. (2000). Preventing congenital toxoplasmosis. *Morbidity and Mortality Weekly Report, 49* (RR02), 57–75. https://www.cdc.gov/mmWR/preview/mmwrhtml/rr4902a5.htm.

46. Hughes, J. M., et al., Preventing congenital toxoplasmosis.

The high estimate is based on two studies from the 1970s that screened 7,500 and 4,048 live births for *Toxoplasma gondii* and found an infection rate of 13 and 7 per 10,000 live births, respectively. The lower estimate is based on a study that was more recent and on a much larger scale: the New England Regional Newborn Screening Program screened 635,000 live births from 1986–1992 and found an infection rate of 1 per 10,000 live births.

47. Buzby, J. C., et al., ERS updates US foodborne disease costs for seven pathogens.

48. Goldenberg, R. L., & Thompson, C. (2003). The infectious origins of stillbirth. *American Journal of Obstetrics and Gynecology, 189* (3), 861–873. http://zoologia.biologia.uasnet.mx/protozoos/protozoa16.pdf.

49. Djurkovic-Djakovic, O. (1995). Toxoplasma infection and pathological outcome of pregnancy. *Gynecologic and Obstetric Investigation, 40* (1), 36–41.

50. Parasites—*Giardia*: general information. (2015, July 21). US Centers for Disease Control and Prevention. https://www.cdc.gov/parasites/giardia/general-info.html.

51. Diseases and conditions: *Giardia* infection (giardiasis). (2015, October 13). Mayo Clinic. www.mayoclinic.com/health/giardia-infection/DS00739/DSECTION=treatments-and-drugs.

52. Smith, J. L., Foodborne infections during pregnancy.

No increased susceptibility; disease may be more severe in pregnancy.

53. US Centers for Disease Control and Prevention, Parasites—*Giardia*: general information.

54. Stenfors Arnesen, L. P., Fagerlund, A., & Granum, P. E. (2008). From soil to gut: *Bacillus cereus* and its food poisoning toxins. *FEMS Microbiology Reviews, 32* (4), 579–606. http://onlinelibrary.wiley.com/doi/10.1111/j.1574-6976.2008.00112.x/full.

55. Ibid.

56. Guinebretière, M. H., & Broussolle, V. (2002). Enterotoxigenic profiles of food-poisoning and food-borne *Bacillus cereus* strains. *Journal of Clinical Microbiology, 40* (8), 3053–3056. http://jcm.asm.org/content/40/8/3053.full.

57. Stenfors Arnesen, L. P., et al., From soil to gut: *Bacillus cereus* and its food poisoning toxins.

58. Workowski, K. A., & Flaherty, J. P. (1992). Systemic *Bacillus* species infection mimicking listeriosis of pregnancy. *Clinical Infectious Diseases, 14* (3), 694–696. http://cid.oxfordjournals.org/content/14/3/694.short.

59. US Centers for Disease Control and Prevention, *E. coli*: general information.

60. Ibid.

61. Tserenpuntsag, B., Chang, H. G., Smith, P. F., & Morse, D. L. (2005). Hemolytic uremic syndrome risk and *Escherichia coli* O157:H7. *Emerging Infectious Diseases, 11* (12), 1955–1957. http://europepmc.org/articles/PMC3367638.

62. Dashe, J. S., Ramin, S. M., & Cunningham, F. G. (1998). The long-term consequences of thrombotic microangiopathy (thrombotic thrombocytopenic purpura and hemolytic uremic syndrome) in pregnancy. *Obstetrics & Gynecology, 91* (5, Part 1), 662–668. www.sciencedirect.com/science/article/pii/S0029784498000313.

63. Egerman, R. S., Witlin, A. G., Friedman, S. A., & Sibai, B. M. (1996). Thrombotic thrombocytopenic purpura and hemolytic uremic syndrome in pregnancy: review of 11 cases. *American Journal of Obstetrics and Gynecology, 175* (4), 950–956. www.sciencedirect.com/science/article/pii/S0002937896800305.

64. Martinez-Roman, S., Gratacos, E., Torne, A., Torra, R., Carmona, F., & Cararach, V. (1996). Successful pregnancy in a patient with hemolytic-uremic syndrome during the second trimester of pregnancy: a case report. *Journal of Reproductive Medicine, 41* (3), 211–214. http://cat.inist.fr/?aModele=afficheN&cpsidt=3030496.

65. Parasites: *Cryptosporidium* (also known as "Crypto"). (Last updated 2017, January 12). US Centers for Disease Control and Prevention. https://www.cdc.gov/parasites/crypto/index.html.

66. Ibid.

67. Smith, J. L., Foodborne infections during pregnancy.

68. *Vibrio* species causing vibriosis: questions and answers. (Last updated 2017, August 31). US Centers for Disease Control and Prevention. https://www.cdc.gov/vibrio/faq.html.

69. Enterotoxigenic *Escherichia coli* (ETEC): frequently asked questions. (Last updated 2014, December 1). US Centers for Disease Control and Prevention. https://www.cdc.gov/ecoli/etec.html.

70. Ibid.

71. US Food and Drug Administration, Bad bug book—foodborne pathogenic microorganisms and natural toxins.

72. Hamborsky, J., Kroger, A., & Wolfe, S., (eds.), & the US Centers for Disease Control and Prevention. (2015). Chapter 19: Rotavirus. *Epidemiology and prevention of vaccine-preventable diseases: the pink book.* Washington, DC: Public Health Foundation, 311–324. https://www.cdc.gov/vaccines/pubs/pinkbook/downloads/rota.pdf.

73. Parashar, U. D., Alexander, J. P., Glass, R. I., & the Department of Health & Human Services, Centers for Disease Control and Prevention. (2006). Prevention of rotavirus gastroenteritis among infants and children: recommendations of the Advisory Committee on Immunization Practices (ACIP). *Morbidity and Mortality Weekly Report, 55* (RR12), 1–13. www.cdc.gov/mmwr/preview/mmwrhtml/rr5512a1.htm?s_cid=rr5512a1_e.

74. Ibid.

75. Chiba, S., Nakata, S., Numata-Kinoshita, K., & Honma, S. (2000). Sapporo virus: history and recent findings. *Journal of Infectious Diseases, 181* (Supplement 2), S303–S308. http://jid.oxfordjournals.org/content/181/Supplement_2/S303.long.

76. Pang, X. L., Honma, S., Nakata, S., & Vesikari, T. (2000). Human caliciviruses in acute gastroenteritis of young children in the community. *Journal of Infectious Diseases, 181* (Supplement 2), S288–S294. http://jid.oxfordjournals.org/content/181/Supplement_2/S288.full.

77. Feng, P., Weagant, S. D., & Jinneman, K. (Last updated 2017, October). Chapter 4A:

Diarrheagenic *Escherichia coli.* In: *Bacteriological analytical manual.* (2011, February). US Food and Drug Administration. www.fda.gov/Food/FoodScienceResearch/LaboratoryMethods/ucm070080.htm.

78. Parasites—cyclosporiasis (*Cyclospora* infection): disease. (2013, January 10). US Centers for Disease Control and Prevention. www.cdc.gov/parasites/cyclosporiasis/disease.html.

79. Parasites—cyclosporiasis (*Cyclospora* infection): cyclosporiasis FAQs for health professionals. (2014, June 13). US Centers for Disease Control and Prevention. www.cdc.gov/parasites/cyclosporiasis/health_professionals/hp-faqs.html.

80. Parasites—cyclosporiasis (*Cyclospora* infection): treatment. (2013, January 10). US Centers for Disease Control and Prevention. www.cdc.gov/parasites/cyclosporiasis/treatment.html.

81. Group A streptococcal (GAS) disease: strep throat—complications. (2016, September 16). US Centers for Disease Control and Prevention. https://www.cdc.gov/groupastrep/diseases-public/strep-throat.html#complications.

82. Strep throat during pregnancy. (Last updated 2017, February 16). American Pregnancy Association. http://americanpregnancy.org/pregnancycomplications/strep-throat-during-pregnancy/.

83. FDA pregnancy categories. (2014). Drugs.com. www.drugs.com/pregnancy-categories.html.

84. Typhoid fever: symptoms and treatment. (2013, May 14). US Centers for Disease Control and Prevention. www.cdc.gov/typhoid-fever/symptoms.html.

85. Mohanty, S., Gaind, R., Sehgal, R., Chellani, H., & Deb, M. (2009). Neonatal sepsis due to *Salmonella* typhi and paratyphi A. *The Journal of Infection in Developing Countries, 3* (08), 633–638. http://jidc.org/index.php/journal/article/viewFile/19801808/292.

86. Hasbun, J., Osorio, R., & Hasbun, A. (2006). Hepatic dysfunction in typhoid fever during pregnancy. *Infectious Diseases in Obstetrics and Gynecology, 2006* (64828), 1–2. www.ncbi.nlm.nih.gov/pmc/articles/PMC1581472/.

87. Buongiorno, R., & Schiraldi, O. (1984). Treatment of typhoid fever in pregnancy. *Chemioterapia: International Journal of the Mediterranean Society of Chemotherapy, 3* (2), 136. www.ncbi.nlm.nih.gov/pubmed/6335838.

88. Sulaiman, K., & Sarwari, A. R. (2007). Culture-confirmed typhoid fever and pregnancy. *International Journal of Infectious Diseases, 11* (4), 337–341. www.sciencedirect.com/science/article/pii/S1201971206001871.

89. Pregnant or older? Be safe with ready-to-eat meats. (2011). US Centers for Disease Control and Prevention. https://www.cdc.gov/media/matte/2011/05_listeriapregnant.pdf.

90. Mylonakis, E., Paliou, M., Hohmann, E. L., Calderwood, S. B., & Wing, E. J. (2002). Listeriosis during pregnancy: a case series and review of 222 cases. *Medicine, 81* (4), 260–269.

91. Roberts, T., & Pinner, R. (1990). Economic impact of disease caused by *Listeria monocytogenes.* In: Miller, A. J., Smith, J. L., and Somkuti, G. A. (eds). *Topics in industrial microbiology: foodborne listeriosis.* New York: Elsevier Science Pub, 137–149.

92. Viral hepatitis: hepatitis A questions and answers for the public. (Last updated 2017, November 2). US Centers for Disease Control and Prevention. https://www.cdc.gov/hepatitis/hav/afaq.htm.

93. Ibid.

94. Smith, J. L., Foodborne infections during pregnancy.

95. Elinav, E., Ben-Dov, I. Z., Shapira, Y., Daudi, N., Adler, R., Shouval, D., & Ackerman, Z. (2006). Acute hepatitis A infection in pregnancy is associated with high rates of gestational complications and preterm labor. *Gastroenterology, 130* (4), 1129–1134. www.sciencedirect.com/science/article/pii/S0016508506000084.

96. Brucellosis: signs and symptoms. (2012, November 12). US Centers for Disease Control and Prevention. https://www.cdc.gov/brucellosis/symptoms/index.html.

97. Smith, J. L., Foodborne infections during pregnancy.

98. Khan, M. Y., Mah, M. W., & Memish, Z. A. (2001). Brucellosis in pregnant women. *Clinical Infectious Diseases, 32* (8), 1172–1177. http://cid.oxfordjournals.org/content/32/8/1172.short.

99. Ibid.

100. Brucellosis: risks for expecting mothers. (2012, November 12). US Centers for Disease Control and Prevention. www.cdc.gov/brucellosis/exposure/expecting-mothers.html.

101. Brucellosis: treatment. (2012, November 12). US Centers for Disease Control and Prevention. www.cdc.gov/brucellosis/treatment/index.html.

102. US National Library of Medicine, Doxycycline (oral route).

103. Rifampin pregnancy and breastfeeding warnings. (2014). Drugs.com. www.drugs.com/pregnancy/rifampin.html.

104. Parasites—trichinellosis (also known as trichinosis): trichinellosis FAQs. (2012, August 8). US Centers for Disease Control and Prevention. www.cdc.gov/parasites/trichinellosis/gen_info/faqs.html.

105. Parasites—trichinellosis (also known as trichinosis): resources for health professionals, treatment. (2018, January 9). US Centers for Disease Control and Prevention. www.cdc.gov/parasites/trichinellosis/health_professionals/index.html#tx.

106. Smith, J. L., Foodborne infections during pregnancy.

107. Bruschi, F., Dupouy-Camet, J., Kociecka, W., Pozio, E., & Bolas-Fernandez, F. (2002). Opinion on the diagnosis and treatment of human trichinellosis. *Expert Opinion on Pharmacotherapy, 3* (8), 1117–1130. http://www.tandfonline.com/doi/abs/10.1517/14656566.3.8.1117.

108. Nuñez, G. G., Costantino, S. N., Gentile, T., & Venturiello, S. M. (2008). Immunoparasitological evaluation of *Trichinella spiralis* infection during human pregnancy: a small case series. *Transactions of the Royal Society of Tropical Medicine and Hygiene, 102* (7), 662–668. www.sciencedirect.com/science/article/pii/S0035920308001077.

109. Dubinsky, P., Böör, A., Kincekova, J., Tomasovicova, O., Reiterova, K., & Bielik, P. (2001). Congenital trichinellosis? Case report. *Parasite, 8* (2), S180–S182. http://europepmc.org/abstract/med/11484349.

110. Taybouavone, T., Hai, T. N., Odermatt, P., Keoluangkhot, V., Delanos-Gregoire, N., Dupouy-Camet, J., Strobel, M., & Barennes, H. (2009). Trichinellosis during pregnancy: a case control study in the Lao Peoples' Democratic Republic. *Veterinary Parasitology, 159* (3), 332–336. www.sciencedirect.com/science/article/pii/S0304401708005889X.

111. US Centers for Disease Control and Prevention, Parasites—trichinellosis (also known as trichinosis): resources for health professionals, treatment.

112. Tuberculosis (TB): fact sheets. (2012, September 1). US Centers for Disease Control and Prevention. www.cdc.gov/tb/publications/factsheets/general/mbovis.htm.

113. Bothamley, G. (2001). Drug treatment for tuberculosis during pregnancy. *Drug Safety, 24* (7), 553–565. http://link.springer.com/article/10.2165/00002018-200124070-00006#.

114. De Snider, J., Layde, P. M., Johnson, M. W., & Lyle, M. A. (1980). Treatment of tuberculosis during pregnancy. *American Review of Respiratory Disease, 122* (1), 65–79. www.atsjournals.org/doi/abs/10.1164/arrd.1980.122.1.65.

115. Figueroa-Damian, R., & Arredondo-Garcia, J. L. (1998). Pregnancy and tuberculosis: influence of treatment on perinatal outcome. *American Journal of Perinatology, 15* (05), 303–306. www.thieme-connect.com/products/ejournals/html/10.1055/s-2007-993948.

116. Botulism. (Last updated 2017, October 25). US Centers for Disease Control and Prevention. https://www.cdc.gov/botulism/.

117. US Centers for Disease Control and Prevention, Botulism.

118. Botulism antitoxin pregnancy and breastfeeding warnings. (2014). Drugs.com. www.drugs.com/pregnancy/botulism-antitoxin.html.

119. Morrison, G. A., Lang, C., & Huda, S. (2006). Botulism in a pregnant intravenous drug abuser. *Anaesthesia, 61* (1), 57–60. http://onlinelibrary.wiley.com/doi/10.1111/j.1365-2044.2005.04434.x/full.

APPENDIX V

Pesticides

*I*n this book, I've focused attention on organophosphate pesticides, as this class of pesticide is both commonly used and definitively linked to problems in pregnancy and therefore is the most pressing threat. However, I arrived at this conclusion only after working through the full list of pesticides in use in the United States.

The most recent data on pesticide usage come from the EPA, which has published a document entitled "Pesticides Industry Sales and Usage 2006 and 2007 Market Estimates."[1] This document provides estimates of the annual volumes of the most commonly used pesticide active ingredients in the Agricultural, Home and Garden, and Industry/Commercial/Government sectors. I added up the volumes from these three sectors and took the average of the high and low estimates. Each of the pesticides is listed below in descending order, with the annual volume in number of pounds provided in parentheses.

Some categories of pesticide are more likely to cause risks to human health than others. For example, herbicides are aimed at killing weeds—i.e., plants—often through mechanisms like inhibiting photosynthesis, so these are less likely than insecticides to have an effect on humans.

Glyphosate (203 million pounds) is the active ingredient in the popular weed killer Roundup and a variety of other herbicides. A recent review of its effects during pregnancy "found no consistent effects of glyphosate exposure on reproductive health or the developing offspring. Furthermore, no plausible mechanisms of action for such effects were elucidated."[2]

Atrazine (78m pounds) is a member of the triazine family of herbicides, and the EPA's cumulative risk assessment for triazines has concluded that the main cause for concern is contamination of drinking water in farming communities.[3] In such communities, there is some evidence that Atrazine may increase the risk of babies being small for gestational age. For example, a study of women in Iowa showed that those who were most heavily exposed to herbicides in their drinking water had almost double the risk of having a child with intrauterine growth retardation,[4] and a study in Indiana looking at data on 24,000 births found that high levels of Atrazine in drinking water during the third trimester caused an ~18 percent increase in the likelihood of having a child small for its gestational age.[5] Atrazine could also potentially cause birth defects in very high doses: according to the CDC, "Chronic high dose toxicity observed in animals includes developmental ossification defects." But the CDC caveats that "estimated human exposures are thousands of times lower than doses that caused effects in animals."[6]

2,4-D (62m) is an herbicide used to control weeds with broad leaves. According to the EPA, 2,4-D did appear to have developmental effects in one study in rats, where "fetal effects (skeletal abnormalities) were observed at a dose level that produced less severe maternal toxicity (decreased bodyweight gain and food consumption)." But similar developmental toxicity studies in rabbits or two generations of rats showed no effect. The EPA has therefore concluded that after applying appropriate uncertainty factors, "the Agency has no residual concerns for the effects seen in the developmental toxicity studies." The only caveat is that "a developmental neurotoxicity study in the rat is required for 2,4-D."[7]

Metam sodium (55m) is a soil fumigant, which is applied to the soil prior to planting crops to control soilborne pests. The California Environmental Protection Agency has evaluated the developmental effects of metam sodium based on the results of six animal studies.[8] One study of the six concluded that "the embryo/fetus may be more sensitive to the toxic effects of metam sodium." Fortunately, the agency also caveated that "exposure of the general public to metam sodium was not anticipated" based on an assessment by the Department of Pesticide Regulation. And the EPA agrees that risks are limited to "handlers, workers, and bystanders who live and work near agricultural fields and greenhouses."[9]

When metam sodium is applied, it breaks down into another product called methyl isothiocyanate, or MITC. Fortunately, according to the California Environmental Protection Agency, "MITC was not considered a developmental toxicant because doses which affected fetal parameters were associated with maternal toxicity." However, according to the EPA, further study is required to ensure there are no developmental effects: a "two generation reproduction study in rat via inhalation with pathological evaluation of the complete respiratory tract in offspring is needed."[10]

Metolachlor-S (32.5m) is an herbicide that inhibits plant protein synthesis. According to the CDC in its National Report on Human Exposure to Environmental Chemicals, although the "general population exposure may occur through the consumption of contaminated food or drinking water"; in fact "urinary levels of metolachlor mercapturate were generally not detectable in the NHANES 2001–2002 subsample" and furthermore "metolachlor did not show developmental or reproductive toxicity in chronic animal studies."[11]

Acetochlor (30.5m) is an herbicide. According to a CDC Biomonitoring Summary, "Acetochlor has not shown developmental or fetal toxicity in chronic animal studies" and "urinary levels of acetochlor mercapturate [which reflect recent exposure] were generally not detectable in the NHANES 2001–2002 subsample."[12]

Dichloropropene (29.5m) is a fumigant, or gaseous pesticide. According to the CDC, "we do not know whether dichloropropenes can cause birth defects in humans. Pregnant rats that inhaled 1,3-dichloropropene gave birth to fewer pups or pups with lower body weight," but "this occurred at exposures high enough to be toxic to the mothers."[13] It's also unclear how likely we are to be exposed to this pesticide. According to the CDC, "1,1-dichloropropene has been detected in drinking water. However, it was found in only 0.01 percent of samples collected nationwide; therefore, exposure to this substance via drinking water is expected to be very low. . . . Individuals with the greatest potential for exposure to 1,3-dichloropropene include bystanders and residents located near fields treated with this fumigant who may inhale 1,3-dichloropropene that has volatilized into the air [EPA 1998]. . . . Although human exposure to these substances is not expected to be important, information would be helpful in verifying this."[14]

Pendimethalin (15m) is an herbicide used to control grasses and certain leafy weeds. According to the EPA, testing in rats showed "no maternal or developmental effects noted at any dose level tested."[15]

Methyl bromide (13m) is a fumigant and pesticide that is highly toxic to humans; direct inhalation can cause severe lung damage. Fortunately, there appears to be little risk during pregnancy. According to the EPA, "Information from animal studies suggest that methyl bromide does not cause birth defects and does not interfere with normal reproduction except at high exposure levels. . . . Inhalation exposure of animals during gestation has not resulted in significant developmental effects, even when there was severe maternal toxicity."[16]

Chlorothalonil (12m) is a fungicide and mildewcide. According to the EPA, "No developmental toxicity was observed at any dose level in a rabbit study, and no maternal toxicity was observed at the highest dose tested. No reproductive effects were observed in any study, and developmental effects occurred only in the presence of significant maternal toxicity."[17]

Chloropicrin (10m) is a pesticide used to clean soil of fungi, microbes, insects, and other pests prior to planting. According to the CDC, "It is unknown whether chronic or repeated exposure to chloropicrin can cause developmental or reproductive toxicity."[18]

Ethephon (8m) is an organophosphate pesticide, the class of pesticide that is discussed in detail in the "Poisonous Produce" section.

Metam potassium (8m) is a soil fumigant applied prior to planting crops to control soilborne pests. Metam potassium has been evaluated jointly by the EPA with the closely related fumigant metam sodium, discussed above, as it also breaks down into MITC, also discussed previously.

Chlorpyrifos (8m) is an organophosphate pesticide, the class of pesticide discussed in detail in the "Poisonous Produce" section.

Trifluralin (8m) is an herbicide. According to the EPA, two animal studies have suggested "no teratogenic effects occurred in rats or rabbits"[19] exposed to trifluralin, and in those studies negative effects were seen only in fetuses at doses higher than those that affected the mothers.

Copper hydroxide (7m) is a fungicide. Fortunately, according to the EPA, "available reproductive and developmental studies by the oral route of exposure generally indicate that the main concern in animals for reproductive and teratogenic effects of copper has usually been associated with the deficiency rather than the excess of copper. Current available data in animals do not show any evidence of upper limit toxicity level."[20]

Simazine (6m) is a member of the triazine family of herbicides, and the EPA's cumulative risk assessment for triazines has concluded that the main cause for concern is contamination of drinking water in farming communities.[21]

Diuron (6m), the trade name of a chemical called DCMU, is an herbicide that inhibits photosynthesis. According to the EPA, this chemical is unlikely to pose any risks during pregnancy: "In a developmental toxicity study in rabbits, there were no developmental effects at the highest dose tested. In the developmental toxicity study in rabbits and in the 2-generation rat reproduction study, developmental/

offspring effects were observed only at maternally/parentally toxic dose levels."[22]

Propanil (5m) is an herbicide. According to the EPA, "the weight-of-evidence supports a receptor-mediated rather than a neurologically-mediated endocrine mode of action. On that basis, it was concluded that a developmental neurotoxicity study was not needed for propanil."[23]

Mancozeb (5m) is a fungicide. Based on the results of animal testing, there is little concern regarding mancozeb itself during pregnancy. According to the EPA, "in the rat developmental study, developmental effects were observed in the presence of severe maternal effects. In the rabbit developmental study, developmental effects (spontaneous abortions) were observed at the same dose at which maternal effects included mortality and clinical signs. In the rat reproduction study, no effects were observed in offspring, while thyroid effects and body weight gain decrements occurred in adults." However, mancozeb's metabolite and environmental degradate, ethylene thiourea (ETU), may be of concern. Again, according to the EPA, the effects on fetuses from ETU "occurred at a dose associated only with decreased maternal food consumption and body weight gain but not with significant maternal toxicity." As a result, the EPA has specified that "a developmental neurotoxicity study with ETU will be required." In the meantime, the EPA does not seem overly concerned about the potential for exposure, stating that "mancozeb dietary risks from food and drinking water sources are low and not of concern" and that "mancozeb risks as a result of residential or recreational exposures are of concern for toddlers" but "risks to toddlers are being mitigated with a pre-harvest interval requirement."[24]

Carbaryl (5m) is an insecticide sold under the brand name Sevin, which does not appear to present any specific risk during pregnancy. The Food and Agriculture Organization of the United Nations concluded based on existing animal studies that "carbaryl induces developmental toxicity, manifested as deaths in utero, reduced fetal weight, and malformations, but only at doses that cause overt maternal toxicity."[25]

MCPP (5m) is a common herbicide, otherwise known as methylchlorophenoxypropionic acid, mecoprop, or MCPP-p (MCPP-p is the active isomer in MCPP, which can now be produced in more pure form). According to the EPA, "there is no evidence of developmental toxicity by dermal routes of exposure," and according to the material data safety sheet issued by Bayer for its Advanced Season Long Weed Control for Lawns, "MCPP-p was not a primary developmental toxicant in rats and rabbits. Developmental effects were observed in rats but were considered secondary to maternal toxicity."[26, 27]

Malathion (5m) is an organophosphate pesticide, the class of pesticide discussed in detail in the "Poisonous Produce" section.

Aldicarb (3.5m) is an insecticide that may pose risks to the health of a fetus. According to the EPA, as of October 2010:

> EPA and Bayer CropScience, the manufacturer, have reached an agreement to end use of the pesticide aldicarb in the United States.... In EPA's August 4, 2010 risk assessment, the Agency concludes that aggregate dietary (food and drinking water) exposure reflecting the current uses of aldicarb exceeds the Agency's level of concern for infants, children ages 1–2, and children ages 3–5.... To address the most significant risks, Bayer has agreed to first end aldicarb use on citrus and potatoes, and will adopt risk mitigation measures for other uses to protect groundwater resources. The company will voluntarily phase out production of aldicarb by December 31, 2014. All remaining aldicarb uses will end no later than August 2018.... During the phase-out, aldicarb will continue to be registered for use on cotton, dry beans, peanuts, soybeans, sugar beets, and sweet potatoes.[28]

Unfortunately, the detailed risk assessment conducted by the EPA is currently unavailable online, so it's unclear if aldicarb poses a specific risk during pregnancy and, if so, what the magnitude of that risk might be.[29] But for the next several years, the continued use of aldicarb on foods may provide another reason to go organic during pregnancy, and its continued presence in groundwater may represent yet another threat that we unfortunately cannot control.

Acephate (3m) is an organophosphate pesticide, the class of pesticide discussed in detail in the "Poisonous Produce" section.

MCPA (3m) is an herbicide. According to the EPA, there's no evidence of developmental toxicity except in one study of susceptibility following in-utero exposure to rats. The Agency therefore concludes that "a developmental neurotoxicity study is necessary," but the Agency believes that "the regulatory endpoints are protective of children despite the need for a DNT study."[30]

Paraquat (3m) is an herbicide. According to the EPA, two animal studies both have indicated that Paraquat poses no significant risks in pregnancy: "In the first study, no developmental effects were found.... In the second study, maternal toxicity was reported at the two highest doses . . . and developmental effects were observed only in the mid-dose and high-dose groups."[31]

Dimethanamid (3m) is an herbicide that appears to represent no threat to pregnancy. According to a registration document submitted to the EPA, "Developmental toxicity studies in rat and rabbit demonstrated no effects on progeny below the maternal lowest effect level."[32]

Pyrethroids (3m) are the active ingredients in many common household insecticides, such as Anvil® and Biomist®. According to the EPA, they pose little risk to human health in general: "Not only does the Agency believe that there are no cumulative estimated risks of concern for the currently registered uses, the Agency also concludes that there is sufficient room in the pyrethroid cumulative risk cup to support consideration of new pyrethroids."[33] However, in their cumulative risk assessment, the EPA cites a review suggesting that there is still uncertainty over the developmental effects of pyrethroids. This review points out that "neonatal rats are at least an order of magnitude more sensitive than adults to two pyrethroids," although cautioning that "to better understand the potential for developmental exposure to pyrethroids to cause neurotoxicity, additional well-designed and well-executed developmental neurotoxicity studies are needed."[34] Furthermore, piperonyl butoxide, a chemical frequently added to pyrethroid insecticides to increase their efficacy, appears to cause developmental effects in preliminary studies.[35, 36] Therefore, the jury remains out on this class of insecticide.

MSMA (3m) is an herbicide that appears to represent no threat to pregnancy. According to the EPA, "Results of developmental and reproductive toxicity studies provided no indication of increased susceptibility."[37]

Triclopyr (3m) is an herbicide that appears to represent no threat to pregnancy. According to the EPA, "The developmental and reproductive data for triclopyr indicate that developmental and reproductive effects occurred only at doses that are the same as or higher than doses which caused maternal or parental effects."[38]

Copper sulfate (3m) is a fungicide. Fortunately, according to the EPA, "available reproductive and developmental studies by the oral route of exposure generally indicate that the main concern in animals for reproductive and teratogenic effects of copper has usually been associated with the deficiency rather than the excess of copper. Current available data in animals do not show any evidence of upper limit toxicity level."[39]

Dicamba (2m) is an herbicide. According to the EPA, it poses little risk during pregnancy: "Developmental studies were conducted on both rats and rabbits, following in-utero and/or prenatal exposure to dicamba. No evidence of increased susceptibility was observed. In addition, no evidence of developmental anomalies of the fetal nervous system were observed in the prenatal developmental toxicity studies in either rats or rabbits at maternally toxic doses of up to 300 or 400 mg/kg/day. Also, no evidence of behavioral or neurological effects on the offspring was observed in the two-generation reproduction study in rats."[40]

Sulfuryl fluoride (2m) is an insecticide used to control insects in stored grains, dried fruits, tree nuts, coffee, and cocoa beans. According to the California Department of Pesticide Regulation, in animal studies, the effects of sulfuryl fluoride on fetuses were seen only at levels that also caused maternal effects, although there hasn't yet been a developmental neurotoxicity study.[41] However, as of 2016, the EPA is considering phasing out use of sulfuryl fluoride anyway, because it breaks down into fluoride: "Although sulfuryl fluoride residues in food contribute only a very small portion of total exposure to fluoride, when combined with other fluoride exposure pathways, including drinking water and toothpaste, EPA has concluded that the tolerance no longer meets the safety standard under the Federal Food, Drug, and Cosmetic Act. . . . EPA is proposing to phase out uses of sulfuryl fluoride over a period of three years."[42]

Notes

1. Grube, A., Donaldson, D., Kiely, T., & Wu, L. (2011). Pesticides industry sales and usage. US Environmental Protection Agency. https://www.epa.gov/sites/production/files/2015-10/documents/market_estimates2007.pdf.

2. Williams, A. L., Watson, R. E., & DeSesso, J. M. (2012). Developmental and reproductive outcomes in humans and animals after glyphosate exposure: a critical analysis. *Journal of Toxicology and Environmental Health, Part B, 15* (1), 39–96. www.tandfonline.com/doi/abs/10.1080/10937404.2012.632361.

3. Triazine cumulative risk assessment. (2006, March 28). US Environmental Protection Agency. http://itrcweb.org/FileCabinet/GetFile?fileID=6880.

4. Munger, R., Isacson, P., Hu, S., Burns, T., Hanson, J., Lynch, C. F., Cherryholmes, K., Van Dorpe, P., & Hausler Jr, W. J. (1997). Intrauterine growth retardation in Iowa communities with herbicide-contaminated drinking water supplies. *Environmental Health Perspectives, 105* (3), 308. https://www.ncbi.nlm.nih.gov/pmc/articles/PMC1470002/.

5. Ochoa-Acuña, H., Frankenberger, J., Hahn, L., & Carbajo, C. (2009). Drinking-water herbicide exposure in Indiana and prevalence of small-for-gestational-age and preterm delivery. *Environmental Health Perspectives, 117* (10), 1619–1624. https://www.ncbi.nlm.nih.gov/pmc/articles/PMC2790519/.

6. Fourth national report on human exposure to environmental chemicals. (2009). US Centers for Disease Control and Prevention, Atlanta, GA. https://www.cdc.gov/exposurereport/pdf/FourthReport.pdf.

7. Reregistration eligibility decision for 2, 4-D. (2005). US Environmental Protection Agency. https://archive.epa.gov/pesticides/reregistration/web/pdf/24d_red.pdf.

8. Rubin, A. L. (2004). Metam sodium (sodium n-methyldithiocarbamate) risk characterization document. Medical Toxicology Branch, Department of Pesticide Regulation, California Environmental Protection Agency, 1–120. www.cdpr.ca.gov/docs/risk/rcd/metam.pdf.

9. Reregistration eligibility decision (RED) for methyldithiocarbamate salts—metam sodium/potassium and MITC. (2008, July 9). US Environmental Protection Agency, Office of Pesticide Programs. https://nepis.epa.gov/Exe/ZyPDF.cgi/P1000VXU.PDF?Dockey=P1000VXU.PDF.

10. Amended reregistration eligibility decision (RED) for the methyldithiocarbamate salts (metamsodium, metam-potassium) and methyl isothiocyanate (MITC). (2009, May). US Environmental Protection Agency. https://nepis.epa.gov/Exe/ZyPDF.cgi/P1004V9Z.PDF?Dockey=P1004V9Z.PDF.

11. Centers for Disease Control and Prevention, Fourth national report on human exposure to environmental chemicals.

12. National Biomonitoring Program, biomonitoring summary: acetochlor. (2014, December 4). US Centers for Disease Control and Prevention. www.cdc.gov/biomonitoring/Acetochlor_BiomonitoringSummary.html.

13. Agency for Toxic Substances & Disease Registry. (2008, September). Toxic substances portal—dichloropropenes: ToxFAQs for dichloropropenes. US Centers for Disease Control and Prevention. www.atsdr.cdc.gov/toxfaqs/tf.asp?id=835&tid=163.

14. Agency for Toxic Substances & Disease Registry. (2008, September). Toxicological profile for dichloropropenes. US Centers for Disease Control and Prevention. https://www.atsdr.cdc.gov/toxprofiles/tp.asp?id=836&tid=163.

15. Rate, Deborah. (2007, August 22). Pendimethalin: human health risk assessment for the proposed food uses of the herbicide on artichoke, globe; asparagus; *Brassica* head and stem vegetables, subgroup 5A; and grape (PP#6E7129). US Environmental Protection Agency. http://citeseerx.ist.psu.edu/viewdoc/download?doi=10.1.1.168.6162&rep=rep1&type=pdf.

16. Methyl bromide (bromomethane). (2000, January). US Environmental Protection Agency. https://www.epa.gov/sites/production/files/2016-09/documents/methyl-bromide.pdf.

17. R.E.D. Facts: chlorothalonil pesticide reregistration. (1999, April). US Environmental Protection Agency. https://archive.epa.gov/pesticides/reregistration/web/pdf/0097fact.pdf.

18. The Emergency Response Safety and Health Database. (2014, October 7). Chloropicrin (PS): lung damaging agent. US Centers for Disease Control and Prevention. www.cdc.gov/niosh/ershdb/EmergencyResponseCard_29750034.html.

19. Reregistration eligibility decision (RED): trifluralin. (1996, April). US Environmental Protection Agency. https://nepis.epa.gov/Exe/ZyPDF.cgi/20000IVJ.PDF?Dockey=20000IVJ.PDF.

20. Reregistration eligibility decision (RED) for coppers. (2009, May). US Environmental Protection Agency. https://nepis.epa.gov/Exe/ZyPDF.cgi/P1004513.PDF?Dockey=P1004513.PDF.

21. Triazine cumulative risk assessment. (2006, March 28). US Environmental Protection Agency. http://itrcweb.org/FileCabinet/GetFile?fileID=6880.

22. Reregistration eligibility decision (RED) for diuron. (2003, September 30). US Environmental Protection Agency. https://archive.epa.gov/pesticides/reregistration/web/pdf/diuron_red-2.pdf.

23. Amendment to reregistration eligibility decision (RED) for propanil (March 2006) and the propanil RED (September 2003). (2006, March). US Environmental Protection Agency. https://archive.epa.gov/pesticides/reregistration/web/pdf/propanil_red_combined.pdf.

24. Reregistration eligibility decision for mancozeb. (2005, September). US Environmental Protection Agency. https://archive.epa.gov/pesticides/reregistration/web/pdf/mancozeb_red.pdf.

25. 4.4 Carbaryl (008) (T). (n.d.). FAO Corporate Document Repository. www.fao.org/docrep/w3727e/w3727e0a.htm.

26. Reregistration eligibility decision (RED) for mecoprop-p (mcpp). (2007, August 29). US Environmental Protection Agency. https://archive.epa.gov/pesticides/reregistration/web/pdf/mcpp_red.pdf.

27. Material safety data sheet: Bayer Advanced Season Long Weed Control for Lawns concentrate. (2005, December 5). Bayer Environmental Science. http://www.kellysolutions.com/erenewals/documentsubmit/KellyData%5CAK%5Cpesticide%5CMSDS%5C72155%5C72155-87%5C72155-87_Bayer_Advanced_Season_Long_Weed_Control_for_Lawns_Concentrate_7_16_2009_5_50_04_PM.pdf.

28. Pesticides: reregistration—agreement to terminate all uses of aldicarb. (2010, October). US Environmental Protection Agency. https://archive.epa.gov/pesticides/reregistration/web/html/aldicarb_fs.html.

29. Office of Chemical Safety and Pollution Prevention. (2010, August 4). Aldicarb: revised acute probabilistic aggregate dietary (food and drinking water) exposure and risk assessment incorporating revised FQPA factor. US Environmental Protection Agency. www.beyondpesticides.org/documents/Aldicarb%20Revised%20Dietary%20Risk%20Assessment.pdf.

30. Reregistration eligibility decision (RED) for MCPA (2-methyl-4-chlorophenoxyacetic acid) List A Case 0017. (2004, September 30). US Environmental Protection Agency. https://archive.epa.gov/pesticides/reregistration/web/pdf/mcpa_red.pdf.

31. Reregistration eligibility decision (RED), paraquat dichloride. (1997, August). US Environmental Protection Agency. https://archive.epa.gov/pesticides/reregistration/web/pdf/0262red.pdf.

32. Registration of SAN 582H / Frontier* Herbicide. (1993, March 5). US Environmental Protection Agency. https://archive.epa.gov/pesticides/chemicalsearch/chemical/foia/web/pdf/129051/129051-048.pdf.

33. Pyrethrins/pyrethroid cumulative risk assessment. (2011, October 4). US Environmental Protection Agency. https://www.regulations.gov/document?D=EPA-HQ-OPP-2011-0746-0003.

34. Shafer, T. J., Meyer, D. A., & Crofton, K. M. (2005). Developmental neurotoxicity of pyrethroid insecticides: critical review and future research needs. *Environmental Health Perspectives, 113* (2), 123. www.ncbi.nlm.nih.gov/pmc/articles/PMC1277854/.

35. Williams, M., Barr, D., Camann, D., Rundle, A., Rauh, V., & Whyatt, R. (2009). Prenatal exposure to pyrethroid insecticides and infant neurocognitive development at 3 years of age. *Epidemiology, 20* (6), S222–S223. http://journals.lww.com/epidem/Citation/2009/11001/Prenatal_Exposure_to_Pyrethroid_Insecticides_and.669.aspx.

36. Horton, M. K., Rundle, A., Camann, D. E., Barr, D. B., Rauh, V. A., & Whyatt, R. M. (2011). Impact of prenatal exposure to piperonyl butoxide and permethrin on 36-month neurodevelopment. *Pediatrics, 127* (3), e699–e706. http://pediatrics.aappublications.org/content/127/3/e699.short.

37. Revised reregistration eligibility decision for MSMA, DSMA, CAMA, and cacodylic acid. (2006, August 10). US Environmental Protection Agency. https://nepis.epa.gov/Exe/ZyPDF.cgi/P10013JM.PDF?Dockey=P10013JM.PDF.

38. Reregistration eligibility decision (RED), triclopyr. (1998, October). US Environmental Protection Agency. https://nepis.epa.gov/Exe/ZyPDF.cgi/20000PDW.PDF?Dockey=20000PDW.PDF.

39. US Environmental Protection Agency, Reregistration eligibility decision (RED) for coppers.

40. Reregistration eligibility decision for dicamba and associated salts. (2006, June 8). US Environmental Protection Agency. https://nepis.epa.gov/Exe/ZyPDF.cgi/P10049M3.PDF?Dockey=P10049M3.PDF.

41. Medical Toxicology Branch, Department of Pesticide Regulation. (2006, July). Sulfuryl fluoride (Vikane*) risk characterization document, volume I, health risk assessment. California Environmental Protection Agency. www.cdpr.ca.gov/docs/emon/pubs/tac/tacpdfs/sulfluor/final_rcd_vol1.pdf.

42. Pesticides: registration review; EPA proposes to withdraw sulfuryl fluoride tolerances. (2016, February 20). US Environmental Protection Agency. https://archive.epa.gov/opps-rrd1/registration_review/web/html/evaluations.html.

APPENDIX VI

Threats or Benefits
Unsubstantiated

*I*n my attempt to be exhaustive, as discussed in Appendix II, I researched a wide variety of topics. In the following cases, I concluded that either the particular substance represented no material threat/benefit or there was insufficient information currently to make a judgment one way or the other.

Acrylamide is a water-soluble thickener most commonly used in wastewater treatment. According to a National Toxological Profile published by the US Government Office of Health Assessment and Translation, "Considering the low level of estimated human exposure to acrylamide derived from a variety of sources, the Expert Panel expressed negligible concern for adverse reproductive and developmental effects for exposures in the general population."[1] According to the CDC: "Animal studies have shown that acrylamide can cause reproductive effects (reduced litter size, fetal death, male germinal cell injury, dominant lethality)," but "acrylamide is not thought to accumulate in the body at environmental doses," and "estimated intakes are hundreds of times lower than occupational exposures, and well below doses known to cause nerve damage or carcinogenicity in animals."[2]

Alcohol ethoxysulphates (AES) include sodium lauryl sulfate (SLS) and sodium laureth sulphate (SLES), both of which are common ingredients in shampoo to help produce lather. Despite recent media hype, there is little evidence these compounds are harmful to human health. According to a Human Health Risk Assessment in 2003, "Alcohol ethoxysulphates were evaluated for teratogenic or embryotoxic effects mainly in rats, but in a few investigations also in mice and rabbits. . . . There also wasn't any evidence of reproductive toxicity, teratogenic, or developmental effects in animals at the highest doses tested. . . . [T]he human health risk assessment has demonstrated that the use of AES in household laundry and cleaning detergents is safe and does not cause concern with regard to consumer use."[3] And according to the EPA in their evaluation of a consumer product with sodium lauryl sulfate in it, "published reports suggest that sodium lauryl sulfate has low acute mammalian toxicity and no known chronic effects. EPA has no reports of adverse effects resulting from its use. Both exposure and health risks to people using the product are expected to be low."[4]

Aldrin, an organochlorine insecticide, was banned in the United States in 1974 but continues to contaminate the environment. Aldrin was one of the original "dirty dozen" persistent organic pollutants (POPs) outlawed by the Stockholm Convention, an international environmental treaty signed by fifty countries in 2004. For the moment, there's no evidence that aldrin poses any risk in pregnancy, although this topic hasn't been properly studied. According to a CDC report from 2002, "no studies were located regarding developmental effects in humans or animals after inhalation exposure to aldrin."[5] And according to the World Health Organization, "Based on the available data, there is no evidence of a teratogenic potential for aldrin."[6]

Amalgam: Approximately one-third of women in the United States have silver-colored dental fillings made of amalgam (~80% of adults in the United States have a filling,[7] and somewhere between 37 percent and 47 percent of fillings are made of amalgam[8, 9]), which is composed of 50 percent inorganic mercury. (Mercury exists in three different forms. Metallic and organic mercury—i.e., the methylmercury in contaminated fish—are toxic to the central nervous system and the fetus, whereas inorganic forms of mercury released from dental amalgams may affect the kidneys.)

Although amalgam has now been banned in Germany, Sweden, Denmark, and Canada, it's still in use in the United States,[10] partly because it's both cheap and durable.[11] The mercury is technically bound within the amalgam, but over time, small amounts are released due to chewing and grinding. According to the CDC, fillings account for 53 percent of mercury exposure for those with only a few fillings and up to 87 percent of mercury exposure for those with >8 fillings.[12] (Unfortunately, the CDC also cautions that improper removal of dental amalgams can actually increase the risk of exposure, so there's very little you can do about mercury from this source.)

As of 1999, the CDC provided a wishy-washy recommendation regarding dental amalgam during pregnancy: "If you are pregnant, the decision of whether to have dental amalgam or a nonmercury material used for fillings, or whether existing amalgam fillings should be repaired or replaced during pregnancy, should be made in consultation with your dentist."[13] But according to the National Research Council in 2000, "as data become available, exposure to elemental Hg from dental amalgams should be considered in risk assessment of MeHg."[14] Since then, one study from 2005 found no evidence that maternal dental amalgams are linked to low birth weight,[15] but a review from 2006 still caveated that "there is little direct evidence that can be used to assess reproductive hazards. . . . Better designed studies are needed, particularly for investigation of neurodegenerative diseases and effects on infants and children."[16] Fortunately, one further study from 2011 has since found no evidence of later neurobehavioral consequences in children of mothers with amalgam fillings.[17]

Aniline is a manufactured chemical used by a number of industries. According to the Agency for Toxic Substances and Disease Registry, "significant exposure may occur only if you work with aniline. . . .

The general population may be exposed to aniline by eating food or drinking water containing aniline, but these amounts are usually very small. . . . We do not know if exposure to aniline will result in birth defects or other developmental effects in people. The studies on developmental effects in animals are not conclusive."[18]

Aspartame is an artificial sweetener that in the United States is most frequently consumed in diet soft drinks. According to a review citing studies submitted to the Food and Drug Administration and World Health Organization for aspartame's food additive petition and safety evaluation, "aspartame is considered to have no reproductive or teratogenic activity."[19]

Bisphenol A (BPA) is used to produce the most common form of polycarbonate plastic, which is clear and shatterproof and used in a variety of household products, such as water bottles and CDs. Since 2008, there has been heightened public concern about the safety of BPA, particularly its use in baby bottles, and the FDA ultimately ended its authorization of the use of BPA in baby bottles, sippy cups, and infant formula packaging—but based on market abandonment rather than safety.[20] The hype surrounding BPA appears to be disproportionate to the threat it poses. In terms of its effect during pregnancy, preliminary studies suggest there may be a link, for example, between prenatal exposure and later child behavior.[21] But according to the CDC, the evidence is still inconclusive: "Some reproductive or developmental changes are observed at high doses in standard experimental animal studies," and "animal studies suggest possible low dose effects include altered development of the fetal prostate and mammary gland, inhibition of postnatal testosterone production, and changes in neurodevelopment."[22] According to a report from the National Toxicology Program (NTP), "The NTP has negligible concern that exposure of pregnant women to bisphenol A will result in fetal or neonatal mortality, birth defects, or reduced birth weight and growth in their offspring. . . . The NTP has some concern for effects on the brain, behavior, and prostate gland in fetuses, infants, and children at current human exposures to bisphenol A. . . . Recognizing the lack of data on the effects of bisphenol A in humans . . .

the possibility that bisphenol A may alter human development cannot be dismissed."[23]

1-bromopropane, also known as n-propyl bromide (nPB), is an organic solvent used in a variety of applications, including degreasing, adhesives, and dry cleaning. According to a National Toxological Profile published by the US Government Office of Health Assessment and Translation, the risk to the general population from 1-bromopropane is unknown, but there may be risk to those occupationally exposed: "Although there is no direct evidence that exposure of people to 1-BP adversely affects reproduction or development, recent studies in rats show that exposure to 1-BP can adversely affect reproduction and development. . . . There are no data on 1-BP exposure of the general US population. . . . Based on the occupational exposure data and studies in humans and laboratory animals, the NTP concurs with the CERHR Bromopropanes Expert Panel that there is serious concern for reproductive and developmental effects at the upper end of the human occupational exposure range."[24]

Cadmium is a metal that has historically been used in coating iron and steel to prevent corrosion and making yellow paint but is now most commonly used in batteries. It primarily enters the environment as a result of mining activities and is spread by wind and rain, absorbed by plants, and then ingested in trace amounts in our diets.[25] According to the CDC, "animal studies have demonstrated reproductive and teratogenic effects. Small epidemiologic studies have noted an inverse relationship between cadmium in cord blood, maternal blood, or maternal urine and birth weight and length at birth."[26] According to a 2012 Toxicological Profile from the Agency for Toxic Substances and Disease Registry, "Studies in animals exposed to high enough levels of cadmium during pregnancy have resulted in harmful effects in the young," but "there are few human data on developmental effects from exposure to cadmium. Some studies indicate that maternal cadmium exposure may cause decreased birth weight in humans, but most of these studies are of limited use. . . . A number of other studies did not find a significant relationship between maternal cadmium levels and newborn body weight. . . . Russian women occupationally exposed to cadmium had offspring with decreased birth weights compared to unexposed controls, but without congenital malformations."[27]

Carbofuran is a pesticide that was banned by the EPA in 2010.[28] Fortunately, carbofuran does not appear to be particularly harmful during pregnancy. According to the World Health Organization, carbofuran didn't cause birth defects in any of the available developmental studies in animals.[29] The CDC concurs that carbofuran doesn't cause birth defects, although the report caveats that "high chronic doses in animals produced nonspecific developmental effects, such as reduced weight gain and pup survival."[30]

Carbon disulfide is an industrial chemical used to manufacture products such as rayon and cellophane film. According to the EPA, "Laboratory studies show that exposure to large amounts of carbon disulfide during pregnancy adversely affects the developing fetus of animals."[31] But according to a National Toxological Profile published by the Agency for Toxic Substances and Disease Registry, "human exposure to carbon disulfide is expected to be highest among certain occupational groups (e.g., rayon plant workers)" and those "living in the vicinity of industrial point emission sources" rather than the general population.[32] Furthermore, occupational studies in humans haven't shown any negative effects in pregnancy.[33, 34]

Carbon monoxide is a colorless, odorless, tasteless gas that is emitted by fuel-burning appliances and can therefore represent a dangerous source of indoor air pollution. "There are reports of carbon monoxide poisoning in pregnant women causing fetal death or damage to the developing baby's brain. This is thought to be from the large amounts of carbon monoxide in the mother's blood. This causes the baby to receive less oxygen . . . [but] a small study has shown that fetal death and brain damage only happen when carbon monoxide levels in the mother are high enough to make her lose consciousness."[35]

Carbon tetrachloride is a clear liquid that was used for many years as a refrigeration fluid, an aerosol propellant, a cleaning fluid, and a pesticide. It has been gradually phased out of use after being found to affect the ozone layer.

Fortunately, it does not appear to cause significant problems in pregnancy. According to the CDC, "No studies were located regarding reproductive effects in humans after exposure to carbon tetrachloride, and the available human data for developmental effects are limited to epidemiological studies of pregnancy outcomes in women exposed to carbon tetrachloride and other halogenated hydrocarbons in drinking water. These data are inadequate for establishing a causal relationship between carbon tetrachloride exposure and developmental toxicity in humans.... In developmental studies in animals exposed by inhalation or ingestion, no fetal toxicity was observed in the absence of maternal toxicity and morphological defects were not observed in offspring."[36]

Chlordane is an organochlorine pesticide that was banned in the United States in 1988 but continues to contaminate the environment.[37] Chlordane was one of the original "dirty dozen" persistent organic pollutants (POPs) outlawed by the Stockholm Convention. Chlordane doesn't appear to represent a material threat to pregnancy. According to the CDC, feeding studies with animals "have demonstrated neonatal mortality and alterations in immune function of offspring," but "epidemiologic studies have not demonstrated teratogenic or developmental effects."[38] Furthermore, according to the World Health Organization, "Chlordane exposure may occur through food, but due to its highly restricted uses, this route does not appear to be a major pathway of exposure."[39]

Chlordecone is an insecticide that was banned in the United States in 1978 and was added to the list of persistent organic pollutants banned by the Stockholm Convention in 2009.[40] Chlordecone exposure may pose a risk to pregnancy. According to the CDC, "We do not know if harmful developmental effects occur in people. However, it is possible that if parents are exposed to enough chlordecone, their children's development may be harmed." This is based on the fact that "animal studies show that chlordecone harms the offspring of exposed animals"; for example, "gestational exposure of rats and mice to chlordecone resulted in increased stillbirths and decreased postnatal viability."[41] And according to a more recent addendum to the same CDC report, "chlordecone may interfere with estrogen-dependent events during sexual differentiation of the brain that impact later activation of hormone-dependent behavior."[42] Fortunately, "most people are exposed to very low levels of chlordecone." Because chlordecone does not dissolve or evaporate easily, people are not likely to be exposed to it by drinking water or by inhaling air. The only people likely to be exposed are those who "live near hazardous waste sites" or eat "fish caught in Lake Ontario" or "fish or shellfish caught in the lower 113 miles of the James River."[43]

1,2-dibromo-3-chloropropane (DBCP) is a soil fumigant pesticide that hasn't been used in the continental United States since 1979. According to the CDC, any exposure to DBCP today is likely to be minimal: "Levels where the chemical has not been used or discarded are either low or nonexistent. In areas where the chemical has been used as a soil fumigant, it may still be present in soil and groundwater at low levels," but "the limited use of DBCP in recent years suggests that exposure is minimal and infrequent." Furthermore, DBCP does not appear to pose a high risk during pregnancy: "Studies in animals show that DBCP may cause birth defects in the offspring of rats exposed to large amounts. However, human exposure to DBCP that occurred at work or by drinking contaminated water has not been linked with birth defects."[44]

Dichlorodiphenyltrichloroethane (DDT), an insecticide, was banned in the United States in 1972 after the book *Silent Spring* brought it to public attention and helped launch the modern environmental movement. Nevertheless, DDT continues to contaminate the environment and is one of the original "dirty dozen" persistent organic pollutants (POPs) limited by the Stockholm Convention. "People in the United States are exposed to DDT mainly by eating foods containing small amounts," with the largest fraction coming from "meat, poultry, dairy products, and fish, including sport fish." Fortunately, DDT appears to pose minimal risk to pregnancy in the United States. According to the CDC, "reproductive effects in humans affecting birth weight . . . have not been consistently demonstrated," and "there is no evidence that exposure to DDT at levels found in the environment causes birth defects in people."[45] Although one study did find an increased risk of preterm birth, this was only at levels of exposure higher than currently found in women in the United States.[46]

Dieldrin, an insecticide, was banned in the United States for most uses in 1987 and is no longer produced in the United States, but it continues to contaminate the environment.[47] Dieldrin was one of the original "dirty dozen" persistent organic pollutants (POPs) outlawed by the Stockholm Convention. For the moment, there's no evidence that Dieldrin poses any risk in pregnancy, although this topic hasn't been fully studied. For example, according to a CDC report from 2002, "no studies were located regarding developmental effects in humans or animals after inhalation exposure to dieldrin."[48] And according to the World Health Organization, the only studies finding evidence of birth defects involved doses that were also toxic to the mothers.[49]

Diquat is an herbicide that is not used in sufficient volume to appear on the list of the top 30 pesticides used in the United States. According to the EPA, "diquat dibromide causes developmental and reproductive toxicity at the highest dose levels tested," but "although people may be exposed to residues of diquat dibromide through their diets, the chronic dietary risk from such exposure is minimal."[50]

Disinfection by-products (DBPs) form when the chlorine added to public water systems to prevent microbial contamination reacts with organic matter in the water (decomposing leaves, etc.) to form unwanted by-products, including haloacetic acids and trihalomethanes (THMs) such as chloroform.[51] Over 84 percent of US households receive water from public water systems, most of which use chlorine. Fortunately, according to the CDC, these DBPs appear to pose little risk to pregnancy: "DBPs did not produce reproductive or developmental effects in animals unless maternal toxicity was present. . . . [E]pidemiologic studies of the relationships between chlorinated water source and adverse reproductive outcomes have been inconclusive."[52]

Endrin is an organochlorine insecticide that was banned in the United States in 1986 but continues to contaminate the environment. Endrin was one of the original "dirty dozen" persistent organic pollutants (POPs) outlawed by the Stockholm Convention. Endrin can cause problems in pregnancy; according to the CDC, "birth defects, especially abnormal bone formation, have been seen in some animal studies. While there are no human data on birth defects, evidence in rodents suggests that exposure to high doses of endrin during pregnancy could be a health risk to developing fetuses."[53] Fortunately, the risk from exposure is low. Again according to the CDC, "since endrin is no longer produced or used in the United States, you can probably be exposed to it only in areas where it is concentrated, such as a hazardous waste site," and "residues on imported foods are the main source of potential human exposure in food."[54] The World Health Organization also agrees that "the main source of endrin exposure to the general population is residues in food," and "contemporary intake is generally below the acceptable daily intake."[55]

Endosulfan is an organochlorine insecticide currently in the process of being phased out globally. Endosulfan and its related isomers were added to the list of persistent organic pollutants banned by the Stockholm Convention in 2009.[56] In the United States, use of endosulfan has been fully banned as of 2016. Endosulfan may pose a threat to pregnancy. According to the CDC in 2013, "exposure of pregnant animals to endosulfan can produce abnormalities in the skeleton and organs in the offspring and reduced pup weight during lactation," although "this often occurred with doses that were also toxic to the mothers." In humans, the evidence is suggestive but not conclusive: "We do not know whether endosulfan can produce birth defects in children. Studies have examined possible associations between maternal exposure to endosulfan and autism, thyroid function, and development of the nervous system in newborn children. Studies also have examined potential associations between direct exposure of children to endosulfan and blood cancer and sexual maturation in males. In all cases, the results were suggestive but not conclusive due to study limitations." Fortunately, exposure is likely to be minimal: "The main route of exposure to endosulfan for the general population is ingestion of food containing residues of endosulfan. . . . A dietary exposure assessment for endosulfan was conducted by both the EPA and the California Department of Pesticide Regulation. . . . [B]oth assessments concluded that calculated risks of dietary exposure of endosulfan are below protective benchmarks for all subgroups."[57]

Ethylene oxide is a poisonous gas used to make products such as detergents, thickeners, solvents, and plastics. According to a 1990 Toxicological Profile from the Agency for Toxic Substances and Disease Registry, "There is limited evidence in both animal and human studies that inhalation exposure to ethylene oxide can result in adverse reproductive effects, although there is currently no clear pattern in the nature of those effects."[58] But according to the EPA, the threat from ethylene oxide is primarily from occupational exposure: "The major use for ethylene oxide is as a chemical intermediate in industry. . . . Some evidence exists indicating that inhalation exposure to ethylene oxide can cause an increased rate of miscarriages in female workers."[59]

Fluoride is a naturally occurring mineral that is also added to public water supplies and toothpastes for its ability to prevent tooth decay. Based on studies in China, where "widespread dental fluorosis indicates the prevalence of high exposures," there's evidence that prolonged exposure to high levels of fluoride can reduce IQ in children.[60] But for the moment, "there's no evidence of adverse effects of consuming fluoride during pregnancy, although there's also no evidence of benefit"[61]: according to the CDC, "use of fluoride supplements by pregnant women does not benefit their offspring. . . . The only randomized controlled trial[62] to assess fluoride supplements taken by pregnant women provides evidence of no benefit for their children."[63]

Formaldehyde is a gas that was formerly used dissolved in water as a disinfectant and to preserve biological specimens. According to a review from 2001, "Formaldehyde is unlikely to reach the reproductive system in humans in concentrations sufficient to cause damage since it is rapidly metabolized and detoxified upon contact with the respiratory tract. . . . When biases were taken into account, we found no evidence of increased risk of spontaneous abortion among workers exposed to formaldehyde. . . . Information from experimental studies and studies of metabolism indicate reproductive impacts are unlikely at formaldehyde exposure levels observed in the epidemiology studies."[64]

Genistein is a phytoestrogen (or dietary estrogen) naturally occurring in soybeans, among other plants. According to an expert panel report published by the US Government Office of Health Assessment and Translation, "Even though there is a paucity of available human data on exposure to purified genistein, the Expert Panel expresses negligible concern for reproductive and developmental effects from exposure of adults in the general population. The most highly reported exposed human population is Japanese adults with ingestion of approximately 0.43 mg/kg bodyweight/day. However, adverse effects in rodent studies were not observed at levels below 35–44 mg/kg bodyweight/day. Therefore, the Expert Panel feels that under current exposure conditions, adults would be unlikely to consume sufficient daily levels of genistein to cause adverse reproductive and/or developmental effects."[65]

Heptachlor is an organochlorine insecticide that was banned in the United States in 1988 for all uses except the control of fire ants. Heptachlor was one of the original "dirty dozen" persistent organic pollutants (POPs) outlawed by the Stockholm Convention. Food is the major source of exposure,[66] with potentially contaminated foods including fish, shellfish (such as clams), dairy products, meat, and poultry.[67] According to the CDC, animal studies suggest heptachlor may have negative effects during pregnancy: "Chronic feeding studies with heptachlor have demonstrated neonatal mortality, and alterations in immune function of offspring," and "subtle neurodevelopmental effects have been observed in rodents after prenatal exposure to heptachlor," although "epidemiologic studies have not demonstrated teratogenic or developmental effects."[68] However, the evidence remains inconclusive in humans: "there is some evidence that similar effects may occur in humans, but a study that found some changes in performance on some tests that measure nervous system function is not conclusive and exposure to other chemicals cannot be ruled out."[69]

Hexachlorobenzene (HCB), a fungicide, was banned in the United States in 1966 and hasn't been in use since 1984, but it continues to contaminate the environment.[70] HCB was one of the original "dirty dozen" persistent organic pollutants (POPs) outlawed by the Stockholm Convention. According to the CDC, humans are primarily exposed to hexachlorbenzene through food, "including fish caught in contaminated areas."[71] Studies of the effects of hexachlorbenzene in pregnancy are inconclusive. According to the World Health Organization, "HCB was associated with cleft palate and some kidney malformations in mice."[72] And according to the CDC, "higher levels of hexachlorobenzene were found in the fat of boys with undescended testes," but "we don't know if hexachlorobenzene caused the birth defect." Fortunately, "other investigators found little evidence for associations between hexachlorobenzene levels and preterm birth, birth weight, postpartum growth, or results of infant intelligence testing."

Hexachlorocyclohexane, or HCH, is a chemical that has eight different forms. One of these forms, gamma-HCH, commonly called lindane, is an insecticide. Lindane has not been produced in the United States since 1976, but is still imported and used as an insecticide and also as the active ingredient in prescription shampoos and creams used to treat lice and scabies. Lindane and the two additional forms of HCH that are by-products of lindane production (alpha- and beta-HCH) were all added to the list of persistent organic pollutants banned by the Stockholm Convention in 2009, with the exception of use against lice and scabies.[73] The effects of exposure to lindane during pregnancy have not been thoroughly studied. According to a CDC report, "It is not known whether HCH causes birth defects in humans," although "γ-HCH does not cause significant birth defects in animals" and "a single report of an association with intrauterine growth retardation is insufficient to draw any conclusion regarding developmental effects of HCH in humans, particularly since other organochlorine pesticides were also present." Again according to the CDC, "no studies were located regarding developmental effects in humans or animals" following inhalation or dermal exposure to HCH. The lack of research on dermal exposure is surprising, given that head lice treatment involves lindane coming in contact with the skin, and according to the CDC, the most common source of exposure is using the prescription medication for lice/scabies (although you could also technically be exposed if an unqualified person applied pesticides around your home). Lindane treatments are available over the counter, and the CDC says they are "normally safe if used as directed."[74] However, the FDA cautions: "Tell your doctor if you are pregnant. Lindane Shampoo can reach your baby and may harm it. Ask your doctor for a safer medicine. Use Lindane Shampoo only if needed."[75]

Lymphocytic choriomeningitis virus (LCMV) can be caught from mice: as many as 5 percent of house mice in the United States are infected with the disease.[76] LCMV can cause miscarriage if contracted during pregnancy. However, this is fortunately very rare: "There have been 54 cases of congenital LCMV reported since 1955, with 34 of the cases diagnosed since 1993."[77]

Manganese is a metal that occurs naturally in rocks and soil and is used in the production of steel. It's also required by the human body in trace amounts. Several studies have suggested that children with long-term exposure to elevated levels of manganese (e.g., living in Bangladesh and Quebec, Canada, where manganese is naturally present in drinking water, or living next to manganese mining and processing facilities) exhibit impairments of various kinds.[78, 79, 80, 81] But the evidence is less conclusive regarding the effects during pregnancy. According to the CDC, "studies of manganese workers have not found increases in birth defects or low birth weight in their children. No birth defects were observed in animals exposed to manganese. Developmental studies involving the use of laboratory animals have detected subtle changes in growth."[82] A few preliminary studies suggest that high levels of exposure in utero could reduce birth weight[83] and affect early psychomotor development and neurodevelopment.[84, 85] But according to the CDC, in the United States, exposure is likely to be minimal for the majority of the population: "The primary way you can be exposed to manganese is by eating food . . . [but] children are not likely to be exposed to harmful amounts of manganese in the diet."[86]

Marine toxins: Certain baby websites caution against eating sushi in part because of potential exposure to marine toxins. How common is such poisoning? According to the CDC, "Every year, approximately 30 cases of poisoning by marine toxins are reported in the United States."[87] That would be a chance of 1 in 10 million of getting fish poisoning. To put this into context, according to the National Weather Service, there are approximately 40 deaths each year in the United States due to people being struck by lightning.[88] The CDC does caveat that more cases may go unreported, but the very reason they would go unreported is because the illness tends to be so mild. There is also little evidence that marine toxins pose a specific risk for pregnancy. For example, of eight published cases of ciguatera poisoning during pregnancy, only one baby showed symptoms at birth, and even that baby doesn't appear to have suffered any lasting problems.[89, 90, 91, 92]

Methanol, also known as methyl alcohol, is a type of simple alcohol that is used primarily in the production of other chemicals. It's poisonous when consumed in large quantities and is therefore often added to ethanol used for industrial purposes to exempt it from liquor taxes. According to a National Toxological Profile published by the US Government Office of Health Assessment and Translation: "Are current exposures to methanol high enough to cause concern? Probably not. The general US population presently appears to be exposed to methanol at levels that are not of immediate concern for causing adverse reproductive or developmental effects. However, there are studies to suggest that maternal exposure to acutely toxic doses of methanol may produce developmental effects in children."[93]

Methylene chloride, also known as dichloromethane, is an industrial solvent with applications in stripping paint, degreasing, and decaffeinating coffee, among others. According to the CDC, although "a retrospective study of pregnancy outcomes among Finnish pharmaceutical workers reported a slightly increased risk of spontaneous abortion associated with inhalation exposure to methylene chloride ... methylene chloride is not likely to cause developmental effects or behavioral changes at levels normally encountered in the environment ... with current standards and procedures, workplace exposure of pregnant women is unlikely to be hazardous to the fetus."[94]

Mirex, an insecticide, was banned in the United States in 1978, but it continues to contaminate the environment. Mirex was one of the original "dirty dozen" persistent organic pollutants (POPs) outlawed by the Stockholm Convention. Mirex may cause problems in pregnancy. According to the CDC, "developmental abnormalities including cataracts and edema in the offspring [of laboratory animals fed high doses] have been reported,"[95] and a recent addendum to a CDC report cites a study in humans in which mirex levels were "inversely associated with cognitive development at 4 years of age."[96]

Fortunately, "most people are exposed to very low levels of mirex." Because mirex does not dissolve or evaporate easily, people are not likely to be exposed to it by drinking water or by inhaling air. The only people likely to be exposed are those who "live near hazardous waste sites" or eat "fish caught in Lake Ontario" or "fish or shellfish caught in the lower 113 miles of the James River."[97]

Molybdenum is a metal that humans require in trace amounts for certain enzymes to function. The CDC references adverse reproductive effects in rats and mice at high levels of exposure to molybdenum,[98] but according to the EPA, "human health effects from molybdenum at low environmental doses are unknown."[99]

Nickel is a common metal used to produce steel and other metal alloys as well as magnets and five-cent coins. Trace amounts can also be found in drinking water. According to the CDC, "Animal studies have found increases in newborn deaths and decreases in newborn weight after ingesting nickel. [But] these doses are 1,000 times higher than levels typically found in drinking water."[100]

Parabens are chemicals used primarily as preservatives in the cosmetic and pharmaceutical industries. Despite recent media hype, there is little evidence that parabens present any harm to human health in general and no evidence of harm specific to pregnancy. According to the CDC, "At levels producing maternal toxicity, parabens were not teratogenic in animal studies. . . . Safety assessments of maximum estimated paraben exposures have concluded that estrogenic effects are unlikely in humans."[101] According to the FDA, "The Cosmetic Ingredient Review (CIR) reviewed the safety of methylparaben, propylparaben, and butylparaben in 1984 and concluded they were safe for use in cosmetic products at levels up to 25 percent. Typically parabens are used at levels ranging from 0.01 to 0.3 percent. . . . In December 2005, after considering the margins of safety for exposure to women and infants, the [CIR] Panel determined that there was no need to change its original conclusion that parabens are safe as used in cosmetics. . . . In a review of the estrogenic activity of parabens,[102] the author concluded that based on maximum daily exposure estimates, it was implausible that parabens could increase the risk associated with exposure to estrogenic chemicals . . . FDA believes that at the present time there is no reason for consumers to be concerned about the use of cosmetics containing parabens."[103]

Pentachlorobenzene (PeCB) used to be included in products containing PCBs; now it's used as a fire retardant and as an ingredient in a fungicide.[104] In 2009, it was added to the list of persistent organic pollutants banned by the Stockholm Convention.[105] Pentachlorobenzene is unlikely to pose a threat during pregnancy. According to two studies cited by both the Canadian government and the United Nations Environment Programme,[106, 107] the evidence from animal studies is inconclusive, with fetal effects seen in rats but not mice (no studies have been done in humans). Furthermore, it's also unlikely that we're exposed to PeCB in harmful quantities. The Canadian government has estimated that intakes are 5 to 1000 times less than the tolerable daily intake derived from animal studies, based on dietary information from the United States.[108]

Pentachlorophenol used to be one of the most heavily used pesticides in the United States. Now it can only be used for treating wood for utility poles, railroad ties, and wharf pilings, but unfortunately it had already become a pervasive environmental contaminant by the time its use was restricted.

According to the CDC, exposure to pentachlorophenol during pregnancy has been shown to be harmful in animal studies: "Animal studies provide strong evidence that pentachlorophenol is a developmental toxicant following oral exposure. Developmental effects are frequently observed at doses that cause decreases in maternal body weight gain. However, decreases in fetal or pup body weight have been observed at doses that do not result in maternal toxicity . . . we do not know if pentachlorophenol produces all of the same effects in humans that it causes in animals."[109]

In terms of sources of exposure, "for most people, food is the most important source of intake of pentachlorophenol, and most of this intake is from root vegetables," but "based on analyses of foods representative of the diets of different age/gender population groups, daily intakes of pentachlorophenol from the diet are low overall" and "daily intakes of pentachlorophenol from food have decreased over time." The CDC concludes, "though pentachlorophenol has been found in some foods, its levels are low." [110]

Perchlorates are salts that are naturally occurring and also produced for rocket fuel and fireworks, and they have become contaminants in the water supply. According to the CDC, "Animal and human studies have shown that perchlorate can inhibit thyroid hormone production" and "maternal and congenital hypothyroidism adversely effects neurological development and decreases learning capability." But fortunately, "studies of elevated perchlorate in the regional drinking water have indicated no increased prevalence of this disorder. Also, altered thyroid function was not found in Chilean pregnant women or their newborns with mean urinary perchlorate levels about 40-fold higher than average US levels,[111] although iodine intake was higher than US levels."[112]

Perchlorethylene (also called tetrachloroethylene, tetrachlorothene, PCE, pert, perclene, and perchloris) is a solvent used in dry cleaning and for degreasing metal. It evaporates easily and as a result is a pervasive contaminant in air, soil, and water. For example, tetrachloroethylene was found in 38 percent of surface water sampling sites throughout the United States.[113]

According to the CDC, PCE can have negative effects in pregnancy. For example, "results from some studies suggest that women who work in dry cleaning industries where exposures to tetrachloroethylene can be quite high may have more menstrual problems and spontaneous abortions than women who are not exposed. However, it is not known for sure if tetrachloroethylene was responsible for these problems because other possible causes were not considered. . . . Because of its pervasiveness in the environment, the general public can be exposed to tetrachloroethylene through drinking water, air, or food." Fortunately, "the levels of exposure are probably far below those causing any adverse effects."[114]

Perfluorochemicals (PFCs) are used to make coatings and products that resist heat, oil, stains, grease, and water and are found in such varied products as clothing, furniture, adhesives, food packaging, heat-resistant nonstick cooking surfaces, and electrical wire insulation.[115] Certain chemicals in this group have recently begun to cause concern because they don't break down in the environment; as of 2009, perfluorooctane sulfonic acid (PFOS), its salts, and perfluorooctane sulfonyl fluoride (POSF) were added to the list of persistent organic pollutants limited by the Stockholm Convention.[116] The effect of these chemicals during pregnancy remains uncertain. According to the CDC, in animal studies, "at high but non-toxic maternal doses of PFOS, development in offspring was stunted. . . . Late gestational exposure to PFOS in animal studies has also demonstrated early neonatal lethality, possibly related to lung immaturity."[117] Studies in humans are inconclusive, however: "Three studies of pregnant women found that as the levels of PFOA in the mother's blood increased, there was a tendency for the newborn babies to have slightly lower birth weight. However, another study that looked at exposure to PFOA in drinking water did not find such an association."[118]

Periodontal therapy: There is preliminary evidence suggesting there may be a link between preterm birth and maternal periodontal disease, although further research is needed. According to one review, "There is evidence of an association between periodontal disease and increased risk of preterm birth and low birth weight, especially in economically disadvantaged populations, but potential biases (especially in terms of inconsistent definitions of periodontal disease) and the limited number of randomized controlled trial studies prevent us from offering a clear conclusion. Several randomized controlled trials are under way to test the hypothesis that periodontal treatment can reduce rates of certain adverse pregnancy outcomes."[119] Similarly, another review concludes, "findings indicate a likely association, but it needs to be confirmed by large, well-designed, multicenter trials."[120]

However, periodontal therapy does not appear to improve pregnancy outcomes. According to a report by the American Academy of Periodontology, "Although periodontal therapy has been shown to be safe and leads to improved periodontal conditions in pregnant women, case-related periodontal therapy, with or without systemic antibiotics, does not reduce overall rates of preterm birth and low birth weight."[121] This could be because poor pregnancy outcomes and periodontal disease could both be caused by the same underlying factor—for example, a genetic predisposition towards a heightened inflammatory response to infection.

Phenol is a chemical used to make plastics (a key ingredient in bisphenol A). According to the CDC, "The primary way you can be exposed to phenol is by breathing air containing it. Releases of phenol into the air occur from industries using or manufacturing phenol, automobile exhaust, cigarette smoke, and wood burning. Recent data on levels of phenol in air are lacking." Fortunately, there's little evidence that phenol is harmful during pregnancy: "Two studies of women exposed to phenol and other chemicals during pregnancy did not provide evidence of birth defects. Some birth defects have been observed in animals born to females exposed to phenol during pregnancy," but "this generally occurred at exposure levels that were also toxic to the mothers."[122]

Polybrominated diphenyl ethers (PBDEs) are flame retardants that are added to a variety of consumer products. There are many types of PBDEs; several of them (tetrabromodiphenyl ether, pentabromodiphenyl ether, hexabromodiphenyl ether, and heptabromodiphenyl ether) were added to the list of persistent organic pollutants banned by the Stockholm Convention in 2009.[123] Nevertheless, PBDEs are still produced and widely used in the United States; in fact, according to the CDC, "concentrations of lower brominated PBDEs have been increasing in tissues and body fluids," with levels now higher in the United States than in other regions of the world. Although there have been no definitive studies, people appear to be primarily exposed through food, particularly foods with high fat content, such as fatty fish.[124] Fortunately, PBDEs don't appear to pose a threat to pregnancy: although no studies have been conducted in humans, "none of the commercial BDE mixtures have been shown to be overtly teratogenic in animals," and in two studies of PDBE in rats, there were no indications of developmental toxicity.[125]

Probiotics are "live micro-organisms which, when administered in adequate amounts, confer a health benefit on the host," according to the World Health Organization.[126] Probiotics are present in yogurt and fermented foods, among others. Probiotics appear to be safe to consume during pregnancy, and a recent meta-analysis has suggested that consuming lactobacilli during pregnancy reduced the risk of eczema in offspring by ~6 percent,[127] although consuming a mixture of various bacterial strains did not.[128] This result is intriguing, and the topic is worthy of further study, given the dramatic and as yet unexplained recent increase in the prevalence of childhood allergies and eczema.

Protein: There doesn't appear to be a need to specifically increase protein intake during pregnancy. According to a review, women who are undernourished may benefit from balanced energy/protein supplements. But this same review cautions that high protein supplements for pregnant women may actually be harmful.[129] Given the frequent concern that vegetarian diets might be deficient in protein, it's also worth pointing out here that the American Dietetic Association cites an "evidence-based review" showing that "vegetarian diets can be nutritionally adequate in pregnancy and result in positive maternal and infant health outcomes."[130]

Soy: Soybeans are legumes that are high in protein and are a globally important crop. According to the National Institute of Environmental Health Sciences, as of 2010, there are no studies of the effects of soy during pregnancy in humans, but in animal studies, "evidence is insufficient to conclude that a soy-based diet produces or does not produce developmental toxicity."[131] (Incidentally, there has been more extensive research on the effects of feeding infants soy-based formula. According to the National Toxicology Program, "the NTP concurred with the expert panel that there is minimal concern for adverse effects on development in infants who consume soy infant formula."[132]) See also genistein, a key component of soy.

Toxaphene, an insecticide, was banned in the United States in 1990, but it continues to contaminate the environment. Toxaphene was one of the original "dirty dozen" persistent organic pollutants (POPs) outlawed by the Stockholm Convention. According to the CDC, animal studies suggest that toxaphene may cause minor changes in fetal development: "Toxaphene is not teratogenic [capable of causing birth defects]," but "some studies reported treatment-related effects on development," although only at doses that were also toxic to the mother, and "the perinatal immunological system may be at risk for toxaphene toxicity." The effect of exposure in humans, however, is unknown: "We do not know if toxaphene would cause developmental effects in humans. . . . No studies were located regarding developmental effects in humans following oral exposure to toxaphene."[133] Fortunately, according to the World Health Organization, "exposure of the general population is most likely through food; however, levels detected are generally below maximum residue limits."[134] And, according to the CDC, only very specific populations are likely to be at risk, including "northern Native American groups that eat toxaphene-contaminated aquatic mammals, recreational or subsistence hunters in the southern United States that consume significant amounts of game animals (especially species like raccoons), and people who consume certain types of sport-caught fish (such as trout, salmon, herring, smelt, and walleye) from the Great Lakes."[135]

Tributyltin (TBT) is a type of persistent organic pollutant. Tributyltin and other similar compounds are used in making plastics, food packages, plastic pipes, pesticides, paints, wood preservatives, and rat and mice repellents. According to the CDC, "You may be exposed to butyltin compounds by eating seafood from coastal waters or from contact with household products that contain organotin compounds (polyurethane, plastic polymers, and silicon-coated baking parchment paper)." Fortunately, "there are no reports of adverse developmental effects in humans exposed to tin or its compounds. . . . Exposure of rodents to some organotins during pregnancy has produced birth defects in the newborn animals," but "the results of several studies suggest that this may occur only at high exposure levels that cause maternal toxicity," although "further research is needed to clarify this issue."[136]

Trichloroethylene (TCE) is a solvent used primarily by factories to remove grease from metals. It evaporates into the air and disperses, ultimately contaminating soil and groundwater: "Between 9 percent and 34 percent of the drinking water supply sources that have been tested in the United States may have some trichloroethylene contamination."[137]

According to the CDC, "There is some evidence that exposure to trichloroethylene in drinking water may cause certain types of birth defects. However, this body of research is still far from conclusive and there is insufficient evidence to determine whether or not there is an association between exposure to TCE and developmental effects. . . . Because of the pervasiveness of trichloroethylene in the environment, most people are exposed to it through drinking water, air, or food," but fortunately, "the levels of exposure are probably far below those causing any adverse effects."[138]

2,4,5-Trichlorophenoxyacetic acid (2,4,5-T) was used as an herbicide until it was banned by the EPA in 1985. (It also was one of two ingredients in Agent Orange, the defoliant used in the Vietnam War.) The effects of exposure to 2,4,5-T in pregnancy are uncertain. According to the CDC, birth defects and developmental effects have been reported in rodents treated with high doses.[139] 2,4,5-T is also metabolized by the body into chlorophenols, and according to another CDC report, "in one study animals exposed to chlorophenols showed delayed hardening of some bones"; however, "we do not know whether chlorophenols cause birth defects in humans."[140] Fortunately, women are no longer likely to be exposed: "given the unavailability of 2,4,5-T, the general population is unlikely to be exposed to 2,4,5-T."[141]

Ultrasound: An ultrasound machine creates images by sending high-frequency sound waves through your body. As the sound waves bounce off your organs and tissues, they create echoes.[142] According to a review conducted by the World Health Organization in 2009 that considered the results of more than sixty publications, "ultrasonography in pregnancy was not associated with adverse maternal or perinatal outcome, impaired physical or neurological development, increased risk for malignancy in childhood, subnormal intellectual performance or mental diseases. According to the available clinical trials, there was a weak association between exposure to ultrasonography and non–right handedness in boys." The review concludes that exposure to diagnostic ultrasonography during pregnancy appears to be safe.[143]

Uranium is a metallic chemical element that is weakly radioactive and is naturally occurring in rock, soil, and water in addition to being used for nuclear power. According to the EPA, "It is not known if exposure to uranium has effects on the development of the human fetus. Very high doses of uranium in drinking water can affect the development of the fetus in laboratory animals. One study reported birth defects, and another reported an increase in fetal deaths. However, we do not believe that uranium can cause these problems in pregnant women who take in normal amounts of uranium from food and water, or who breathe the air around a hazardous waste site that contains uranium."[144]

Zika virus dominated the news for a period of time due to its ability to cause birth defects, including microcephaly. Fortunately, residents of the continental United States have nothing to fear. While the CDC reported 224 cases of local transmission in the continental United States in 2016, the number has dropped to 0 for the half-year to June 21, 2017, as was predicted by experts who suggested infections would peak in 2016.[145, 146] Furthermore, according to data from the World Health Organization, the peak of the epidemic has now passed across the Americas,[147] in line with recent predictive models.[148]

Zinc is a metallic chemical element that is an essential mineral for the human body. According to a review that examined studies of zinc supplementation during pregnancy, "The reduction in preterm birth for zinc compared with placebo was primarily in the group of studies involving women of low income. . . . There was no convincing evidence that zinc supplementation during pregnancy results in other useful and important benefits. Since the preterm association could well reflect poor nutrition, studies to address ways of improving the overall nutritional status of populations in impoverished areas, rather than focusing on micronutrient and or zinc supplementation in isolation, should be an urgent priority."[149]

Notes

1. Manson, J., Brabec, M. J., Buelke-Sam, J., Carlson, G. P., Chapin, R. E., Favor, J. B., Fischer, L. J., Hattis, D., Lees, P. S. J., Perreault-Darney, S., Rutledge, J., Smith, T. J., Tice, R. R., & Working, P. (2005). NTP-CERHR Expert Panel report on the reproductive and developmental toxicity of acrylamide. *Birth Defects Research Part B: Developmental and Reproductive Toxicology, 74* (1), 17–113. http://onlinelibrary.wiley.com/doi/10.1002/bdrb.20030/full.

2. Fourth national report on human exposure to environmental chemicals. (2009). US Centers for Disease Control and Prevention, Atlanta, GA. https://www.cdc.gov/exposurereport/pdf/FourthReport.pdf.

3. Human Environmental Risk Assessment on ingredients of European household cleaning products: alcohol ethoxysulphates. (2003, January). Human & Environmental Risk Assessment (HERA), Edition 1. www.heraproject.com/files/1-HH-04-HERA%20AES%20HH%20web%20wd.pdf.

4. R.E.D. Facts: lauryl sulfate salts. (1993, September). US Environmental Protection Agency. https://archive.epa.gov/pesticides/reregistration/web/pdf/4061fact.pdf.

5. Agency for Toxic Substances and Disease Registry (ATSDR). (2002). Toxicological profile for aldrin/dieldrin. US Department of Health and Human Services, Public Health Service. https://www.atsdr.cdc.gov/toxprofiles/tp.asp?id=317&tid=56.

6. Ritter, L., Solomon, K. R., Forget, J., Stemeroff, M., & O'Leary, C. (1995). A review of selected persistent organic pollutants. International Programme on Chemical Safety (IPCS). PCS/95.39. Geneva: World Health Organization, 65, 66. http://cdrwww.who.int/entity/ipcs/assessment/en/pcs_95_39_2004_05_13.pdf.

7. Richardson, G. M., Wilson, R., Allard, D., Purtill, C., Douma, S., & Graviere, J. (2011). Mercury exposure and risks from dental amalgam in the US population, post-2000. *Science of the Total Environment, 409* (20), 4257–4268. www.sciencedirect.com/science/article/pii/S0048969711006607.

8. Beazoglou, T., Eklund, S., Heffley, D., Meiers, J., Brown, L. J., & Bailit, H. (2007). Economic impact of regulating the use of amalgam restorations. *Public Health Reports, 122* (5), 657. www.ncbi.nlm.nih.gov/pmc/articles/PMC1936958/.

9. Rosenstiel, S. F., Land, M. F., & Rashid, R. G. (2004). Dentists' molar restoration choices and longevity: a web-based survey. *The Journal of Prosthetic Dentistry, 91* (4), 363–367. www.sciencedirect.com/science/article/pii/S0022391304000502.

10. Agency for Toxic Substances and Disease Registry. (1999). Toxicological profile for mercury. US Department of Health and Human Services, Public Health Service. www.atsdr.cdc.gov/toxprofiles/tp.asp?id=115&tid=24.

11. Dental amalgam: overview. (Last updated 2017, August 25). American Dental Association. www.ada.org/en/advocacy/advocacy-issues/dental-amalgam.

12. Agency for Toxic Substances and Disease Registry, Toxicological profile for mercury.

13. Ibid.

14. National Research Council. (2000). Toxicological effects of methylmercury. National Academies Press. https://www.nap.edu/catalog/9899/toxicological-effects-of-methylmercury.

15. Hujoel, P. P., Lydon-Rochelle, M., Bollen, A. M., Woods, J. S., Geurtsen, W., & Del Aguila, M. A. (2005). Mercury exposure from dental filling placement during pregnancy and low birth weight risk. *American Journal of Epidemiology, 161* (8), 734–740. http://aje.oxfordjournals.org/content/161/8/734.full.

16. Bates, M. N. (2006). Mercury amalgam dental fillings: an epidemiologic assessment. *International Journal of Hygiene and Environmental Health, 209* (4), 309–316. www.sciencedirect.com/science/article/pii/S1438463906000034.

17. Watson, G. E., Lynch, M., Myers, G. J., Shamlaye, C. F., Thurston, S. W., Zareba, G., Clarkson, T. W., & Davidson, P. W. (2011). Prenatal exposure to dental amalgam: evidence from the Seychelles Child Development Main Cohort. *Journal of the American Dental Association (1939), 142* (11), 1283. www.ncbi.nlm.nih.gov/pmc/articles/PMC3245741/.

18. Agency for Toxic Substances and Disease Registry. (2002, April). Toxic substances portal—aniline: ToxFAQs for aniline. US Department of Health and Human Services, Public Health Service. www.atsdr.cdc.gov/toxfaqs/tf.asp?id=449&tid=79.

19. Magnuson, B. A., Burdock, G. A., Doull, J., Kroes, R. M., Marsh, G. M., Pariza, M. W., Spencer, P. S., Waddell, W. J., Walker, R., & Williams, G. M. (2007). Aspartame: a safety evaluation based on current use levels, regulations, and toxicological and epidemiological studies. *CRC Critical Reviews in Toxicology, 37* (8), 629–727. http://www.tandfonline.com/doi/abs/10.1080/10408440701516184.

20. FDA regulations no longer authorize the use of BPA in infant formula packaging based on abandonment; decision not based on safety. (2013, July 11). US Food and Drug Administration. www.fda.gov/food/newsevents/constituentupdates/ucm360147.htm.

21. Braun, J. M., Kalkbrenner, A. E., Calafat, A. M., Yolton, K., Ye, X., Dietrich, K. N., & Lanphear, B. P. (2011). Impact of early-life bisphenol A exposure on behavior and executive function in children. *Pediatrics, 128* (5), 873–882. http://pediatrics.aappublications.org/content/128/5/873.short.

22. US Centers for Disease Control and Prevention, Fourth national report on human exposure to environmental chemicals.

23. Chapin, R. E., Adams, J., Boekelheide, K., Gray, L. E., Hayward, S. W., Lees, P. S., McIntyre, B. S., Portier, K. M., Schnorr, T. M., Selevan, S. G., Vandenbergh, J. G., & Woskie, S. R. (2008). NTP-CERHR Expert Panel report on the reproductive and developmental toxicity of bisphenol A. *Birth Defects Research Part B: Developmental and Reproductive Toxicology, 83* (3), 157–395. http://onlinelibrary.wiley.com/doi/10.1002/bdrb.20147/full.

24. Shelby, M. D. (2004). NTP-CERHR Expert Panel report on the reproductive and developmental toxicity of 1-bromopropane. *Reproductive Toxicology, 18* (2), 157–187. http://www.sciencedirect.com/science/article/pii/S0890623804000139.

25. National Biomonitoring Program: cadmium factsheet. (2016, December 23). Centers for Disease Control and Prevention. https://www.cdc.gov/biomonitoring/Cadmium_FactSheet.html

26. US Centers for Disease Control and Prevention, Fourth national report on human exposure to environmental chemicals.

27. Agency for Toxic Substances and Disease Registry. (2012, September). Toxicological profile for cadmium. US Department of Health and Human Services, Public Health Service. https://www.atsdr.cdc.gov/ToxProfiles/TP.asp?id=48&tid=15.

28. Pesticides: reregistration: carbofuran cancellation process. (2011, June). US Environmental Protection Agency. https://archive.epa.gov/pesticides/reregistration/web/html/carbofuran_noic.html.

29. Carbofuran in drinking-water: background document for development of WHO guidelines for drinking-water quality. (2004). World Health Organization. www.who.int/water_sanitation_health/dwq/chemicals/carbofuran.pdf.

30. US Centers for Disease Control and Prevention, Fourth national report on human exposure to environmental chemicals.

31. Chemicals in the environment: carbon disulfide. (1994, August). US Environmental Protection Agency, Office of Pollution Prevention and Toxics. https://nepis.epa.gov/Exe/ZyPDF.cgi/9101D90W.PDF?Dockey=9101D90W.PDF.

32. Sciences International, Inc., & Research Triangle Institute. (1996). Toxicological profile for carbon disulfide. US Department of Health and Human Services, Public Health Service, Agency for Toxic Substances and Disease Registry. https://www.atsdr.cdc.gov/ToxProfiles/TP.asp?id=474&tid=84.

33. Zhou, S. Y., Liang, Y. X., Chen, Z. Q., & Wang, Y. L. (1988). Effects of occupational exposure to low-level carbon disulfide (CS2) on menstruation and pregnancy. *Industrial Health, 26* (4), 203–14.

34. Bao, Y. S., Cai, S., Zhao, S. F., Xhang, X. C., Huang, M. Y., Zheng, O., & Jiang, H. (1991). Birth defects in the offspring of female workers occupationally exposed to carbon disulfide in China. *Teratology, 43* (5), 451–452.

35. Carbon monoxide and pregnancy. (2013, November). Organization of Teratology Information Specialists. https://mothertobaby.org/fact-sheets/carbon-monoxide-pregnancy/.

36. Agency for Toxic Substances and Disease Registry. (2005). Toxicological profile for carbon tetrachloride. US Department of Health and Human Services, Public Health Service. www.atsdr.cdc.gov/toxprofiles/tp.asp?id=196&tid=35.

37. Chlordane: hazard summary. (2000, January). US Environmental Protection Agency. https://www.epa.gov/sites/production/files/2016-09/documents/chlordane.pdf.

38. US Centers for Disease Control and Prevention, Fourth national report on human exposure to environmental chemicals.

39. Ritter, L., et al., A review of selected persistent organic pollutants.

40. Stockholm Convention. (2017). The new POPs under the Stockholm Convention. http://chm.pops.int/TheConvention/ThePOPs/TheNewPOPs/tabid/2511/Default.aspx.

41. Agency for Toxic Substances and Disease Registry. (1995, August). Toxicological profile for mirex and chlordecone. US Department of Health and Human Services, Public Health Service. www.atsdr.cdc.gov/ToxProfiles/tp.asp?id=643&tid=118.

42. Ibid.

43. Ibid.

44. Agency for Toxic Substances and Disease Registry. (1992). Toxicological profile for 1,2-dibromo-3-chloropropane. US Department of Health and Human Services, Public Health Service. www.atsdr.cdc.gov/toxprofiles/tp.asp?id=852&tid=166.

45. US Centers for Disease Control and Prevention, Fourth national report on human exposure to environmental chemicals.

46. Harris, M. O., Llados, F., Swarts, S., Sage, G., Citra, M., & Gefell, D. (2002). Toxicological profile for DDT, DDE, and DDD. US Department of Health and Human Services, Public Health Service, Agency for Toxic Substances and Disease Registry. www.atsdr.cdc.gov/ToxProfiles/tp.asp?id=81&tid=20.

47. Persistent Bioaccumulative and Toxic (PBT) Chemical Program. (2011, April 18). Aldrin/dieldrin. US Environmental Protection Agency. http://archive.is/Fy4V.

48. Agency for Toxic Substances and Disease Registry. (2002). Toxicological profile for aldrin/dieldrin. US Department of Health and Human Services, Public Health Service. https://www.atsdr.cdc.gov/toxprofiles/tp.asp?id=317&tid=56.

49. Ritter, L., et al., A review of selected persistent organic pollutants.

50. R.E.D. Facts: diquat dibromide. (1995, July). US Environmental Protection Agency. https://archive.epa.gov/pesticides/reregistration/web/pdf/0288fact.pdf.

51. Bove, F., Shim, Y., & Zeitz, P. (2002). Drinking water contaminants and adverse pregnancy outcomes: a review. *Environmental Health Perspectives, 110* (Suppl 1), 61. https://www.ncbi.nlm.nih.gov/pmc/articles/PMC1241148/.

52. US Centers for Disease Control and Prevention, Fourth national report on human exposure to environmental chemicals.

53. Agency for Toxic Substances and Disease Registry. (1996). Toxicological profile for endrin. US Department of Health and Human Services, Public Health Service. www.atsdr.cdc.gov/ToxProfiles/tp.asp?id=617&tid=114.

54. Ibid.

55. Ritter, L., et al., A review of selected persistent organic pollutants.

56. Stockholm Convention, The new POPs under the Stockholm Convention.

57. Agency for Toxic Substances and Disease Registry. 2013. Toxicological profile for endosulfan. US Department of Health and Human Services, Public Health Service. www.atsdr.cdc.gov/ToxProfiles/tp.asp?id=609&tid=113.

58. Agency for Toxic Substances and Disease Registry. (1990). Toxicological profile for ethylene oxide. US Department of Health and Human Services, Public Health Service. https://www.atsdr.cdc.gov/ToxProfiles/TP.asp?id=734&tid=133.

59. Ethylene oxide: hazard summary. (2000, January). US Environmental Protection Agency. https://www.epa.gov/sites/production/files/2016-09/documents/ethylene-oxide.pdf.

60. Choi, A. L., Sun, G., Zhang, Y., & Grandjean, P. (2012). Developmental fluoride neurotoxicity: a systematic review and meta-analysis. *Environmental Health Perspectives, 120* (10), 1362. www.ncbi.nlm.nih.gov/pmc/articles/pmc3491930/.

61. Aschengrau, A., Zierler, S., & Cohen, A. (1993). Quality of community drinking water and the occurrence of late adverse pregnancy outcomes. *Archives of Environmental Health: An International Journal, 48* (2), 105–113. www.tandfonline.com/doi/abs/10.1080/00039896.1993.9938403.

62. Leverett, D. H., Adair, S. M., Vaughan, B. W., Proskin, H. M., & Moss, M. E. (1997). Randomized clinical trial of the effect of prenatal fluoride supplements in preventing dental caries. *Caries Research, 31* (3), 174–179. www.karger.com/Article/Abstract/262394.

63. Kohn, W. G., Maas, W. R., Malvitz, D. M., Presson, S. M., & Shaddix, K. K. (2001, August 17). Recommendations for using fluoride to prevent and control dental caries in the United States. *Morbidity and Mortality Weekly Report, 50* (RR14), 1–42. www.cdc.gov/mmwr/preview/mmwrhtml/rr5014a1.htm.

64. Collins, J. J., Ness, R., Tyl, R. W., Krivanek, N., Esmen, N. A., & Hall, T. A. (2001). A review of adverse pregnancy outcomes and formaldehyde exposure in human and animal studies. *Regulatory Toxicology and Pharmacology, 34* (1), 17–34. www.ncbi.nlm.nih.gov/pubmed/11502153.

65. Rozman, K. K., Bhatia, J., Calafat, A. M., Chambers, C., Culty, M., Etzel, R. A., Flaws, J. A., Hansen, D. K., Hoyer, P. B., Jeffery, E. H., Kesner, J. S., Marty, S., Thomas, J. A., & Umbach, D. (2006). NTP-CERHR Expert Panel report on the reproductive and developmental toxicity of genistein. *Birth Defects Research Part B: Developmental and Reproductive Toxicology, 77* (6), 485–638. https://www.ncbi.nlm.nih.gov/pmc/articles/PMC2020434/.

66. Ritter, L., et al., A review of selected persistent organic pollutants.

67. Agency for Toxic Substances and Disease Registry. (2007). Toxicological profile for heptachlor and heptachlor epoxide. US Department of Health and Human Services, Public Health Service. www.atsdr.cdc.gov/ToxProfiles/tp.asp?id=746&tid=135.

68. US Centers for Disease Control and Prevention, Fourth national report on human exposure to environmental chemicals.

69. Agency for Toxic Substances and Disease Registry, Toxicological profile for heptachlor and heptachlor epoxide.

70. Agency for Toxic Substances and Disease Registry. (2013). Toxicological profile for hexachlorobenzene. US Department of Health and Human Services, Public Health Service. www.atsdr.cdc.gov/ToxProfiles/tp.asp?id=627&tid=115.

71. Ibid.

72. Ritter, L., et al., A review of selected persistent organic pollutants.

73. Stockholm Convention, The new POPs under the Stockholm Convention.

74. Agency for Toxic Substances and Disease Registry. (2005). Toxicological profile for hexa-chlorocyclohexane. US Department of Health and Human Services, Public Health Service. www.atsdr.cdc.gov/toxprofiles/tp.asp?id=754&tid=138.

75. Medication guide: lindane shampoo, USP 1%. (2007, August). US Food and Drug Administration. http://www.pdr.net/pdrcontent/PDRe_201407180931/mg/pdf/5360.PDF.

76. Lymphocytic choriomeningitis (LCM). (2014, May 6). US Centers for Disease Control and Prevention. www.cdc.gov/vhf/lcm/.

77. Jamieson, D. J., Kourtis, A. P., Bell, M., & Rasmussen, S. A. (2006). Lymphocytic cho-riomeningitis virus: an emerging obstetric pathogen? *American Journal of Obstetrics and Gynecology, 194* (6), 1532–1536. www.sciencedirect.com/science/article/pii/S0002937805026025.

78. Khan, K., Wasserman, G. A., Liu, X., Ahmed, E., Parvez, F., Slavkovich, V., Levy, D., Mey, J., Van Geen, A., Graziano, J. H., & Factor-Litvak, P. (2012). Manganese exposure from drinking water and children's academic achievement. *Neurotoxicology, 33* (1), 91–97. www.ncbi.nlm.nih.gov/pmc/articles/PMC3282923/.

79. Bouchard, M., Laforest, F., Vandelac, L., Bellinger, D., & Mergler, D. (2007). Hair man-ganese and hyperactive behaviors: pilot study of school-age children exposed through tap water. *Environmental Health Perspectives, 115* (1), 122. www.ncbi.nlm.nih.gov/pmc/articles/PMC1797845/.

80. Riojas-Rodríguez, H., Solís-Vivanco, R., Schilmann, A., Montes, S., Rodríguez, S., Ríos, C., & Rodríguez-Agudelo, Y. (2010). Intellectual function in Mexican children living in a min-ing area and environmentally exposed to manganese. *Environmental Health Perspectives, 118* (10), 1465. www.ncbi.nlm.nih.gov/pmc/articles/PMC2957930/.

81. Lucchini, R. G., Guazzetti, S., Zoni, S., Donna, F., Peter, S., Zacco, A., Salmistraro, M., Bontempi, E., Zimmerman, N. J., & Smith, D. R. (2012). Tremor, olfactory and motor changes in Italian adolescents exposed to historical ferro-manganese emission. *Neurotoxicology, 33* (4), 687–696. http://europepmc.org/articles/PMC3360122.

82. Agency for Toxic Substances and Disease Registry. (2012). Toxicological profile for manga-nese. US Department of Health and Human Services, Public Health Service. www.atsdr.cdc.gov/toxprofiles/tp.asp?id=102&tid=23.

83. Zota, A. R., Ettinger, A. S., Bouchard, M., Amarasiriwardena, C. J., Schwartz, J., Hu, H., & Wright, R. O. (2009). Maternal blood manganese levels and infant birth weight. *Epidemiology, 20* (3), 367. www.ncbi.nlm.nih.gov/pmc/articles/PMC3113478/.

84. Takser, L., Mergler, D., Hellier, G., Sahuquillo, J., & Huel, G. (2003). Manganese, mono-amine metabolite levels at birth, and child psychomotor development. *Neurotoxicology, 24* (4), 667–674. www.sciencedirect.com/science/article/pii/S0161813X03000585.

85. Lin, C. C., Chen, Y. C., Su, F. C., Lin, C. M., Liao, H. F., Hwang, Y. H., Hsieh, W. S., Jeng, S. F., Su, Y. N., & Chen, P. C. (2013). *In utero* exposure to environmental lead and manga-nese and neurodevelopment at 2 years of age. *Environmental Research, 123*, 52–57. www.sciencedirect.com/science/article/pii/S0013935113000625.

86. Agency for Toxic Substances and Disease Registry. (2014, March 20). Toxic substances por-tal—manganese: ToxFAQs for manganese. US Department of Health and Human Services, Public Health Service. www.atsdr.cdc.gov/toxfaqs/tf.asp?id=101&tid=23.

87. Marine toxins. (2005, October 12). US Centers for Disease Control and Prevention. www.cdc.gov/ncidod/dbmd/diseaseinfo/marinetoxins_g.htm.

88. Lightning safety: medical aspects of lightning. (n.d.). National Weather Service. http://www. lightningsafety.noaa.gov/medical.shtml.

89. Pearn, J. H., Harvey, P., De Ambrosis, W., Lewis, R., & McKay, R. (1982). Ciguatera and pregnancy. *Medical Journal of Australia, 1* (2), 57–58.

90. Rivera-Alsina, M. E., Payne, C., Pou, A., & Payne, S. (1991). Ciguatera poisoning in pregnancy. *American Journal of Obstetrics & Gynecology, 164,* 397.

91. Geller, R. J., Olson, K. R., & Senécal, P. E. (1991). Ciguatera fish poisoning in San Francisco, California, caused by imported barracuda. *Western Journal of Medicine, 155* (6), 639. https://www.ncbi.nlm.nih.gov/pmc/articles/PMC1003121/.

92. Senecal, P. E., & Osterloh, J. D. (1991). Normal fetal outcome after maternal ciguateric toxin exposure in the second trimester. *Clinical Toxicology, 29* (4), 473–478. http://www. tandfonline.com/doi/abs/10.3109/15563659109025743.

93. National Toxicology Program, US Department of Health and Human Services, Center for the Evaluation of Risks to Human Reproduction. (2003, September). NTP-CERHR Expert Panel on the reproductive and developmental toxicity of methanol. *Reproductive Toxicology, 18* (3), 303–390. http://www.sciencedirect.com/science/article/pii/ S0890623803001618.

94. Agency for Toxic Substances and Disease Registry. (1998). Toxicological profile for methylene chloride. US Department of Health and Human Services, Public Health Service. https://www.atsdr.cdc.gov/toxprofiles/tp.asp?id=234&tid=42.

95. "According to the CDC, 'developmental abnormalities including cataracts and edema in the offspring [of laboratory animals fed high doses] have been reported . . .'" US Centers for Disease Control and Prevention, Fourth national report on human exposure to environmental chemicals.

96. Agency for Toxic Substances and Disease Registry, Toxicological profile for mirex and chlordecone.

97. Ibid.

98. Centers for Disease Control and Prevention, Fourth national report on human exposure to environmental chemicals.

99. Biomonitoring summary: molybdenum. (2016, December 23). US Environmental Protection Agency. https://www.cdc.gov/biomonitoring/Molybdenum_ BiomonitoringSummary.html.

100. Agency for Toxic Substances and Disease Registry. (1997). Toxicological profile for nickel. US Department of Health and Human Services, Public Health Service. https://www.atsdr. cdc.gov/toxprofiles/tp.asp?id=245&tid=44.

101. "According to the CDC, 'at levels producing maternal toxicity, parabens were not teratogenic in animal studies . . .'" National Biomonitoring Program, biomonitoring summary, parabens. (2013, December 4). Centers for Disease Control and Prevention. www.cdc.gov/biomonitoring/Parabens_BiomonitoringSummary.html.

102. Golden, R., Gandy, J., & Vollmer, G. (2005). A review of the endocrine activity of parabens and implications for potential risks to human health. *CRC Critical Reviews in Toxicology, 35* (5), 435–458. http://informahealthcare.com/doi/abs/10.1080/10408440490920104.

103. Cosmetics: products & ingredients—ingredients, parabens. (2007, October 31). US Food and Drug Administration. www.fda.gov/cosmetics/productsingredients/ingredients/ ucm128042.htm.

104. Pentachlorobenzene factsheet. (n.d). US Environmental Protection Agency. https:// archive.epa.gov/epawaste/hazard/wastemin/web/pdf/pentchlb.pdf.

105. Stockholm Convention, The new POPs under the Stockholm Convention.

106. Government of Canada. (1993). Canadian Environmental Protection Act priority substances list assessment report: pentachlorobenzene. Environment Canada and Health Canada, Ottawa, Ontario. www.hc-sc.gc.ca/ewh-semt/pubs/contaminants/psl1-lsp1/pentachlorobenzene/index-eng.php.

107. Stockholm Convention. (2007). Report of the Persistent Organic Pollutants Review Committee on the work of its second meeting: risk profile on chlordecone. United Nations Environment Programme. http://chm.pops.int/Convention/POPsReviewCommittee/PreviousMeetingsDocuments/POPRC2/POPRC2ReportandDecisions/tabid/349/Default.aspx.

108. Government of Canada, Canadian Environmental Protection Act priority substances list assessment report: pentachlorobenzene.

109. Agency for Toxic Substances and Disease Registry. (2001). Toxicological profile for pentachlorophenol. US Department of Health and Human Services, Public Health Service. https://www.atsdr.cdc.gov/toxprofiles/tp.asp?id=402&tid=70.

110. Agency for Toxic Substances and Disease Registry, Toxicological profile for pentachlorophenol.

111. Téllez, R. T., Chacón, P. M., Abarca, C. R., Blount, B. C., Landingham, C. B. V., Crump, K. S., & Gibbs, J. P. (2005). Long-term environmental exposure to perchlorate through drinking water and thyroid function during pregnancy and the neonatal period. *Thyroid, 15* (9), 963–975. http://online.liebertpub.com/doi/abs/10.1089/thy.2005.15.963?journalCode=thy.

112. Centers for Disease Control and Prevention, Fourth national report on human exposure to environmental chemicals.

113. Agency for Toxic Substances and Disease Registry. (1997). Toxicological profile for tetrachloroethylene. US Department of Health and Human Services, Public Health Service. www.atsdr.cdc.gov/toxprofiles/tp.asp?id=265&tid=48.

114. Ibid.

115. Perfluorochemicals (PFCs). (2009, November). Centers for Disease Control and Prevention. https://www.cdc.gov/biomonitoring/PFCs_FactSheet.html.

116. Stockholm Convention, The new POPs under the Stockholm Convention.

117. Centers for Disease Control and Prevention, Fourth national report on human exposure to environmental chemicals.

118. Agency for Toxic Substances and Disease Registry. (2009). Toxicological profile for perfluoroalkyls. (Draft for public comment.) US Department of Health and Human Services, Public Health Service. www.atsdr.cdc.gov/toxprofiles/tp.asp?id=1117&tid=237.

119. Xiong, X., Buekens, P., Fraser, W. D., Beck, J., & Offenbacher, S. (2006). Periodontal disease and adverse pregnancy outcomes: a systematic review. *BJOG: An International Journal of Obstetrics & Gynaecology, 113* (2), 135–143. http://onlinelibrary.wiley.com/doi/10.1111/j.1471-0528.2005.00827.x/full.

120. Vergnes, J. N., & Sixou, M. (2007). Preterm low birth weight and maternal periodontal status: a meta-analysis. *American Journal of Obstetrics and Gynecology, 196* (2), 135–e1. www.sciencedirect.com/science/article/pii/S0002937806012257.

121. Sanz, M., & Kornman, K. (2013). Periodontitis and adverse pregnancy outcomes: consensus report of the Joint EFP/AAP Workshop on Periodontitis and Systemic Diseases. *Journal of Clinical Periodontology, 40* (s14), S164–S169. http://onlinelibrary.wiley.com/doi/10.1111/jcpe.12083/full.

122. Agency for Toxic Substances and Disease Registry. (2008). Toxicological profile for phenol. US Department of Health and Human Services, Public Health Service. www.atsdr.cdc.gov/ToxProfiles/tp.asp?id=148&tid=27.

123. Stockholm Convention, The new POPs under the Stockholm Convention.

124. Agency for Toxic Substances and Disease Registry. (2004). Toxicological profile for polybrominated biphenyls and polybrominated diphenyl ethers. US Department of Health and Human Services, Public Health Service. www.atsdr.cdc.gov/ToxProfiles/tp.asp?id=529&tid=94.

125. Agency for Toxic Substances and Disease Registry, Toxicological profile for polybrominated biphenyls and polybrominated diphenyl ethers.

126. Schlundt, J. (2001). Health and nutritional properties of probiotics in food including powder milk with live lactic acid bacteria: report of a joint FAO/WHO expert consultation. Food and Agriculture Organization of the United Nations/World Health Organization. http://www.fao.org/3/a-a0512e.pdf.

127. Dugoua, J. J., Machado, M., Zhu, X., Chen, X., Koren, G., & Einarson, T. R. (2009). Probiotic safety in pregnancy: a systematic review and meta-analysis of randomized controlled trials of *Lactobacillus*, *Bifidobacterium*, and *Saccharomyces* spp. *Journal of Obstetrics and Gynaecology Canada, 31* (6), 542. www.ncbi.nlm.nih.gov/pubmed/19646321.

128. Doege, K., Grajecki, D., Zyriax, B. C., Detinkina, E., zu Eulenburg, C., & Buhling, K. J. (2012). Impact of maternal supplementation with probiotics during pregnancy on atopic eczema in childhood—a meta-analysis. *British Journal of Nutrition, 107* (01), 1–6. http://journals.cambridge.org/action/displayAbstract?fromPage=online&aid=8474017.

129. "But this same review cautions that high protein supplements for pregnant women may actually be harmful."

   Ota, E., Hori, H., Mori, R., Tobe-Gai, R., & Farrar, D. (2015). Antenatal dietary education and supplementation to increase energy and protein intake. *Cochrane Database of Systematic Reviews 2015*, (6), CD000032. http://onlinelibrary.wiley.com/doi/10.1002/14651858.CD000032.pub3/full.

130. Craig, W. J., & Mangels, A. R. (2009). Position of the American Dietetic Association: vegetarian diets. *Journal of the American Dietetic Association, 109* (7), 1266–1282. http://europepmc.org/abstract/MED/19562864.

131. Center for the Evaluation of Risks to Human Reproduction. (2010, January 15). Final CERHR Expert Panel report on soy infant formula, Appendix II. National Toxicology Program, US Department of Health and Human Services. https://ntp.niehs.nih.gov/ntp/ohat/genistein-soy/soyformula/soymonograph2010_508.pdf.

132. McCarver, G., Bhatia, J., Chambers, C., Clarke, R., Etzel, R., Foster, W., Hoyer, P., Leeder, J. S., Peters, J. M., Rissman, E., Rybak, M., Sherman, C., Toppari, J., & Turner, K. (2011). NTP-CERHR Expert Panel report on the developmental toxicity of soy infant formula. *Birth Defects Research Part B: Developmental and Reproductive Toxicology, 92* (5), 421–468. www.ncbi.nlm.nih.gov/pubmed/21948615.

133. Agency for Toxic Substances and Disease Registry. (2010). Toxicological profile for toxaphene. US Department of Health and Human Services, Public Health Service. https://www.atsdr.cdc.gov/toxprofiles/tp.asp?id=548&tid=99.

134. Ritter, L., et al., A review of selected persistent organic pollutants.

135. Agency for Toxic Substances and Disease Registry, Toxicological Profile for toxaphene.

136. Agency for Toxic Substances and Disease Registry. (2005). Toxicological profile for tin. US Department of Health and Human Services, Public Health Service. https://www.atsdr.cdc.gov/ToxProfiles/tp.asp?id=543&tid=98.

137. Agency for Toxic Substances and Disease Registry. (1997). Toxicological profile for trichloroethylene. US Department of Health and Human Services, Public Health Service.

www.atsdr.cdc.gov/toxprofiles/tp.asp?id=173&tid=30.

138. Agency for Toxic Substances and Disease Registry, Toxicological profile for trichloroethylene.

139. US Centers for Disease Control and Prevention, Fourth national report on human exposure to environmental chemicals.

140. Agency for Toxic Substances and Disease Registry. (1999). Toxicological profile for chlorophenols. US Department of Health and Human Services, Public Health Service. www. atsdr.cdc.gov/ToxProfiles/tp.asp?id=941&tid=195.

141. National Biomonitoring Program, biomonitoring summary, 2,4,5-trichlorophenooxy-acetic acid. (2013, December 4). Centers for Disease Control and Prevention. www.cdc.gov/biomonitoring/2,4,5-TrichlorophenoxyaceticAcid_BiomonitoringSummary.html.

142. Ultrasound for cancer. (2015, November 30). American Cancer Society. https://www.cancer.org/treatment/understanding-your-diagnosis/tests/ultrasound-for-cancer.html.

143. Torloni, M. R., Vedmedovska, N., Merialdi, M., Betrán, A. P., Allen, T., González, R., & Platt, L. D. (2009). Safety of ultrasonography in pregnancy: WHO systematic review of the literature and meta-analysis. *Ultrasound in Obstetrics & Gynecology, 33* (5), 599–608. http://onlinelibrary.wiley.com/doi/10.1002/uog.6328/full.

144. Biomonitoring summary: molybdenum. (2016, December 23). US Environmental Protection Agency. https://www.cdc.gov/biomonitoring/Molybdenum_BiomonitoringSummary.html.

145. Zhang, Q., Sun, K., Chinazzi, M., Pastore-Piontti, A., Dean, N. E., Rojas, D. P., Merler, S., Mistry, D., Poletti, P., Rossi, L., Bray, M., Halloran, M. E., Longini, I. M., & Vespignani, A. (2016). Projections of Zika spread in the Continental US. www.zika-model.org/files/projectedZikaContinentalUS.pdf.

146. Davis, N. (2016, July 14). Zika epidemic has peaked and may run its course within 18 months, say experts. *The Guardian.* www.theguardian.com/world/2016/jul/14/zika-epidemic-has-peaked-and-will-run-its-course-within-18-months-say-experts.

147. Regional Zika epidemiological update (Americas): August 25, 2017. (2017, May 25). World Health Organization. www.paho.org/hq/index.php?option=com_content&id=11599&Itemid=41691.

148. Zhang, Q., Sun, K., Chinazzi, M., Pastore y Piontti, A., Dean, N. E., Rojas, D. P., Merler, S., Mistry, D., Poletti, P., Rossi, L., & Bray, M., Halloran, M. E., Longini, I. M., & Vespignani, A. (2017). Spread of Zika virus in the Americas. *Proceedings of the National Academy of Sciences, 114* (22), E4334–E4343. www.pnas.org/content/114/22/E4334.full.pdf.

149. "According to a review that examined studies of zinc supplementation during pregnancy, 'The reduction in preterm birth for zinc . . .'"

Ota, E., Mori, R., Middleton, P., Tobe-Gai, R., Mahomed, K., Miyazaki, C., & Bhutta, Z. A. (2015). Zinc supplementation for improving pregnancy and infant outcome. *Cochrane Database of Systematic Reviews 2015* (2), CD000230. http://onlinelibrary.wiley.com/doi/10.1002/14651858.CD000230.pub5/full.

ABOUT THE AUTHOR

DAPHNE ADLER holds an undergraduate degree in theoretical mathematics from Harvard College and an MBA from Harvard Business School. She has spent her professional career working in management consulting. She grew up in Norwich, Vermont, and now lives in London, England, with her husband and three young children.

ABOUT FAMILIUS

Visit Our Website: www.familius.com

Join Our Family

There are lots of ways to connect with us! Subscribe to our newsletters at www.familius.com to receive uplifting daily inspiration, essays from our Pater Familius, a free ebook every month, and the first word on special discounts and Familius news.

Get Bulk Discounts

If you feel a few friends and family might benefit from what you've read, let us know and we'll be happy to provide you with quantity discounts. Simply email us at orders@familius.com.

Connect

- Facebook: www.facebook.com/paterfamilius
- Twitter: @familiustalk, @paterfamilius1
- Pinterest: www.pinterest.com/familius
- Instagram: @familiustalk

FAMILIUS

The most important work you ever do will be within the walls of your own home.

CPSIA information can be obtained
at www.ICGtesting.com
Printed in the USA
LVOW03s0218060418
572486LV00001B/12/P